ALLERGIES

THE COMPLETE GUIDE TO DIAGNOSIS, TREATMENT, AND DAILY MANAGEMENT

NEW AND REVISED 3RD EDITION

ALLERGIES

THE COMPLETE GUIDE TO DIAGNOSIS, TREATMENT, AND DAILY MANAGEMENT

NEW AND REVISED 3RD EDITION

BRUCE S. DOBOZIN MD. & STUART H. YOUNG MD.

FOREWORD BY LYNN M. TAUSSIG, MD, FORMER PRESIDENT AND CEO, NATIONAL JEWISH MEDICAL AND RESEARCH CENTER

A NOTE TO THE READER

The ideas, procedures, and suggestions contained in this book are not intended as a substitute for consulting with your physician. All matters regarding your health require medical supervision.

Also every effort has been made to verify dosages of medications but we cannot guarantee the dosages of medications and the facts contained in this book. Any dosing of medications should be verified with your doctor or pharmacist. And facts and opinions stated in this book may change as new scientific research is published.

To order additional copies of this book, contact:
Xlibris Corporation
1-888-795-4274
www.Xlibris.com
Orders@Xlibris.com
97605

CONTENTS

Dedication

To my wife, Devorah Sperber, who inspires me to live life passionately.

Bruce S. Dobozin

To the memory of my mother, Sylvia, who taught me the meaning of life.

To my wife Ronnie who gave my life meaning and to

Michael, Jacqueline, Jeff, Steven, Stacey and Ethan

Stuart H. Young, MD

Foreword

People of all ages have suffered from allergies for centuries, but it was not until 1906 that the term *allergy* was introduced by Clemens von Pirquet. Since then, scientists have done extensive research to figure out what causes allergies and the best ways to treat them. The discovery at National Jewish Medical and Research Center in the 1960s of the allergy molecule immunoglobulin E (IgE) was a singularly important observation that helped to explain the cascade of events that lead to an allergic reaction. Over the past thirty years, we have learned much more about allergies and how to treat them.

In spite of these research efforts, the number of people who have developed allergies has risen markedly worldwide over the past several decades. In the United States, nearly fifty million people now have allergies; this represents more than 15 percent of the population.

The reasons for the increase in allergic disorders are unclear. Hypotheses include changes in the ozone layer, new chemicals in the environment, air pollution, and the fact that, in some ways, young children may be "healthier" (because of immunizations, fewer siblings, and other factors), which alters the maturing immune system in favor of the development of allergies. These theories have not been proven. In fact, allergies appear to be rising in areas where air pollution is low or decreasing. Allergies are less common in parts of the world (e.g., the former East Berlin) where there has been considerable air pollution, in contrast to adjacent areas (e.g., the former West Berlin) where there have been lower levels of air pollution but higher rates of allergies. Genetic factors do not appear to be the cause of this rise in allergies, as the changes have occurred too rapidly.

The social, economic, physical, and psychological burdens of allergy-related conditions are huge and immeasurable. The direct medical costs for caring for patients with allergic rhinitis and asthma exceed 10.3 billion dollars per year. Billions of dollars are also lost each year in work productivity due to absenteeism or decreased efficiency; for asthma alone, this indirect cost approaches 3 billion dollars. More than three million workdays are lost each year due to asthma, and the number of school days missed by children due to allergies or asthma exceeds ten million per year. And more than five thousand American children and adults die each year from allergy-related conditions such as asthma and anaphylaxis.

One of the most important aspects of the management of allergies is education of the patient (and appropriate family members). This concise and well-written book achieves that. A thorough reading, and rereading, of the relevant chapters will provide the individual patient (or family member) with an easily understood explanation of the medical problem, therapeutic principles, the pros and cons of various therapies, and self-management strategies. The authors have provided a comprehensive review of a complicated topic in an easily readable way. Used, and used appropriately, this book will improve the health and lives of all patients who suffer from the plague of allergies.

Lynn M. Taussig, MD former President and CEO
National Jewish Medical and Research Center
(now known as National Jewish Health)
Denver, Colorado
Professor of Pediatrics
University of Colorado School of Medicine
Denver, Colorado

Preface to the Third Edition

Since we published the previous editions of this book, Bruce and I have utilized it to help educate our patients and various community groups. Our book has always been very informative and well received by all. Last year, Bruce contacted me to see if I had any books I could loan, give, or sell him, as our publisher had stopped printing the book. Since I was completely out of them as well, it was obvious to both of us what we needed to do.

So after a year of laborious but enjoyable work of a labor of love, here is the latest version of our book. We reviewed our previous prefaces, and they are still relevant to what we hope our book will do for you and have included them as well.

Since this book's publication twelve years ago all our predictions have come true. Research in the field of allergy and immunology has increased exponentially so that evidence based medicine has provided us the knowledge to discard or verify current methods, whereas methods that worked were improved and new lifesaving technologies—such as omalizumab (Xolair)—emerged.

Medicine as well as communication has changed in the twelve years. In our last book, we guided our reader to relevant sections in other books. In this edition we will guide you to resources on the Internet that supplement our book.

So read on about how to utilize all these miraculous treatments in our field. And of course, tune in to the new miracles that we expect to be available shortly. We hope you enjoy reading our book as much as we enjoyed writing it.

Stuart H. Young, MD
Bruce S. Dobozin, MD
New York, New York
April 2011

Prefaces to the Second Edition

Bruce Dobozin and I decided to write this book because of the lack of a comprehensive basic text for the general reader that we could recommend to patients who wanted more information. We particularly wanted to offer a text that is as free as possible of ideological bias. Perhaps because allergies are so complex and affect so many people—at least fifty million U.S. residents—they have been blamed for every imaginable disorder, from malaise and head¬aches to fatigue and hyperactivity. Responsible allergists in recent years have had to sort through a plethora of speculative theories and questionable treatments, some worthy of further research, others clearly fraudulent.

Our intention is to describe accepted scientific and medical practice and treatment, discuss those lines of speculation that may prove fruitful in the future, and warn about undertaking tests and treatment based on unproven or disproven claims.

Since our last book was published just seven years ago, there have been extraordinary advances in the diagnosis and treatment of allergies. I have practiced allergy medicine for thirty years and suffered from allergies for fifty years. The medications currently being used for the treatment of allergies were not even developed at the time that I started to practice allergy medicine.

So, in planning and writing this book we aimed to provide information in as useful a form as possible. We do not expect readers to go straight through the text from beginning to end. Most people naturally tend to look up the symptoms or treatments with which they are most concerned. We have tried, therefore, to make each section as self-contained as possible, and to refer readers to other relevant chapters as necessary.

The purpose of this book is to give you, the reader, information about what is known today about the causes and treatments of allergies. We hope you will use this information to better compre¬hend and follow a competent physician's state-of-the-art advice to you. Equally important, this information should prevent you from spending money on useless tests or treatment or on doctors who take advantage of your credulity. We hope you will benefit from the information in this book written from our lifelong experience with allergies—from both sides of the doctor's desk.

Stuart H. Young, M.D.
New York City
September 1, 1998

The rise in consumerism, spearheaded by Ralph Nader's pursuit of the auto industry in the early 1960s, led to a general sense that the consumer was not totally powerless in the face of big business. Since then, consumer advocacy has percolated through many industries. In medicine, the situation is somewhat different since there are no guarantees issued when a consumer purchases health care from a provider. Still, I believe that medical consumers, or patients, would receive better care if they educated themselves in such a way as to be able to participate fully in health-care decisions affecting themselves or family members.

Education may be especially important in the field of allergy medicine, since there are many factors playing into allergies that patients should know about. Our aim in writing this book is to bring these factors to readers' attention.

As we approach the millennium, there are numerous new sources of information, many just a mouse-click or phone call away. However, one has to be sure that these sources are reliable. This book provides a context for understanding and assessing new information and claims. We have also added a list of Internet sites that can be used to supplement this book.

There are many misconceptions about allergies—I hear a new one almost every day. We trust that this book will clarify such misconceptions, and prove useful to you, the consumer.

Bruce S. Dobozin, M.D.
New York City and Woodstock
September 1, 1998

Chapter 1

ALLERGY: WHAT IS IT?

Allergy afflicts millions of people worldwide, including about fifty million in the United States. If you sniffle in the summertime or sneeze when you clean the house, you may be allergic.

Many snifflers and sneezers go through life more or less contentedly without seeking a definitive diagnosis or medical treatment. Their symptoms just don't bother them much. But for many others, allergies seriously interfere with their ability to enjoy life and get their work done. These people usually want some kind of treatment,for these troubling symptoms if only an over-the-counter remedy. For a few patients, allergy is a serious, even dangerous, condition that requires expert medical attention and constant vigilance to prevent a life-threatening allergic reaction.

As common as allergies are, however, they are not always easy to diagnose. The first step is to find out whether your symptoms are caused by an allergy or some other problem, such as a chronic respiratory or intestinal infection.

Most patients visit an allergy doctor with one or more of the following kinds of complaints:

- Nasal and respiratory symptoms of the sort usually associated with a head cold or hay fever—that is, runny nose, sneezing, watery eyes, sinus headaches (pain in the forehead).
- **Wheezing (especially on exhaling), shortness of breath, chest tightness, difficulty in exhaling completely.** These are typical symptoms of asthma but may be caused by other conditions as well. Asthma is often but not always associated with allergy.
- **Itchy hives or rashes or other skin irritations.** The patient may suspect a food allergy or skin sensitivity to some chemical substance, such as suntan lotion.

- **Diarrhea, indigestion, nausea.** Food allergies are often suspected by the patient.
- **Headache, irritability, fatigue, malaise.** The patient may feel that a food or something in the air at home or in the office is causing the problem. It's ordinarily much easier to find the causes of the symptoms at the top of the list than of those toward the end. In fact, until recently, patients suffering from fatigue, headaches, or jumpiness probably would not have thought of going to an allergist. In the past few years, however, there has been considerable speculation that a wide range of ills may be caused by allergy or allergy like sensitivities and intolerances.

Some physicians (identified as clinical ecologists) diagnose and treat an extraordinary number of so-called allergies. As a consumer, you should be wary of any doctor who regularly detects extremely unusual allergies, such as allergies to all synthetic materials or to many different kinds of foods. Such a doctor may be relying more on speculation than science. In particular, watch out for so-called cytotoxic testing; it does not work. (See chapter 19.)

Luckily, most allergy sufferers report symptoms and histories that fit a common pattern, and a doctor who asks the right questions can quickly make a pretty shrewd guess as to the identity of the guilty allergen or allergens. Normally, it does not take long to confirm the diagnosis and begin treatment.

The chances that you are allergic to something are increased if one or both of your parents are or were allergic. There are certain physical signs that indicate allergy; for example, swollen, darkened eyes (almost like black eyes) are likely to appear in allergies affecting the respiratory tract. Also, many patients have noticed a pattern to their symptoms that suggests an allergy is at work. This is often the case when the symptoms are seasonal, or are related to a particular locale, or are associated with eating certain foods. By trial and error, patients sometimes find that antihistamines (which block allergic reactions) are helpful when they feel sick. If antihistamines help, the ailment is probably caused by an allergy.

THE ALLERGIC REACTION

Allergic reactions are triggered by the immune system, the complex system that recognizes and combats outside substances or organisms that get into the body. An allergy is a mistake by the immune system. The system reacts vigorously, even violently, to some harmless substance.

For example, a family gets a cat; and everyone is fine except for one daughter, Alice, who after a few weeks or months begins to sneeze and wheeze anytime she is around the cat. Alice, it turns out, is sensitive to cat dander.

The dander from one cat is essentially harmless. Nevertheless, Alice gets sick because her body reacts to a few specks of dander as if this were an invasion of pneumonia bacteria or some other dangerous organism.

Allergic reactions, these mistakes by the immune system, appear to arise from the body's protective reaction against parasites. There are several similarities in the way that the body fights parasites and allergens. In both cases, the body produces a large amount of immunoglobulin E (IgE) antibodies. In other immune system reactions, different antibodies take the lead.

For a person living in an undeveloped country and is exposed to numerous parasites, the tendency to produce IgE is protective and valuable. For our young friend Alice, who gets sick around cats, IgE production is a problem.

The first stage of allergy development is called sensitization. In this stage, the person is free of symptoms. Alice is playing with the cat and feeling fine, but unfortunately, cells in her immune system are engaged in a complex process that results in the production of numerous IgE antibody molecules.

These antibodies attach themselves to mast cells, which come from the bone marrow. Mast cells are found in connective tissues throughout the body, especially near the small blood vessels and near the epithelial tissue (which is tissue that covers or lines, such as skin and the lining of the intestines). IgE antibodies also attach to basophils, a type of white blood cell that can exit the small blood vessels and congregate around invading molecules.

The antibodies remain attached to the mast cells and basophils, which now resemble mobile grenades, packed with ammunition (histamine and other allergy mediators). It requires only the trigger of a new invasion of the allergen, in this instance, cat dander, to activate these grenades and set off all those miserable symptoms of cat allergy—burning eyes, sneezing, and so on. This is the second stage of the allergy process, and it is characterized by acute symptoms.

The IgE antibodies are especially designed to recognize and attach to the specific allergen that led to their creation. Like all antibodies, IgE molecules are Y-shaped. Their base attaches to the mast or basophil cells; their arms extend outward. When invading allergens attach to at least two IgE antibodies, the grenade is triggered and a cascade of substances is released. These cause allergy symptoms. (See illustration.)

The most important of these substances is histamine, which (1) dilates blood vessels, causing redness and, in extreme cases, shock; (2) constricts the bronchial tubes, impairing breathing; 3) irritates nerve endings, causing itching and pain; and 4) stimulates the production of mucus in the respiratory system.

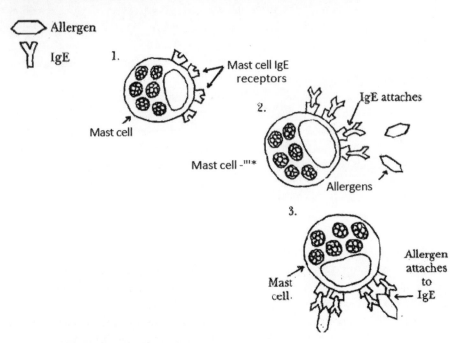

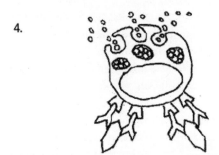

Histamines and
other chemical
mediators release

A third stage of allergy development, a delayed, sometimes prolonged period of immune activity, is called the late-phase reaction. In this stage, white cells including eosinophils plus other inflammatory cells and various chemical mediators play a role, and an elevated eosinophil count can help to diagnose the presence of allergy. Basophils, eosinophils, and other white blood cells may cause ongoing inflammation and may damage tissue in their vicinity.

IGE AND ALLERGY MEDICINE

The allergy antibody, IgE, was not actually detected until the 1960s at National Jewish Medical and Research Center in Denver, but researchers had hypothesized for many years that there must exist a special type of immunoglobulin that would account for allergy reactions. The term *allergy* was coined in 1906, by two physicians, Clemens von Pirquet and Bela Schick, who were struggling to understand the occasional sudden, deaths among patients who had received immunization injections against diphtheria, a frequently fatal disease. *Allergy* roughly means "altered reaction," and the doctors devised the term to refer to the unusual, sometimes fatal reaction of some patients to the immunization shots.

Strictly speaking, an allergic reaction is one produced by IgE antibodies. *Allergy medicine,* however, is often defined more widely to include all disorders of the immune system that involve a heightened sensitivity to substances.

You may be sensitive to or intolerant of some substances, and react badly to them, without being allergic. The distinction may be of no practical importance since you must avoid the substance in any case. But sometimes the distinction makes an enormous difference. If you are intolerant of penicillin, for example, it may give you diarrhea. But if you are allergic to it, it may kill you. (See chapter 8.)

ALLERGENS GET AROUND

An antigen is any foreign substance capable of causing an immune system reaction that produces antibodies. An allergen is a special kind of antigen that causes an allergic reaction. Common allergens include animal dander, pollen, bee venom, mold spores, and various foods and drugs, such as peanuts and penicillin.

Allergens are invaders. To affect their victims, they must find a way into the body. It is not easy to enter through the skin (including the lining of the eyes—the conjunctiva), which offers pretty good protection. Molecules of an allergen—say, cat dander—in contact with the skin usually have a limited, local effect, if any. You may get a rash and feel itchy. Various chemicals, however, can penetrate the skin and travel through the body. For example, an antibiotic cream used topically may sensitize you, causing the production of allergy antibodies. If you later take the drug orally, you may experience an allergic reaction in the form of a rash or fever or other symptoms.

The respiratory and alimentary tracts are much-better ports of entry for allergens. Substances breathed in or swallowed may affect the entire respiratory tract (from nose to lungs) or alimentary tract (from lips and mouth to intestines). Ragweed pollen, for example, breathed in through the nose of someone sensitive to it causes hay fever or, if it reaches the lungs, may cause an asthma attack. Animal dander can also provoke asthma as well as hay feverlike complaints.

Allergen molecules can escape the systems by which they enter, traveling widely in the body via the bloodstream. Thus, an allergen in food may activate mast cells in the skin, causing hives or a rash. Moreover, the histamine and other chemicals produced in an allergic response can cause a general, widespread reaction.

Often people overlook this traveling habit of allergens and look for local causes of symptoms. For example, if a baby has a rash, the parents often guess that the baby is sensitive to soap used in the wash. This may be true. But it is equally likely that the baby is allergic to milk. A baby with milk allergy will often also get diarrhea, a sign that the allergen is indeed in the alimentary tract.

In rare cases, an allergen can cause problems in remote organs, including the liver and kidneys. A patient at a large metropolitan hospital, who had been receiving penicillin for strep throat, developed fever, a rash, and blood in the urine. This kidney failure was evidently associated with an allergic sensitivity to penicillin. The penicillin was stopped, and prednisone (a steroid drug used to reduce swelling and suppress the reaction of the immune system in allergy reactions) was administered. The kidneys returned to normal function.

TREATING ALLERGIES

Supermarkets and drugstores carry dozens of medicines for treating allergies, including antihistamines and decongestants to be taken orally or as nasal sprays. With many allergies, particularly those that are seasonal or sporadic and also mild, you can safely endure most of the more common symptoms or treat them with over-the-counter medications. However, it is also important to know when it may not be safe to use these over-the-counter drugs. For all but the mildest symptoms, we recommend that you consult a doctor before starting to medicate yourself for allergies, although that doctor need not be an allergist. A conscientious family physician should be able to help and may also be able to provide a more cost-effective and medically effective treatment than you can manage by buying over the counter. And a physician will be able to warn you if there is any reason you should not take a particular drug. You may also want to know how to keep a mild allergy in check so that you avoid major flare-ups in the future.

Of course, you should not medicate yourself if you know or suspect that you have any important medical problem, such as heart disease, circulatory disease, kidney or liver disease, diabetes, or any serious chronic condition.

Finally, a child or a person over seventy years old should not use over-the-counter medicines except with careful medical monitoring. Both young and old often experience unusual reactions to drugs.

For more, see chapter 5.

Chapter 2

A Brief Overview
Of Allergic Diseases

Allergic diseases include those diseases caused directly by an allergy and those that result indirectly from allergy. For example, an ear infection may arise as a result of chronic hay fever, especially in children. (In youngsters, the immature Eustachian tube is more open, allowing material from the back of the nose and the throat to enter the ear.) Here is a list of the most common allergic diseases:

- Allergic rhinitis triggers include pollen such as tree, grass and ragweed, dust mite, animal dander, as well as other allergens affecting the respiratory tract. Sniffling, sneezing, and watery eyes are typical symptoms. At least 15 percent of the population of North America is affected with allergy of this type. (See chapter 10. Related problems in the sinuses, eyes, and ears are discussed in chapter 11.)
- Asthma, characterized by shortness of breath and wheezing, is a major health problem. Not all cases of asthma are caused by allergy, but many are or have an allergic component. (See chapter 9.)
- Food allergies range from acute, sometimes fatal, sensitivities to particular foods to mild reactions that are little more than a nuisance. (See chapter 7.)
- Drug allergies and intolerances affect some 10 percent of the population treated with drugs. (See chapter 8.)
- Urticaria, better known as hives, and angioedema, which is soft-tissue swelling, can be associated with a wide range of allergic conditions, including allergic shock (anaphylaxis). Hives are sometimes caused by food or drug allergies or sensitivity to bee stings. The so-called physical allergies, such as sensitivity to cold, can give rise to hives in the absence of an outside allergen. In most cases

of chronic hives, the cause cannot be identified, but hives can also be caused by serious medical illnesses—especially thyroiditis. (See chapter 12.)

- Dermatitis, including eczema and other types of rashes, often occurs as a result of allergies. (See chapter 12.)
- Anaphylaxis is an overwhelming, sometimes fatal allergic reaction. (See chapter 13.)

HAY FEVER AND OTHER SEASONAL ALLERGIES

The most common seasonal allergy is popularly called hay fever, although the culprit is usually ragweed. A variety of pollens (grass, tree and weed) can cause sneezing, sniffling, and burning eyes, typically in the spring and summer.

Plants, trees, or grasses in the immediate vicinity of your home can be a major cause of seasonal allergies, and it is a good idea to be familiar with what's growing near you. Some plants are far more likely than others to cause allergies. Your local hospital or doctor should be able to get you information on the most allergenic plants in your locality (see chapter 10). You can also follow the news on pollen counts through your local radio and television broadcasts as well as in many daily newspapers. In the appendix, we list websites where you may obtain reliable pollen counts.

SNIFFLES AND SNEEZES THAT AREN'T HAY FEVER

Respiratory symptoms that are not associated with the spring or summer seasons and that are worse indoors than outdoors are usually due to allergens around the house. The most common household allergens are animal dander, house dust, dust mites, cockroach fragments, and feathers.

Technically, if these things make you sneeze or blow your nose, you suffer from allergic rhinitis, a term that also covers hay fever symptoms.

Sometimes a thorough bedroom cleaning or housecleaning is enough to cure allergic rhinitis (see chapter 4). But if the symptoms persist or you find yourself frequently resorting to antihistamines or cold remedies to get some relief, then you should see an allergist. If an allergist determines that you are allergic to mite, then very effective methods of protecting your bedding against mites exist (see chapter 4).

SERIOUS RESPIRATORY AND EAR, NOSE, AND THROAT SYMPTOMS

Certain symptoms are suggestive of a problem serious enough that you should not rely on home treatment. See a doctor for diagnosis and specific treatment for any of the following:

- Wheezing, difficulty exhaling, shortness of breath, frequent coughing because of excess mucus, tightness or pain in the chest.

- One or more of these symptoms may indicate asthma, emphysema, a serious respiratory infection, or a heart disorder.

- Coughing up mucus that is discolored (gray, yellow, green, or brown, or even worse, bloody or blood-streaked). Such symptoms suggest an infection or lung disease.

- Coughing up mucus as small strings or plugs means that the mucus has been shaped by remaining too long in the airways. This may be a sign of asthma. (See chapter 9.)

- Persistent sinus pain, or chronic postnasal drip, or the production of discolored mucus when you blow your nose warrants a doctor's attention. You may have an infection that needs treatment. Sinus pain can occur in the forehead (over the eyes), near the top of the nose, and in the cheeks (under the eyes). It can also radiate to other areas of the head.

- Persistent headaches may indicate sinus disease or a number of other problems. Well-meaning friends may dismiss your headaches as "only" sinus headaches, as if they pose no risk to health. This is not so. Sinus headaches should be diagnosed by an expert. (See chapters 10 and 11.)

- Redness of the sclera (white) of the eyes without itching, or any kind of discharge from the eyes, may be a sign of an underlying disease of the eyes or of disease elsewhere, for example, of the joints or connective tissue.

- Persistent itching of the eyes, even if it seems just to be part of a hay fever syndrome, should be checked with an eye doctor. A sensation that there is something in the eye, when accompanied by sensitivity to light, may be associated with an allergy but should be checked if at all bothersome to be sure it isn't something more serious, such as a scratched cornea.

- If you use contact lenses and have any of the above eye symptoms, you should tell your eye doctor. A variety of problems can arise from contact lenses, with a possibility of long-term damage to the eyes.

- Ear pain or diminished hearing. See a doctor. Do not try to self-diagnose or self-treat.

- *If you are a smoker of middle age or older or if you have emphysema, diabetes, heart disease, kidney disease, or other chronic illness, do not try to diagnose or treat allergy symptoms by yourself,* even those you may have had for many years. Your allergist and regular doctor should be in communication, in particular on the subject of effects of drugs you may be advised to take. Even if you do not have an allergist, it is important that you let your doctor know of any over-the-counter remedies you are considering taking for an allergy flare-up, even those you may have taken in the past with no problem.

Nonrespiratory Allergies

Rashes

Allergies can express themselves in a variety of itchy rashes, hives, and swelling. The cause can be allergens in the air, such as pollen; something eaten, such as watermelon or an antibiotic taken orally; or something in contact with the skin, such as nickel or cosmetics.

Atopic dermatitis (often called eczema) is an allergic rash that usually occurs without any allergen having been in contact with the skin at the location of the rash. It is typically associated with allergic rhinitis or asthma. Often, there is a family history of other relatives with similar illnesses, and the patient with any of the three atopic diseases (allergic rhinitis, asthma, atopic dermatitis) tends to have at least one of the other two as well. For example, a patient with hay fever may also tend to develop atopic dermatitis; somebody with either hay fever or atopic dermatitis is much more likely to have asthma.

Atopic dermatitis is troubling because the agent causing it may be difficult to identify. Furthermore, it itches, and repeated scratching can cause infections that over time badly traumatize the skin.

Contact dermatitis is a rash caused by contact with some allergen or irritant. The reaction may be relatively mild, as it usually is with jewelry containing nickel, or dramatic, as with poison ivy.

Avoidance is the key to relief of contact dermatitis. If the rash is relatively mild and you are pretty sure you know what caused it, treatment with antihistamine (orally) and/or an over-the-counter cortisone cream may be all that is needed.

The following kinds of rashes need medical attention:

- If the rash is eczema—that is, if it progresses to a thickening and scaling of the skin—consult an allergist or dermatologist.
- Any rash on an infant or toddler should be seen by a physician immediately. If that is difficult to arrange, at least call your pediatrician and describe the problem. Innumerable cases of so-called diaper rash have turned out to be eczema resulting from a milk allergy. (See chapter 12.)
- An itchy rash on the eyelids that does not respond to mild antihistamine treatment should get a definite diagnosis and specific treatment.
- A rash that follows treatment with penicillin, sulfa, or some other drug, or a rash that seems to be caused by eating certain foods, should be brought to a doctor's attention at once, even if the rash was mild and of short duration. Allergic sensitivity to drugs, food, or beestings can progress rapidly to a dangerous stage, so that on your next exposure the reaction may be more violent. (See chapter 13.)

HIVES AND SWELLING

Hives, or urticaria, are itchy swellings, something like mosquito bites and always deserve attention, if not immediate medical treatment. Often, people take them too casually. Hives need a professional diagnosis, even though in the end they sometimes must just be endured.

- If hives persist for more than a few days, if you feel sick when you have them or if they are accompanied by swelling—for example, of the fingers or lips—see a doctor. Individual hives that last more than one day can on rare occasions indicate a circulatory autoimmune disease (vasculitis) or other serious medical conditions. Normally, each hive will disappear in a matter of minutes to several hours.

- Hives rarely may be the first sign of the deadly allergic reaction called anaphylaxis (see chapter 13). If they appear suddenly and are associated with rapid swelling of the throat, tongue, lips, or fingers and an all-over feeling of sickness, *you are in a medical emergency and must get help immediately.* An emergency shot of Adrenalin (epinephrine) may be needed within fifteen or twenty minutes.

- Other kinds of swelling, whether or not the swelling seems to be associated with an allergy, should also be seen by a doctor. Swelling in the ankles and legs may be related to heart disease.

NAUSEA, DIARRHEA, ACHES, AND PAINS

There is a wide range of commonly reported symptoms that are sometimes caused by allergies but more often have other causes. Stomach and intestinal ailments may be due to allergy (especially in infants) but more often have other causes. Headaches and fatigue may stem from allergic conditions but also may arise from dozens of other causes. Aches in the muscles or joints usually are not related to allergy. Arthritis, to the best of our knowledge, is not caused by allergy, although certain drug allergies may temporarily cause arthritic-like symptoms.

If you are seriously bothered by any of these symptoms, you should see a doctor to determine the cause. If your doctor cannot give you a definite diagnosis or you are dissatisfied with the results of treatment, consider getting another opinion, preferably from a physician with a different specialty.

Chapter 3

A Visit To The Doctor: Examination And Tests

Choosing any physician should be done with care to find someone who is not only competent but also with whom you have a good rapport. Of course, now that HMOs dominate our system of medical service, choice is often restricted. Still, in most geographic areas, you should have at least some choice.

First, you want to avoid unscrupulous practitioners. These people, whether they are licensed physicians or not, typically have a history of finding abundant "allergies" in all patients, prescribing unusual treatments, and failing to return their patients to normal, healthy living.

When we were first preparing this book, an allergist active in the northeast did a general mailing of a flier with a checklist of questions, including, "Do you feel you are carrying too much weight although you don't eat too much?" For those who answer yes, and there are likely to be many who do, this physician offers a "metabolic allergy blood test" and a "personalized diet plan" that will take care of the problem.

If you feel that it is time for professional advice on symptoms that may be caused by allergy, we recommend a skeptical attitude toward dramatic promotional claims. You can ask your physician to recommend a board-certified allergist. The appendix lists organizations that provide information on qualified allergists and allergy-treatment centers.

You can also turn to people at your best local hospital or hospitals. A teaching hospital is often a most-useful source because doctors in a teaching hospital typically must keep up-to-date with the latest developments in the field of allergy medicine, a field in which new findings are occurring quite rapidly.

If you have a friend who's a well-informed hospital nurse, she or he may be able to suggest an effective, reliable specialist. Often a nurse will feel freer to comment frankly on a physician's work than another physician would.

A hospital's consulting specialist in allergy or the head of the department of allergy is likely to be competent. If not free to take on more patients themselves, physicians in such positions are able to make informed recommendations about other doctors.

Many people choose doctors on the advice of friends. It is certainly smart to talk to people who have been to the doctor you are considering seeing. But keep in mind that even a mediocre physician may have reasonably good results in most cases, so a favorable recommendation from a single patient may not mean much in terms of establishing medical competence. Nevertheless, in one area, other patients may be a better source of accurate information than medical experts: how pleasant the physician is to work with. Allergy treatments often extend over months and even years—basically, allergies are not cured; they are managed—so you want to like your doctor.

There are questions you should ask before committing yourself to long-term treatment with an allergist. Unfortunately, there is no one source for answers to all these questions. Former patients may be able to answer some. Some are best asked of the doctor or the office staff. Some you will have to answer for yourself after meeting the doctor and the staff.

- Is the doctor a board-certified allergist? Depending on the severity of your symptoms, how long you have had them, and what success your family practitioner has had in treating them, you may be at the point where you want to be seen by a specialist. Your local medical society can confirm for you that a particular doctor who claims to specialize in treating allergies is in fact board certified.

- Does the doctor seem to be a good listener? Does he or she pay close attention to what patients report? It is nice to tell your friends that you are seeing the busiest allergist in the county, the one the local news reporters always interview when the pollen count skyrockets. But if the doctor hasn't the time for you, it's not likely that you'll get the individual treatment you deserve.

- Does the doctor have someone to cover the practice if she or he is unavailable?

- Is the doctor responsive in an emergency? That means, for example, will the doctor work with the school nurse if a child has an allergy flare-up at school or at least accept a call from the school nurse? Will the doctor arrange for an ambulance if a patient calls in with apparent symptoms of anaphylaxis?

- Is the doctor affiliated with a good hospital? If you are not familiar with the reputation of hospitals in your area, a good rule of thumb is to choose a teaching hospital, that is, a hospital affiliated with a university. A call to that hospital's physician-referral number will immediately confirm the doctor's affiliation.

- Are the doctor's office staff and telephone service pleasant to deal with? A good staff is essential to good medicine but especially to good allergy medicine, for here the doctor's assistants often do some of the procedures.

- Do the doctor's patients seem to function fairly well, despite allergies or asthma? The purpose of allergy treatments is to help people to function normally in the world. Some doctors are especially good at teaching patients to care for themselves; they encourage patients to live as fully as possible. All other things being equal, this is the kind of doctor you want.

- Are the fees in line with what other doctors charge? Though some top specialists do elevate their fees, medicine is one field in which it is not necessarily true that you get what you pay for. Sky-high rates do not necessarily mean you have found the most competent doctor.

- Fee levels vary not only according to medical training, reputation, and years of experience but also according to geographical area, the personality of the doctor, the doctor's own financial needs, and so on. All in all, fees are not a particularly reliable indicator of quality one way or another.

- If you do want to factor in cost when selecting a doctor, ask about charges at the outset of treatment. After all, many doctors ask their patients to demonstrate their ability to pay, and what is fair on one side of the equation is fair on the other.

- Once the doctor has given you an estimate of what your treatment is likely to include and cost, you can then turn to your insurance company, which should be able to tell you not only which procedures are covered by your policy but also whether or not your physician's fees for those procedures are in the normal range. As a matter of fact, at the time of the writing of this edition, almost all fees are dictated to the physician by the HMO that you and he are in. If possible, it is a good idea to consult a physician covered by your plan. In that case, which is most cases, the relevant question is whether or not the procedures to be done and treatments to be offered are covered by your plan.

- Finally, if punctuality is important to you, inquire about the average office waiting time. Many doctors overbook their calendars because otherwise, they are left waiting by patients who show up late or not at all. So if your doctor does schedule appointments realistically, you should be particularly careful not to go late or miss appointments.

SERVICE TO EXPECT FROM YOUR DOCTOR

If you call your doctor with an urgent problem, you should be able to get an appointment promptly. If you are in the middle of an asthma attack, for example, you may be told to go to the nearest emergency room, preferably in a hospital with which the doctor is affiliated. The doctor should be able to meet you there or see you soon after the emergency treatment is rendered.

If the problem is not an emergency—say, you have experienced a gradual worsening of your asthma over the past week—a doctor ordinarily should be able to see you within a couple of days.

Similarly, if you have had an adverse reaction to a beesting, a doctor should be willing to see you within several days to plan a diagnostic workup and treatment and to prescribe epinephrine (Adrenalin) for you to carry with you. After all, bees are more social than humans; and where there is one around, there are usually many more in the neighborhood.

If you call in with a flare-up of hay fever or eczema, you may be asked to wait a week or so for an appointment.

Any possible allergy in an infant should be seen promptly by a pediatrician for diagnosis and treatment. The signs of allergy may include wheezing, persistent nasal obstruction, diarrhea, and rashes. For a first appointment, especially a nonemergency, a conscientious doctor will usually allot at least an hour to get background information, do an examination, and conduct initial tests. The doctor may not be present the entire time, but between filling out forms and waiting for test results, the first evaluation might last longer than two hours. Use the time to evaluate the doctor and his staff, even as they are evaluating you and your condition.

Subsequent visits will usually be shorter—say, fifteen to thirty minutes. If your treatment includes a series of desensitization shots, you may not see the doctor during these visits. But any time that you have questions, you should be able to reach your doctor in person or on the telephone to get answers.

A careful doctor should explain any test to be done and what to expect from medicines prescribed, including side effects. You should be encouraged to call if you experience certain specified side effects and to call about any side effects outside the range of what has been described to you.

Your doctor should have literature for you explaining how to avoid allergens that may be causing you a problem and how to medicate yourself effectively. For example, there are several wrong ways and one right way to use an inhaler.

A good doctor does everything possible to convey to the patient a sense of self-sufficiency. For youngsters with allergies or asthma, it is especially important that they not get the impression that they are invalids. The message they need is that they can lead normal lives. For example, a football coach who is willing to carry around inhalers for players with asthma, and who praises those players, goes a long way toward convincing youngsters that they can lead active lives.

Finally, the most-important service you should expect from a doctor is that you get better as a result of treatment. This seems obvious, but it is sometimes overlooked. Whenever a course of treatment is recommended to you, ask when results should be expected. If you do not experience improvement on schedule, ask if it might be time for a new approach. If nothing the doctor tries seems to work, consider getting a second opinion from another doctor. Your first doctor may simply have missed something.

In one case, for instance, a woman living in New York had developed asthma. She was treated for a year without improvement and without getting a clear explanation of what had caused the asthma. At last, dissatisfied with this result, she decided to try another doctor. In taking her history, the new doctor noted that the woman's husband was a baker. Not only was he a baker, the bakery was also below their apartment and she often spent time there. Further questioning showed that when she was away from the bakery, she improved.

The woman suffered from baker's asthma, a form of allergic asthma caused by sensitivity to certain proteins in grains and flour. This had been missed by her first physician. Avoidance of the bakery took care of the problem. (See chapter 14.)

You should feel comfortable enough with any doctor to ask frankly whether he or she thinks you are seeking the impossible. But you should not be too easily talked out of your own convictions. There are, unfortunately, many examples of people wrongly dismissed by their physicians as misguided or hysterical, who have turned out to have genuine medical problems that required treatment.

To sum up, you are entitled to competent, courteous treatment and, in most cases, to treatment that works. If you are not satisfied with the results you are getting from your treatment, or if you simply do not like the doctor you are seeing, it might be time to consider changing to another.

PREPARING FOR THE FIRST VISIT

To make the most of your first visit to an allergist, ask how long the visit is likely to last. It can run two hours or more, so you may have to make arrangements to be free for that time. If you are restless because you have to get to work or back to a babysitter, you cannot get your money's worth out of this meeting.

If you are taking a young child, try to bring someone with you who can help watch the child. Distractions are not helpful during an initial interview. Even if the child is the patient, it is advisable to have a babysitter on hand. You need to be able to concentrate on your conversation with the doctor.

Go to the first visit with as much information as possible concerning your medical history. There is a saying in medical school that 80 percent of the diagnosis comes from the history, the other 20 percent from the physical exam and laboratory testing.

You will be asked about major illnesses affecting close relatives, and of course you'll be asked whether anyone in your family has had allergies. It's surprising how often it is worthwhile to check with your relatives about this. Many times the questions jog long-forgotten memories. Among allergies, the atopic diseases—hay fever, asthma, and atopic dermatitis (eczema)—tend to be inherited and tend to occur together. So if you have asthma, for example, and there is a question of whether the asthma is caused by allergy, it is helpful to know if other people in your family have had hay fever or eczema, even if you are sure nobody has ever had asthma.

If you are bringing a child for treatment, be sure that you know your spouse's family history as well as your own.

Be prepared to answer questions on your own medical history. People usually recall ailments that require attention every day, such as diabetes, but may forget to mention diseases that flare up only occasionally, such as ulcers or migraine headaches.

You should have a complete list of medicines you take regularly—over-the-counter medicines, even aspirin, as well as prescribed ones.

Try to recall in detail any previous treatment that you may have had for allergies. If tests, such as a pulmonary-function test, were done or X-rays were taken, make an effort to get the results for your doctor. These records are yours by right.

If you have been treated for an allergy in the past, you will be asked how well you responded to the treatment.

DESCRIBING YOUR SYMPTOMS

Think very carefully about your current symptoms. Arrange in your mind or, better yet, write down on paper the answers to the following questions:

- What is your chief complaint? Try to narrow the problem to the most troublesome feature—sinus pain, wheezing, runny nose, or whatever. The doctor will ask you about a whole range of symptoms too, but it's helpful for the doctor to know right off what brought you to the doctor's office.
- Be ready for detailed follow-up questions. If you have a cough, you will be asked whether you cough up mucus and, if so, what color it is. If you have ear pain, you will be asked whether you have run a fever in connection with it. If you complain of wheezing, you will be asked whether this happens more when you exercise or sleep.
- How often do you experience difficulty? Do the symptoms occur daily? weekly? seasonally?
- When did the symptom first appear? If possible, give an exact date. At least try to give the time of year and how many months or years ago.
- Is the problem always of the same severity, or are some episodes much worse than others? Do you tend to be worse off at certain times of the day or night? after exercise? after eating? Do you feel better on weekends or workdays? on vacation or at home?
- In what way does your illness interfere with your life? Does it affect your work? your ability to exercise? your ability to get along with people?
- What happened when the symptom first appeared? What were the circumstances? How sick were you? What other symptoms occurred?
- Do certain foods trigger your allergies? What kinds of food do you eat a lot of?
- Do your allergies get worse when you drink alcoholic beverages? (The answer to this question, by the way, is frequently yes.)
- You will be asked about your environment; whether you have pets and, if so, when they were acquired; whether you have down comforters and feather pillows in the bedroom; what soaps you use; what kind of heating system you have; whether your apartment or house is damp or whether there is a damp basement; and so on.

Checklist For The First Visit

- Find out how long the visit will last.
- Collect medical records.
- Be prepared to answer questions about any family history of allergy.
- Prepare written or mental notes on your symptoms, especially when they first appeared and when they are most severe.
- If possible, arrange for child care if a child is going on the visit.

Examination And Tests

A physical examination done by an allergist will be relatively complete, although usually it will focus on the head, ears, eyes, nose, throat, neck, lungs, heart, rarely the abdomen and usually concerning the size of the liver and spleen, as well as the skin. It will ordinarily exclude gynecological or rectal examination.

In the physical, the doctor looks for characteristic signs of allergy as well as other possible causes of the patient's symptoms. For example, in the interior of the nose a pale, boggy gray-blue lining is characteristic of allergic rhinitis. However, a polyp or evidence of infection may point to a nonallergic cause of the trouble.

In one case, a little girl was brought in with a severe summer cold or possible allergy. The problem turned out to be caused by a piece of cotton that had lodged up her nose, causing infection.

X-Rays And Safety

X-ray procedures and some common tests ordered by allergists are described below. You should feel free to question recommendations for tests, on the basis of both cost and safety.

If you have had many X-rays in your life and want to have as few as possible in the future, tell this to your doctor. Your doctor will probably not be surprised that you want to eliminate unnecessary X-rays. If cost is a concern, ask what the price of the X-rays or other tests will be and whether one or more of them might be safely skipped or postponed until the need for them has been fully confirmed. If you are generally healthy and the tests are not essential to the initial diagnosis, the doctor may agree that some can be deferred.

For patients with respiratory difficulties, chest X-rays and/or a CT scan of the sinuses are sometimes necessary. The chest X-ray may be done in the office, or you may be asked to go to a hospital or laboratory to have it done. As far as the CT scan is concerned, you almost always will have to go to a hospital or laboratory to have them done.

If you have had X-rays done recently, be sure to mention this, as they may still be useful. You have a right to copies of your X-rays, although the office holding the X-rays may charge a fee for copying them.

It is wise to keep a record of when and where X-rays and other tests are done. The information can be useful later, sometimes years later. You can ask for copies of the X-rays or test results, although it may be simpler just to record the findings, with the date of the tests and the name of the hospital or office where they were done.

Modern X-ray techniques, using a highly focused, low dosage of radiation, are much safer than the X-ray procedures of a generation ago. Exterior shielding still should be applied to protect areas not to be X-rayed. But actually, today, much of the unwanted exposure to radiation during X-rays comes from internal scatter of the rays—that is, from X-rays bouncing around among internal structures.

Everyone should have the abdomen shielded during the X-ray procedure, especially a chest X-ray. Shielding is most important for children (male or female) and women of a childbearing age. If a woman of childbearing age is being scheduled for an X-ray, she should always tell her doctor if she is pregnant or if there is any chance that she is pregnant. If there is any possibility of pregnancy, nonemergency X-rays should be postponed.

For sinus CT scan, it is advisable to shield the neck to protect the thyroid gland. This is especially important for children.

A conscientious doctor will refer patients only to a radiology laboratory known to be safe and reliable. If for some reason your doctor does not recommend a specific laboratory (for example, if you are using an out-of-town specialist and you will be going back home for your X-rays), ask your family physician for a reference. If you have no regular doctor, then use the X-ray facility in the best nearby hospital—again, preferably a teaching hospital.

It is difficult for a layperson to judge the quality of a radiology lab. Obvious clues such as holes in the wall, bumbling personnel, and X-rays that need to be redone should alert you to the possibility of lax safety procedures. One might also be wary of a hospital or medical center near bankruptcy.

If you want to know more about the facility you are using, you can check the qualifications of the personnel. The physicians who read the X-rays should be board-certified radiologists. Especially in radiology, which involves rapidly increasing risks if procedures are done improperly, the technologists must be properly trained and have passed a nationally administered examination and been licensed by the state. Proper positioning of patients for the X-ray, for example, especially for sinus CT scan, not only ensures clear pictures on the first try but also minimizes the hazard at each exposure. When are X-rays needed? In general, whenever breathing is affected, it is important to have a baseline chest X-ray. (Baseline means that the X-ray will be used for the purpose of future comparison as well as present diagnosis.) People who smoke and are over forty years of age should have a chest X-ray every year or so. The chest X-ray is called a CXR.

In allergy medicine, patients who have difficulty breathing typically are asthmatic. But it is important to do a CXR to be sure the diagnosis is correct. X-ray images help to distinguish between asthma and other possible causes of breathing problems, such as emphysema (in adults) or cystic fibrosis (in children). If the asthma reported is of recent origin or has suddenly become more severe, X-ray examination helps to rule out the remote possibility that the symptoms are related to cancer. In the rare cases when cancer is present, it is most likely to be in the form of bronchogenic carcinoma, but other benign or malignant types of tumor may affect the lungs. Hodgkin's disease or lymphoma (a tumor of the lymph glands) is also occasionally found.

Apart from the possibility of a tumor, allergists look for signs of pneumonia, chronic bronchitis, or a foreign body. In adults, especially smokers, we look for lung damage due to emphysema. In young children, we must consider the possibility of cystic fibrosis, which is characterized by excess production of mucus and collapse of air sacs in the lungs. Such a finding in a patient who goes in complaining of wheezing is extremely rare, affecting less than 1 percent of patients, and usually there are other symptoms that signal this trouble even before the X-ray is taken. Nevertheless, it is important not to assume or rule out the diagnosis without viewing the lungs.

The CXR is also used to check for enlargement of the heart, although in cases where this is the cause of wheezing, the doctor will usually have found other indications of cardiac involvement.

A CXR may occasionally be recommended if a patient reports chronic hives and generalized itching. Patients with hives often find it strange that a doctor would ask for a CXR, but hives are occasionally associated with Hodgkin's disease, lymphoma, or other tumors (in descending order of frequency).

Allergists request sinus X-rays when symptoms such as facial pain suggest sinus disease or if there are nasal polyps. Sometimes in severe, unrelenting asthma, as well as chronic unexplained cough, silent sinus disease is triggering the asthma.

Children under age ten who have sinus disease sometimes do not experience facial pain but instead develop a harsh, chronic cough. If no other cause for the cough can be found, a doctor will want to have a view of the sinuses. Rarely silent, sinus disease can also cause hives. If a patient with hives of unknown cause also has some sign of sinus disease, then the doctor might ask for a sinus X-ray to rule out sinus infection.

To avoid exposing patients to unnecessary risk, many allergists today ask for fewer and less frequent follow-up X-rays than in the past. If the main symptoms are hives and itching, there is rarely any need for a follow-up X-ray. For asthmatic patients, follow-up X-rays can often be omitted unless the patients are on systemic steroids. In such cases, follow-up X-rays should be done every couple of years or so. Of course, if the asthma takes a turn for the worse and doesn't respond to treatment, a CXR should be done to try to find the cause of the problem. Typically, the doctor would be looking for some complication of asthma, such as pneumothorax (air in the pleural cavity—the space between the lungs and the chest wall, which normally contains no air and a minimal amount of fluid). Air in the pleural cavity prevents the lung from expanding. Mediastinal emphysema (air in the space between the lungs) has the same effect. The X-ray also might show evidence of pneumonia. Instead of an X-ray, your doctor may ask for a CT (computerized tomography) scan. This gives a much-clearer picture of what is going on internally.

OTHER DIAGNOSTIC TESTS YOUR DOCTOR MAY RECOMMEND

Sweat test for cystic fibrosis. To distinguish between asthma and cystic fibrosis, doctors will do a "sweat test" on children below age five who have asthma, on children below age ten who have severe asthma, and children aged fifteen or younger with nasal or sinus polyps or severe sinus disease.

The sweat test is painless, safe, and not expensive. It is based on the fact that with cystic fibrosis there is increased production of sodium and chloride by the sweat glands. In the test, the patient is given a drug (pilocarpine) to induce sweating, and then the sweat is tested for these salts. The test is far more reliable today than it was in the past, but for accurate results, it remains important to use a good laboratory.

EKG. For most patients past forty who go to an allergist with complaints about shortness of breath, the doctor may order an EKG (electrocardiogram, the *K* in the middle is a holdover from when the procedure was spelled the German way), especially if the patient has not had a recent EKG. The EKG checks heart function.

Pulmonary-function test. Most doctors who treat patients with asthma or others with breathing difficulties have the apparatus to do pulmonary-function tests right in the office. This test is done with any patient who reports a frequent cough or complains of problems with breathing.

Basically you are asked to breathe into a machine that can measure your lungs' ability to move air in and out. The measurements made are then compared to normal values for a person of your age, sex, and size.

One of the most important measures is FEVI (forced expiratory volume in one second), in other words, the amount of air you can blow out in one second. You should be able to blow out 80 percent of the exhalable air in your lungs in one second. This ability is reduced in severe asthma, although not necessarily in intermittent asthma.

The pulmonary-function test is often done before and then again after use of a bronchodilator (a drug that expands the bronchial air passages). A marked improvement as a result of taking the bronchodilator is one of the major diagnostic signs of asthma as opposed to, say, emphysema. Doctors also use pulmonary-function tests to assess how a patient is doing on a given medication.

It is very important to be aware that you may have bronchial obstruction without realizing it. To test for obstruction, doctors use a measure called PEFR (peak expiratory flow rate). For moderate to severe asthma, you can purchase a PEFR meter (peak flow meter) for use at home so that lack of airflow does not insidiously approach the danger point without your realizing it. The machine is essentially a tube with a rate-of-airflow sensor. You blow into the tube and the machine gives you a PEFR reading. (The machine is not expensive; it can be as cheap as $20.)

Urine test. Understandably, patients sometimes wonder why a urine test is relevant to allergies. Actually, hives are sometimes caused by a urinary-tract infection. Moreover, a urine test is an important indicator of basic health, helping the physician to rule out problems in kidney function, kidney infection, or in the urinary system generally that may be undermining the patient's health.

BLOOD TESTS

Typically, any patient with allergies is asked to take a basic blood test (a CBC, or complete blood count), unless one has been done recently. This test, which is a count of red and white blood cells per cubic millimeter of blood, is a screen to check for anemia and other blood conditions and is a general index of health. It can also provide an allergist with a great deal of information that may bear on your allergies.

If you have symptoms of asthma, your doctor will check for an excess number of red blood cells (polycythemia). This excess indicates that the body is not getting enough oxygen from the lungs and is trying to compensate by producing more red blood cells to maximize oxygen distribution.

A differential white blood cell count, often done along with the CBC, gives the percentage of the various types of white blood cells that are present. In particular, if you are suffering from asthma or hives, your doctor will be interested in whether there is a high eosinophil count. Eosinophils protect the body from parasitic infections, and they modulate allergic reactions. Elevated levels of eosinophils may suggest the presence of allergy. Very high levels suggest an immune system disease more serious than allergy; a parasitic infection; or exposure to a toxic drug or chemical, producing an allergy-like reaction. For example, a high eosinophil count is characteristic of the disease trichinosis (which comes from eating poorly cooked pork contaminated with Trichinella worms).

ESR. The sed rate test, or ESR (erythrocyte sedimentation rate), is a test for underlying inflammation. The principle is that inflammation changes the amount of proteins in the blood, causing the blood cells to clump together, thus forming a sediment faster than they normally do. If you have hives, a sed rate test might be done to check for an underlying illness, such as Hodgkin's disease.

SMA or SMAC. The SMA (serum metabolic analysis) or SMAC is a blood scan that measures a number of chemical substances related to healthy functioning of the kidneys, liver, and other organs. It also measures electrolytes (e.g., potassium) and blood sugar. A number is added after the SMA or SMAC (e.g. SMA-7 or SMAC-25) to specify the number of tests that are included.

Complement. Patients with hives and angioedema (soft-tissue swelling) may show a deficiency in blood complement. (Complement consists of proteins that bind with antibodies; it is involved in many aspects of immune system functioning.) Complement levels may also indicate whether the problem is hereditary or acquired angioedema—conditions that require entirely different management.

In very rare cases, syphilis is a cause of hives, but a blood test for syphilis would not routinely be done on an allergy patient.

If the problem is hives, itching, and/or swelling, a doctor is likely to run more tests if the patient is either over age fifty or under age five. Angioedema can be related to arthritic diseases in the young and old. Among older patients, it may be related to heart disease or cancer.

Alpha-1 antitrypsin. An important blood test for someone with severe asthma is an assessment of the level of alpha-1 antitrypsin in the blood. A deficiency in this protein is likely to cause early emphysema, which can masquerade as asthma. The deficiency may be inherited, so it is important to test for the protein not only for the treatment of the patient but also as an indicator of whether children or other relatives should be tested too.

The deficiency can be helped by infusions of the alpha-1 antitrypsin protein. If this deficiency is found, it is vitally important not to smoke.

Cholesterol. For patients age thirty or older, it is a good idea to get a reading on blood-cholesterol levels, even though these are not the immediate concern of an allergist.

Skin Tests

Skin tests are extremely important in the diagnosis of allergies. In skin tests, suspected allergens, along with some of their near relatives, are applied to or injected into the skin. The allergist then waits for fifteen to twenty minutes to see if there is a reaction, called a wheal, which resembles a hive.

You must be sure not to use antihistamine prior to a skin test, or the result may be misleading. Some of the new antihistamines can stay in your system for up to a month, so be sure that your allergist knows exactly which medications you have been taking and when you last took any of them.

In skin testing, the allergen is applied to the surface of the skin (an epicutaneous test) or deeper into the skin (an intradermal test).

The surface challenge can be done either by scratching the skin and applying an extract of the allergen (a scratch test) or applying a drop of the allergen extract and pricking a microscopic amount into the skin. The latter (prick) is preferable to a scratch test. With either test, a local reaction—a welt, or hive—may appear within fifteen to twenty minutes. But you must wait at least a half hour after the test in case the reaction is stronger than expected. Most reactions just involve swelling and itching around the scratch or puncture. But very rarely, the whole arm starts to swell, and Adrenalin is needed. An allergist will have Adrenalin and other drugs on hand to treat any dangerous reaction, should there be one.

The surface (epicutaneous) tests done by needle prick or puncture are very specific: if you get a reaction, you are almost certainly allergic to that substance, at least in the sense that you produce IgE antibodies to it. But this positive test result must be interpreted in the light of your entire history, especially when food allergies are being tested. Sometimes a positive result is valid but not clinically significant; in other words, the allergen provokes a skin response but doesn't really make you sick.

Also, although specific, the surface prick or puncture tests are not as sensitive as we would like them to be. So it's possible for no reaction to occur as a result of the test, even though you may be allergic to the substance tested. For example, if you always develop hay fever in August and September, there is a good chance you are allergic to ragweed pollen, even if a surface skin test is negative. One way to check this further would be to use an intradermal test, which is far more sensitive.

The intradermal skin test, which involves injection of the allergen under the skin, has just the opposite qualities of the surface test. The intradermal test is very sensitive: if you are allergic to a substance, a reaction is much more likely to occur. But it is not very specific: you may not really be allergic to the particular allergen that provoked the reaction. In other words, the intradermal test gives more false positives.

Another type of skin test, the patch test, is done with patients who suffer from rashes diagnosed as contact dermatitis. The test is done by applying different chemicals to the skin under adhesive patches. The chemicals are often from a kit that contains the twenty most common causes of contact dermatitis. These are chemicals or materials found in jewelry, hair dyes, shampoos, medicinal creams, clothing, glues, cosmetics, and so on. The patches are left on for forty-eight hours. If you are allergic to what is under the patch, you will usually develop a telltale rash.

Immunoglobulins And Blood Tests

In recent years, a variety of blood tests have been developed to detect the presence of allergy activity, even of specific allergies. The hope was that a convenient, relatively simple blood test could replace the more-irksome skin testing. Unfortunately, we have not reached that point. Skin testing is still the most reliable diagnostic test for specific allergies. It is often the least-expensive method, as well.

Immunoglobulins in the blood do convey information on a person's health with respect to allergies and immunity to infection. Immunoglobulins are proteins that function as antibodies. They come in five classes identified by the letters *G*, *A*, *M*, *D*, and *E*, after the Greek letters *gamma*, *alpha*, *mu*, *delta*, and *epsilon*. There are also subclasses of IgG, the levels of which may be low in patients with asthma and other lung disease. The reason for this is not fully understood.

A test called PRIST (paper radioimmunosorbent test) measures IgE in the blood. A paper disk impregnated with antibody to IgE is first exposed to blood serum from the patient and then exposed to a control solution containing radioactive IgE (the radioactivity makes the IgE easy to measure). The more IgE in the patient's blood, the less radioactive IgE will be bound to the antibody in the paper because the patient's IgE has arrived there first.

However, PRIST is rarely needed in the evaluation of allergic disease. Elevated levels of IgE generally indicate the presence of some disorder related to allergies or parasites, but they do not indicate the specific nature of the problem. An IgE level may be done if you have severe or moderately severe asthma. In this situation, it may be helpful in determining if you are a candidate for, and the dosage, of Xolair (omalizumab). (See chapters 5 and 9.)

That drawback to PRIST appeared to be solved by the development, in the 1960s, of the RAST (radioallergosorbent test), another in vitro blood test, which was designed to detect specific IgE antibodies to particular allergens. RAST tends to miss allergies, but when it gives a positive result, it is usually correct.

Another difficulty common to both RAST and PRIST is that the use of radioactive material poses safety problems. Therefore, other blood tests have been developed that use enzymes as markers; FAST, MAST, and ELISA use enzymes.

For most people, skin tests are the most accurate way to evaluate allergic sensitivities. There are some cases, however, in which RAST or a variant should be used. These are cases in which the patient is at risk of harm if a severe reaction to a skin test were to occur and Adrenalin would have to be administered. Infants and people with heart arrhythmia or who have had a stroke would fall into this category. A doctor may also prefer to avoid skin testing if the patient suffers from extensive skin disease. Anyone taking a long-acting antihistamine is not going to get as reliable results from skin tests as we would normally expect.

RAST may also be helpful in predicting reactions to certain foods such as peanuts and nuts and may avoid the need for challenges as discussed below.

Rarely, physicians combine blood tests and skin tests.

There is no one test or pattern of tests that is infallible. All in all, however, we believe that the evidence shows that at this time, for almost all patients, skin testing is the best choice.

CHALLENGE TESTING

Technically, challenge testing includes skin testing for common inhalant allergens such as pollen, but the term is more often reserved for tests for food or drug allergies. Essentially, this type of test involves exposing a person to a substance to determine if it will cause an allergic reaction.

Challenge testing may be called for in cases of a suspected allergy to penicillin or to a local anesthetic, when skin tests have been negative. With the patient closely monitored in the office or hospital, gradually increasing strengths and doses of the drug are injected or taken orally.

This procedure carries a relatively high risk of severe reaction, requiring immediate treatment. Food and drug allergies can be so violent that it is advisable to challenge such a response in the safest possible circumstances to find out for certain whether or not an allergy is present. (See chapters 7 and 8.)

TESTS ACCORDING TO SYMPTOMS

Exactly which tests an allergist is likely to request on the first or second visit will vary according to the symptoms you describe, your age, medical history, and other factors.

Unfortunately, there is no simple, inexpensive way to diagnose suspected allergies. Many tests are usually necessary, and even the tests do not always give the whole picture. Your own perceptions and your case history are also essential in determining if an allergy is present.

Chapter 4

How To Avoid Allergens At Home

Once you have gone to the doctor and identified the allergen(s) causing you difficulty, the most basic treatment is avoidance. There is a great deal more you can do, of course; but you must avoid contact with the offending allergen or allergens, if at all possible and to the fullest extent possible, even when you are taking allergy shots or other treatment.

The majority of people with allergies need to reduce their exposure to one or more of the following common allergens: dust and dust mites; pollen from weeds, grasses, and trees; animal dander and body fluids of animals (cat saliva is a particularly potent allergen for many people); and cockroaches.

In their offices, allergists usually keep literature for their patients on how to create an allergen-free environment. This material can be overwhelming if you imagine cleaning out the entire house all at once. Luckily, the job can be handled in stages, and often, a few improvements in the home environment can bring significant relief from symptoms.

House Dust

Household dust is a ubiquitous indoor allergen (actually a combination of allergens) with an allergic potency that is much the same worldwide.

House dust is quite different from road dust, which is ordinarily merely an irritant, although at some times of the year mold spores and other allergens may get mixed in with normal road dust.

Good old household dust contains breakdown products of rugs and upholstery, such as down and various kinds of lint and debris, including kapok; cotton and sometimes cottonseed linters (short fibers that cling to the seeds); and animal (dog, cat, horse, cow, and pig) hair. Dust also contains dander (which consists of tiny flakes of human and animal skin), bits of plants, food remnants, cockroach fragments, bacteria, and more. Most notoriously, house dust contains dust mites and their droppings.

Dust Mites

For many years, researchers were mystified as to why house dust appeared to cause similar problems worldwide. After all, cultures varied significantly in types of upholstery, foods, cleaning materials, pets, and so on that would leave traces in the dust.

European scientists suspected but could not prove the role of the dust mite in human allergy until the 1960s and 1970s, when a Dutch scientist, R. Voorhorst, and a Japanese researcher, T. Miyamoto, established the dust mite's almost-worldwide role in causing allergy. The barely visible tiny dust mite is truly the global star of household dust.

There are over fifty thousand species of mites, but the mites that most concern us here are *Dermatophagoides farinae* and *Dermatophagoides pteronyssinus*. (The term *Dermatophagoides* means "skin eaters," and these creatures thrive on their high-protein diet.) A third type of dust mite is *Euroglyphus maynei.*

The specific problem with mites is their feces, which can be breathed into the entire respiratory tract. Breakdown products of these particles, if five microns or less, can enter deep into the lungs. A micron, by the way, is 1/1,000 of a millimeter and a human red blood cell is six to eight microns in diameter.

It is the feces of dust mites that contain the mite allergen. When the feces land on mucus membrane, the antigen is released within thirty seconds.

Mites, having an appetite for protein, are more likely to be found in an environment relatively crowded with people. They also prefer humid conditions (humidity of 50 percent and above). There are far fewer mites in high-altitude Denver, Colorado, where the humidity is low, than in sultry Miami, Florida.

Mites also like mattresses, rugs, upholstery, and natural materials of many kinds. They dislike plastic. Mites normally are not a problem in cribs, which typically are furnished with plastic-covered mattresses.

The revival of interest in natural materials—down comforters, genuine Oriental rugs, English tweeds, and so on—has been a boon to mites. Many people, having invested in these popular products, find that they tend to cause allergy reactions, either directly (as in a sensitivity to feathers) or indirectly (as a haven for mites). Once mites have a foothold in your home, they are difficult to eradicate, producing a new generation every three weeks. (The females put out about twenty-five to fifty eggs at a time.)

Both mites and cockroaches can cause asthma, sometimes in a delayed and often severe reaction.

Cockroaches

Cockroaches have been identified as an important provoker of allergy reactions and are a major cause of asthma, especially in inner cities. Cockroach allergen is found in the body parts of cockroaches and in their saliva and feces.

More than ten million Americans are estimated to be allergic to cockroaches, and about half of inner-city allergy patients react positively to skin tests for cockroach sensitivity. If these patients inhale cockroach allergen in a bronchial-challenge test, they are likely to develop an asthmatic reaction. In homes, restaurants, and grocery stores that are infested with cockroaches, cockroach allergen is sometimes present in food.

Cockroaches like water, food leavings, brown paper and newspaper, glue, insulation—just about anything you can think of, they can eat or nest in.

Immunotherapy (allergy shots) using cockroach serum may prove to be helpful in reducing sensitivity to cockroaches. But the effectiveness of this method of treatment has not yet been fully evaluated in the United States. Many allergists do treat with cockroach antigen and believe that it is an effective treatment modality.

MOLD

Molds are primitive plants that lack chlorophyll and feed on other organic material, which they decompose in order to produce food for themselves. There are many thousands of varieties, and they are very adaptable, surviving both outdoors and indoors. It is the mold spores, which are tiny reproductive cells that cause the difficulty to allergy sufferers. Among common molds is the black slime that appears in humid bathrooms, certain lifesaving antibiotics, and numerous plant parasites.

People who get allergy reactions during humid or rainy weather (especially in summer—for example, when mowing the lawn), are most likely sensitive to molds. In tropical and semitropical regions, mold occurs outdoors all year round.

However, in temperate climates, symptoms of mold-sensitive patients increase markedly after the first frost because the frost kills all the plants but spares the mold. As soon as there is a thaw, the mold will thrive on the dead foliage until the hard frost sets in.

How do molds get into our homes? The answer is blowing in the wind: millions of airborne spores settle on anything even slightly damp and organic. They grow on wood and fabric; they live in the refrigerator and under it, in the drip pan. They settle on house plants. They thrive in foam rubber.

Until recently, it was believed that a certain mold, *Stachybotrys,* found indoors on damp surfaces was toxic and could cause serious illness.

Stachybotrys had been in the news, especially in the 1990s when hysterical news articles reported about severe reactions; and it was believed that *Stachybotrys* could cause symptoms as disparate as infection, headaches, muscle aches, fatigue, respiratory problems, rapid heartbeat, and rashes. In infants, it was believed that it could cause bleeding in the lungs and even death.

As it turns out, *Stachybotrys* hardly ever circulates into the atmosphere as it is a slimy mold and the spores cannot escape the slime. In essence, *Stachybotrys* does not appear to contribute to human disease.

POLLEN

Plant pollen is the notorious culprit in hay fever. Pollen granules can get into your home through open windows and on people's clothing. If you have been out on a windy day when pollen is in the air, you may well transport the enemy in your own hair. A shower when the day's outdoor activities are over is often advisable. Otherwise, when you retreat to your clean, allergen-free bedroom, you may carry a small cloud of allergens with you.

People who suffer from hay fever should pay attention to the prevailing winds and not settle down near an open window with the wind blowing in during hay fever season. If you get rhinitis from pollen, be sure that your bed is not near a window on the windward side of your room.

Tactics for avoiding pollen depend on the time of day and whether you live at ground level or in a high-rise apartment. Dew tends to weigh down pollen; but in the heat of the sun, the pollen dries and begins to rise, peaking usually shortly after sunrise until 10:00 a.m. until noon. But this is variable depending on geographic region and weather conditions. The air in midafternoon is relatively pollen-free. If you want to exercise outdoors, early morning, before sunrise is fairly safe—from an avoiding-pollen point of view.

A heavy rain will wash pollen out of the air, but a thunderstorm may not do the job and may even shatter pollen, making matters worse.

Highly allergic people really need air conditioners throughout the pollen season—at home, at work, and in their cars.

Bouquets of flowers, unfortunately, tend to provoke symptoms in people who are allergic. A brightly colored flower is designed to attract bees and other insects to its rich package of sticky pollen. Putting your nose up to the petals and sniffing the delicious aroma can be like settling down for a picnic in a ragweed field. Flowers can be tolerated if you don't get too close.

PETS

Allergies to animals are common and very troublesome. Some people simply cannot give up their pets or their horseback riding or their farm stock—or their friends who have pets. Yet exposure to certain animals can cause a sensitive person quite a serious reaction. For such people, a combination of treatment and avoidance is often the best approach. In some cases, the allergy is just too strong, and the pet must be placed in a new home.

Allergies to cats can be particularly severe. There are people who, without developing burning eyes, sneezing, and even labored breathing, cannot be in a house or apartment where a cat has lived in the past year. Cat saliva contains a very potent allergen (and cats spend half their waking hours grooming themselves); the same allergen is found in the glands of the cat's skin, at the hair roots.

Almost all breeds of cat can cause a reaction in a cat-sensitive person. With dogs, however, sometimes one breed (not necessarily a long-haired breed) will bother a patient while another will not. Contrary to common belief, there is no such thing as a hypoallergenic breed. Unfortunately, this misconception was recently perpetuated in the media as President Obama was looking for a hypoallergenic breed that his daughter would tolerate. Since all breeds of dogs can cause some degree of allergy, our advice to him, had he asked, might have been to give the dog a six-month trial in the White House to see if his daughter would tolerate it. But even that length of time may not be enough. Also, allergies to dogs occur less frequently than cat allergies do. Dog allergen, incidentally, is in the dander, saliva, and urine.

The dander and allergen of cats and dogs can remain in a home, causing allergic symptoms long after the animal is gone, even years later. Cat allergen is sticky and hard to eradicate. So if you are taking allergy shots for sensitivity to an animal, do not stop the shots when you get rid of the animal. You will probably still need them for up to a year or more afterward.

BIRDS, RODENTS, AND HORSES

Birds, and rodents such as hamsters and gerbils (yes, those cute little beasts are rodents), can cause as much trouble to a sensitive person as a cat or dog.

Pigeon and budgerigar (parakeet) fanciers run the risk of contracting pigeon breeder's disease, which causes shortness of breath, chills, and fever. These symptoms are dramatic enough that the person usually seeks medical help. But with one small parakeet, you may develop the same symptoms in a much-milder, more bearable form. This is actually more dangerous, as you may ignore the discomfort and end up with a severely damaged lung.

Pigeon breeder's disease is a form of hypersensitivity pneumonitis, which is discussed in chapter 14.

Both birds and rodents are messy. Birds molt, preen themselves, and shake feather debris all over the place. Rodents kick up dust. Sometimes a young child in kindergarten or first grade may sneeze and sniffle if seated near a hamster's cage in the classroom. Before getting a bird or rodent as a pet for a child, try a few test visits of at least several hours at a time with the species of your choice. However, even if your child does not react, some children eventually become allergic to furry animals, and this could cause a problem in the future.

Horses are no longer part of most people's daily life as they were prior to the advent of motorcars. Also, horsehair is now used less often in furniture and mattresses. But people still ride or work with horses or use horse manure in gardens. And horses and horse products still cause allergies, which you should be aware of if you have contact with these animals.

ENVIRONMENTAL CONTROL IN THE HOME

At this point we will begin our discussion on what measures should be taken to reduce allergen exposure in your home. This is an extremely controversial area of allergy, as we explain below. It is complicated by the fact that we do not have the advantage of the information that your own physician will have as exactly how ill you are and what your allergy evaluation reveals. We will give advice that is general and should be helpful to most individuals.

Complicating the matter is another problem. Prior to discussing environmental controls that can be useful in reducing exposure to the allergens that one is allergic to, we will have a brief discussion as to how controversial environmental controls are in general. The only maneuver that everyone in the allergy scientific community agrees on is that several months after an animal is completely removed from the premises to which someone is allergic to (and that has been demonstrated by skin testing or RAST) and after intensive cleaning is done, that person's symptoms should be diminished.

It is not clear whether mite removal does any good at all—although we will discuss this further below.

The above issues are the most clear-cut. Now we get to the confusing part, which is the relationship of mold to human disease. Allergists ignore biological classification of molds and for practical reasons divide molds into two main groups, indoor molds and outdoor molds. The types of molds are somewhat similar in these two groups, the most significant difference being the amount of mold outdoors compared to indoors. There is no question that outdoor mold can aggravate existing asthma. It is only outdoor mold that unequivocally can do that for two reasons. First, the amount of mold outdoors is so much greater than indoor mold; and second, mold is kept in the air by atmospheric wind, whereas air currents in homes are much less intense and indoor mold levels available to be breathed into the lungs are much lower.

Mold can also cause hypersensitivity pneumonias. However, even in this case, the far-greater exposure from the outdoor mold so far exceeds the exposure to indoor mold that it is extremely unlikely that indoor mold can be the sole cause of the hypersensitivity pneumonias. The only exception to this would be an industrial exposure where the quantity of the mold spores in the air would exceed any home exposure by a thousandfold.

It is not believed that mold either indoor or outdoor can cause allergic rhinitis or any other upper-airway illness—most importantly, sinusitis.

When the previous edition of this book was written, there was mass hysteria concerning mold, and toxic mold—especially concerning **Stachybotrys (AKA black mold),** a mold with alleged legendary powers to cause all sorts of devastating illness. However, sounder minds prevailed, and now we know that was all nonsense. In addition, the following diseases and symptoms attributed to toxic mold are currently not believed to be caused by airborne mold *and absolutely not caused by indoor mold*, and they are as follows: atopic dermatitis, urticaria, angioedema, or anaphylaxis as well as superficial mold infections of the skin, such as jock itch, athlete's foot, or ringworm—the latter three are caused by opportunistic fungi, but they are caused by contact, not airborne mold.

Mold exposure does not cause headaches, joint pain, memory loss, cognitive difficulties, rheumatoid arthritis, any autoimmune disease, COPD, chronic bronchitis, or any other illnesses except those rare illnesses listed as being caused by mold in this chapter and book.

There is extensive litigation at the time of the publication of this edition concerning "toxic mold" in certain homes where water incursion has occurred, possibly occurred, or never occurred at all; but the plaintiff (person bringing the lawsuit) is positive that toxic mold is the cause of all their ills. One author (SHY) has experience in mold litigation and has never found mold, or excessive moisture that could be found in a home, to be the cause of the problem. This is backed up in the medical literature; and it is clearly stated that the current evidence does not support indoor mold, or excessive moisture as the cause of most, if any, illness. For the interested reader, relevant references are cited in appendix G.

In fact, there is a danger of falling into the trap of blaming all your medical problems on a recent leak in your home or some mold behind the wall in your home. If you do have serious illness, then you need a detailed medical and allergic evaluation, as studies have shown that most people who feel that they are victims of toxic mold or **Stachybotrys** poisoning have other totally unrelated illnesses. Delay of the proper diagnoses can be harmful and, at a minimum, can lead to complications or progression of the disease.

However, all that being said, we now will present a commonsense approach to environmental controls in your home that has been very effective for our patients and we believe will be very helpful to you. So let us begin with the age-old question . . .

Do We Have To Give Away Our Pet?

Every allergist is asked this question or one like it on a regular basis. Often the patient is near tears at the thought of losing the animal.

Some doctors feel strongly that a person who is allergic to an animal should find that creature a new home. This is certainly medically the best treatment. But getting rid of a cat or dog or horse, or even a bird or hamster, can be a draconian remedy when the pet is loved. And unfortunately, people (including children) who have not had much exposure to animals may not develop an allergic reaction for many months, sometimes up to two years. By this time, the pet may have become practically a member of the family.

If the prospect of life without your pet is too painful for you or for an allergic child, see an allergist about treatment and try to keep the animal clean and restrict its range.

You should not brush or wash a cat or dog yourself if you are allergic to it. Nevertheless, the animal should be kept well-groomed, with a good wash or brushing once a week. The undercoat should be clipped or combed out regularly, especially in the spring.

If your local animal groomer is too expensive, washing the animal is a good chore for a teenager or even a young child, whose grooming rates should be more reasonable. The animal can be washed and dried in a bathroom and then the towels put in the laundry. Brushing and combing should be done outside the home. The brush and comb should be washed afterward. If you must brush or wash an animal yourself and this causes a flare-up of allergic symptoms, use a face mask and wash yourself afterward. Remove and clean clothing that has been in contact with the animal. Giving a dog a bath is usually a fairly easy chore. Giving a cat a bath is another matter. If you begin when the cat is a kitten, the process may be easier. With an adult cat, you can try to accustom the cat gradually to the bath. Begin by feeding the cat near running water. Then slightly dampen the cat and follow with its favorite food. Gradually increase the washing, and perhaps eventually the cat will accept a full bath in return for a nice meal.

Studies by indoor-allergen expert Dr. Thomas Platts-Mills at the University of Virginia suggest that cat bathing may not be practical. These studies found that it takes some seventy to one hundred gallons of water to rinse cat allergen off a cat, and the procedure must be repeated every two to three days.

Cat and dog bathing may have some minimal beneficial effects in reducing allergens, but the frequency of bathing necessary makes it impractical for most pets. If you decide to undertake it, you should be aware that it is not a cure-all but just one of many things that may be helpful.

An allergic person should not empty a cat-litter box or should wear a mask while doing so.

As for restricting a pet's range, the first step is to keep the animal out of the bedroom. Next, train it to stay away from your favorite chair or sofa. A cat or dog should have its own bed or one or two resting places of its own in the house. (With firm, consistent training—and strategically closed doors—this usually can be managed.)

If the pet has a particular chair or sofa it rests on, it may help to cover that piece of furniture with a sheet. Wash the sheet daily or at least very regularly.

Some animals do not mind being restricted to one or two rooms of an apartment or house for much of the day. If you live in the country, you may find that you can prepare quarters for the animal on a porch, in a basement, or in a garage or barn. But as a rule, an outdoor home for a pet is successful only if the animal has been conditioned to live outdoors from the beginning.

There is not much benefit to keeping a pet out of doors if you then weaken and let it in occasionally. Once the animal has been inside the home, it may take many cleanings to get rid of the allergen.

Check with a veterinarian or ASPCA representative or other expert on how to keep your pet safely (and hygienically) out of doors. People sometimes overestimate the hardiness of pets and lose them to freezing temperatures.

If an allergy-free person in the family has an office or studio outside the home where the cat can stay, that can solve the problem of how to keep a favorite pet. But remember that cat allergen can stick to your clothes.

If you are at all sensitive to birds or to rodents, such as hamsters or gerbils, do not clean their cages.

After playing with a cat or dog or riding a horse, wash your hands or take a shower, and wash or clean your clothes before wearing them again.

However, the bottom line is if you are allergic to a dog or cat, the only effective way to reduce exposure is to eliminate the pet from the house and then thoroughly clean the entire house afterward, giving particular attention to the bedroom.

CLEANING THE HOUSE

Millions of people are mildly sensitive to dust mites, mold, cockroaches, dander, and so on but do not need to take any special measures to guard against exposure. Others find that their reactions to household allergens are really troublesome, especially at times of year when they may already be bothered by pollen or mold from out of doors.

How do you know if you are sensitive to house dust? An allergy may be indicated by a skin test or RAST. But simple observation may be test enough.

Do you sneeze, and do your eyes itch when you are cleaning house or when you shake out a dusty blanket? Do you have trouble when the heat is turned on in winter? Dust that has settled in the system is blown through the air; and heat currents cause dust, dander, and mite particles to become airborne.

Do you have a severe sneezing attack when you change the bag in the vacuum cleaner?

Frankly, you do not need a medical degree to diagnose the ailment. The question is, what should you do about it? If your symptoms are mild or occasional, simply try to avoid exposing yourself to dust. Wear a mask or ask someone else in the family to help. But if you are affected more severely, and especially if you are asthmatic, you may need to take steps to reduce your exposure to allergens in your home.

The first place that needs attention is the bedroom. People with allergies, who can get a good six to eight hours' sleep in an allergen-free room, often do quite well the rest of the time.

Change or alter bedding. The bed's mattress and box springs should be vacuumed and then encased in a hypoallergenic zippered plastic cover. To be extra safe, seal over the zipper with plastic tape. Mattresses not only attract dust mites, but they may also contain allergenic materials such as horsehair.

This is what we wrote ten years ago, and if you are very cost conscious, then those instructions will work. However, much better materials are available today that can be purchased from companies that we have listed in the appendix. There are many products, and we will discuss the basic principles of how they work. You can order catalogs from those companies that will list their entire product line. You will be able to get information as to what masks to wear, filters to put in your vacuum, vacuums, air cleaners as well as dehumidifiers to use.

Starting from the simplest maneuver, don't bother taping the zipper with plastic tape, as the newer products all have zipper flaps that seal the allergens in. The material is tightly woven microfiber that is strong and lightweight. When placed under pillowcases or sheets, you won't know that it's there. The pore size is two microns (that's two-fifths the size of a red blood cell). So this keeps the bad guys, such as dust mite antigen and small animal-dander antigens that can cause allergic symptoms in your nasal passages and bronchi, inside the mattress or pillows. But the good guys such as air and moisture can get in—these new microfibers can "breathe," as they say in the industry. This is what makes them so comfortable, as anyone who has slept on a plastic cover can attest to.

These covers have varying degrees of comfort and breathability, although they all are very effective as allergen barriers. **See the websites or company brochures for more detail.** Cheaper products often have a pore size of six microns and will not be as effective.

The most important thing to do is to cover your pillows and mattress with the best mite barrier cover you can afford. A tip to save a few bucks: the manufacturers make vinyl box spring covers that are much cheaper, completely effective for the box springs, and will not interfere with your comfort in any way since you are not in contact with the box springs.

In fact, most bedding, such as comforters and mattress covers, can be made of these materials. You can buy comforters that are manufactured with mite-barrier outer covers already in place. Bed skirts should be washable or made of mite-barrier materials and both are available. Blankets that can be washed frequently should be purchased. Comforters with less-than-standard fill that simulate a blanket's warmth but are covered with mite-barrier material are also available.

More good news for the homemaker: these materials are almost impervious to water and only have to be washed occasionally, and certainly not every week—see the manufacturer's instructions.

A person showing symptoms of allergy should preferably not use feather pillows or a down comforter (although comforter and pillow covers are available to cover your favorite down comforter if you so desire—and if you do choose to keep the pillows or comforter, it should be covered). Also, allergy patients should probably avoid wool blankets or mattress pads, as they can be irritants. When you change the bedding, which you should do every week or ten days, vacuum the mattress pad or wash it, and wash the bedding regularly in water 140°F or hotter if possible. Follow the manufacturer's instructions about cleaning the mite-proof encasings.

When you travel, take your pillow covering with you. Recently, some manufacturers have introduced pillows with a built-in mite barrier; so theoretically, these don't have to be covered. One concern of ours is if this barrier gets broken, then either the pillow has to be discarded or at that point covered with a mite-proof encasing.

Remove carpets and rugs. The next step is to remove any carpet or rugs in the bedroom. Carpeting typically is loaded with dust mites and is a major source for reinfesting the bedding.

If you want to try to keep a carpet or rug in the bedroom, it should be dry-cleaned or steam-cleaned every six months or so and then vacuumed every few days. Shaggy rugs are inevitably going to be very difficult to live with. A rug or carpet with a short pile or smooth weave may be tolerable, although vacuuming does not effectively remove dust mite allergen from within the carpet, only from the surface.

If you want to try to keep a carpet, some treatments are available.

Dust mite allergen is broken down (denatured) by tannic acid, which is found in tea. A solution of 3 percent tannic acid is used in a product called Acarosan, which comes as a moist powder that should be brushed into the carpeting and then vacuumed up.

We have not found Acarosan to be useful, and application is a bit tedious. It is no longer recommended by the National Heart, Lung, and Blood Institute asthma guidelines, but it is listed in textbooks on allergy as having some beneficial effect. Therefore, if you want to use it, by all means, purchase it and follow the manufacturer's instructions.

Clean the room. Now, give the room a good cleaning; and if you are allergic to dust, consider getting someone else to do the job. If that is not possible, use a damp or oily mop and damp or oily dust rags to keep the dust from flying up. Wear gloves and a surgical mask while dusting.

These steps are often adequate, but a very allergic person may need an even cleaner environment.

Clear out clutter. In the bedroom and throughout the house, reduce or clear out clutter—that is, dust catchers and debris such as wall hangings; collections of stuffed animals; neglected closets full of old clothes and dusty items on shelves; dust rags in the utility closet. Books should be in glass cases or should be dusted regularly. (Keeping books clean will lengthen their life, by the way.)

Suppose you have invested in Persian rugs or wall-to-wall carpeting for the living room. Luckily, it is not as important to get carpeting out of the living room as out of the bedroom. So try frequent cleaning, perhaps in this situation backed up with use of a mite-allergen-control fluid (tannic acid), but do check with a rug expert to make sure your valuable rug can stand the rigors of this treatment.

Change the furniture. The ideal furniture for an allergic person is modern Danish or something similar, that is, furniture made of sealed wood, plastic, and metal with minimum stuffing. Upholstered furniture with stuffing of animal hair, cottonseed, or kapok is likely to cause trouble. In humid conditions, even foam-rubber stuffing tends to harbor dust mites.

The change in furniture may have to be gradual. But the allergic person should avoid musty sofas and chairs. Treat yourself to a modern recliner with a vinyl cover.

Avoid heavy drapes and venetian blinds. Venetian blinds and heavy lined floor-to-ceiling drapes grab on to dust. You are much better off with thin synthetic washable drapes or curtains.

If you are not willing to discard heavy drapes or curtains, have them cleaned frequently. Venetian blinds can be vacuumed and also washed in the bathtub. Drapes and blinds can be replaced by window shades (which are easier to clean). There are some rather elegant shades now on the market, including thermal shades.

Wash down the area. Wash down the walls and shelves. Wash floors if possible.

CLEANING: CURE OR CURSE?

As you may have gathered by now, cleaning is sometimes unhealthy for the allergic person. Perhaps the only benefit of perennial (year-round) rhinitis is that you have a right to ask someone else to do much of your cleaning. Often it is best for the allergic person to be off the premises while the cleaning is done and for eight hours afterward.

The process of vacuuming fills the air with dust disturbed by the flow of the exhaust and by the movement of furniture. Also, fine particles of dust escape through the bag and the exhaust. The result is that, in the short run at least, you'll inhale more dust while vacuuming than if you just curled up in the dusty room with a good book. (Generally, pollen and mite allergen settle out of the air in a few minutes. Mold spores and dander remain airborne much longer but settle eventually.)

If the allergy-afflicted person is stuck with the job of housecleaning because there is no one else to do it, here are some protective measures worth trying:

Filter paper is available to cover vacuum exhaust vents. If you are buying a new vacuum, you might consider a model that filters the exhaust. There are several brands of vacuum cleaners that purport to reduce emissions. Generally, with these machines you lose some efficiency; but in some cases, they really are cleaner to use. Check with a reliable consumer guide, such as *Consumer Reports,* before making a purchase.

Most but not all the vacuum cleaners with low emissions rely on HEPA (high-efficiency particulate arresting) filters. These filters resemble a paper made with thin pleated glass fibers; they are also used in air cleaners and some heating systems (see below).

- A medical mask or dust mask can be worn while cleaning; the latter is available through dealers that specialize in allergy products or at a hardware store.
- Wear gloves to protect your hands while dusting or during spring cleaning. It is a good idea to cover up while cleaning and wash your clothes afterward.
- To clean surfaces, use single-wipe dust rags or damp or oiled rags. There are also mop covers that attract and hold dust. A damp mop is fine on most floors.

- To clean the oven, open all windows. In winter, use an exhaust fan to disperse fumes. If necessary, wear a vapor mask. These masks are sold by hardware stores for people who work with paints, wood strippers, and so on.
- You can reduce the frequency of oven cleaning by wiping up spills with a damp cloth while they are still hot. A self-cleaning oven is wonderfully convenient but still gives off fumes in the cleaning process. You will probably need to ventilate the kitchen for an hour or more.
- If washing chores irritate your skin, try a mild soap instead of detergent and oxidizing bleach (based on hydrogen peroxide) rather than chlorine bleach.
- Keep as few toxic cleaning products as possible in the home, and use them sparingly.
- One of the real hazards of housecleaning, whether or not you suffer from allergies, is the toxicity of many cleaning substances, such as furniture polishes, metal cleaners, moth balls, and pesticides for indoor plants and cockroaches.

ELIMINATING MOLD

How do you know whether you are allergic to mold spores instead of or in addition to dust? You can be tested, but a few simple questions may indicate the probable answer:

- Do you have problems when leaves fall or when walking through leaves or raking them? Fallen leaves become moldy very quickly. Do you feel uncomfortable on hayrides? Allergy symptoms provoked by grass cutting or exposure to hay are often caused by mold, not pollen.
- Are your symptoms most severe on damp summer days? Very likely, you're allergic to mold.

Most molds in the home originate from outside sources but grow readily indoors in garbage bins; in food-storage areas; in wallpaper and upholstered furniture; on bathroom walls, bath mats, and shower curtains; or in any place affected by standing water.

Damp windowsills and frames and bookcases are attractive to molds.

As we have previously said, the evidence that indoor mold causes illness is less than compelling. The following are suggestions for eliminating mold in your home. To start with, you must eliminate dampness, clean up areas where mold is growing, and sometimes remove a favored mold habitat, such as a bathroom carpet.

- *Cut back shrubs.* If you have evergreens or other trees and shrubs growing close to the house, cut them back. Branches should not touch the house. There should be an eighteen-inch space between foliage and siding. Remove leaves from gutters and around the foundation.

- *Check your house or apartment for leaks.* Put a sump pump in the basement if necessary. Look for leaks affecting closets and walls.
- *Remove old wallpaper.* Paint instead.
- *Check the bathroom for leaks.* In bathrooms, you may need to regrout or recaulk to be sure water isn't seeping under the tiles or tub. Be sure the bathroom is well ventilated.
- *Empty the drip pan under the refrigerator.* Clean out the refrigerator too.
- *Dry damp floors and walls.* Dampness should always be attended to. It is the single most important factor in mold growth.

Mold can sometimes simply be wiped away, using chlorine bleach or another fungicide. Common fungicides include halogen products (such as Clorox), phenolated products (such as Lysol), and benzalkonium chloride (Zephiran Chloride).

Clean mold out of bathrooms or other humid areas in the home every two to four months or more often if the mold visibly returns. But read very carefully the label on any products you use. Some fungicides are highly toxic. Windows should be wide-open during cleaning, and an exhaust fan should be used too. You should limit storage of these products, for seeping fumes do nothing to improve the air you breathe.

TECHNOLOGY TO THE RESCUE

Humidity is essential to the survival of both mites and mold. Cockroaches do not like well-ventilated areas. Any significant airflow tends to make them move on. Therefore, dehumidification and ventilation automatically reduce home-based allergens.

DEHUMIDIFIERS

Dehumidification can be done with an air conditioner (an excellent solution, but only in hot weather) or with a dehumidifier machine. Correct venting and fans can also be helpful. For example, an exhaust fan is a useful tool against localized humidity in a bathroom or laundry room. A fan and vent in an attic or cathedral-ceilinged room can be used to get rid of heat and humidity from a fairly large area.

There is, however, a bit of science to getting the most from fans and vents; so you might want to consult a knowledgeable builder or architect. Libraries usually carry do-it-yourself books and periodicals that offer information on this subject.

The first step in undertaking dehumidification is to assess the extent of the problem. There are some obvious clues to high humidity, such as sweating windowpanes in winter or paint peeling off a house.

For a precise measure of home humidity, you can pick up a humidity gauge at almost any hardware store. A range of 40 percent to no higher than 50 percent is good. Humidity lower than 35 percent can make breathing uncomfortable for people with asthma and some other respiratory conditions, but generally, low humidity is not the health hazard that high humidity is.

Do not overlook a check of humidity in out-of-the-way spots, such as a crawlway, attic, basement, or laundry room. Wrapping cold-water pipes with insulation will prevent them from sweating and decrease dampness in such closed-in areas. Storing firewood in the house imports mold and increases humidity. Wood gives off a surprising amount of moisture as it dries out.

If you decide to buy a dehumidifier, use a reliable retailer who will take the time to help you determine what size machine (or machines) you need for your particular situation. From the physician's point of view, the most important thing about a dehumidifier is that it be kept clean (it should be cleaned daily); otherwise, mold will proliferate in the tank, causing more problems than the dehumidifier cures. One can actually smell mold flourishing in some dehumidifiers. Follow the cleaning directions very scrupulously. The machine should come with a solution that will prevent mold growth.

HUMIDIFIERS

In most parts of the country, through most of the year, humidifiers are not needed; humidity levels seldom drop below 35 percent, and too much humidity promotes mite and mold growth throughout the house. However, depending on your area and your home heating system, a well-heated house can be very dry in the winter.

Some hot-air heating systems have built-in humidifiers. These systems may make the air more comfortable to breathe, but they have drawbacks. A hot-air system tends to blow dust, mold, and so on into the air. And while these systems are often promoted as low maintenance, keeping them completely free of mold and bacteria may prove to be a challenge.

There are also stand-alone humidifiers. These are frequently used in homes with antique furniture or valuable paintings that can be damaged by dry air. Humidifiers and vaporizers are also often recommended for people with allergies, asthma, or other respiratory difficulties and also for patients with atopic dermatitis that is aggravated by dryness.

But humidifiers may do more harm than good.

The most common type of humidifier is evaporative, with a wick or pad that soaks up water from a reservoir and a fan that spreads water vapor into the air. The water can become a breeding ground for bacteria, which can cause "humidifier fever," a flulike infection of the respiratory tract.

Ultrasonic humidifiers, which are now rare, were developed to overcome the problems associated with the standard device. Ultrasonic waves kill the harmful microorganisms in the water. Unfortunately, these machines may then spew fragments of the dead creatures into the air, along with molecules of the minerals and gases in the water, including in some cases harmful materials.

A white dust on the furniture indicates that a humidifier is spreading minerals through the air.

A newer type of humidifier uses vibration to create a vapor but does not solve the problems associated with the distribution of materials in the water.

Vaporizers, in which heated water is the source of the humidity, also may contain problem-causing fragments but usually fewer, as the fragments tend to settle below the heated water. Steam-mist vaporizers, especially when used with distilled water, can give relatively safe relief. They should be cleaned after each use, and all other types of humidifiers should be cleaned daily, following the manufacturer's instructions.

With a frail person or a child, to avoid scalding accidents, someone else should always be in the room when the vaporizer is being used.

By and large it is best to use humidifiers sparingly. The health benefit is limited, except in the case of infants with croup, who may need to spend time in a steamy bathroom with a hot shower running.

We usually recommend small hot-steam humidifiers to be used in the bedroom at night only when an apartment or house is very dry (i.e., below 20 to 30 percent). The advantage is that they can be cleaned easily and therefore will not send harmful particles into the air.

In general, low humidity is not harmful. After all, people with respiratory problems often move to the desert, where the air is very dry indeed. Your body has its own humidifying mechanism in its nostrils and airways. By the time air reaches your lungs, it is usually adequately humidified.

Cutting back on heat in winter ordinarily results in moister air. A pan of water on the radiator will increase humidity, but the pan must be cleaned every day.

CLIMATE CONTROL: AIR CONDITIONERS AND CENTRAL HEATING SYSTEMS

An air conditioner is almost essential to filter summertime air for those sensitive to pollen and other seasonal airborne allergens. It is also an excellent dehumidifier and thus limits the proliferation of dust mites and mold. The airflow discourages cockroaches.

Whether the air-conditioning is a central unit or a window box, the filters must be cleaned frequently, both for maximum efficiency and to prevent mold growth.

Central-system air-conditioning and heating sometimes are equipped with electrostatic filters that catch smaller particles, such as dander, which may get through an ordinary filter. The filters work by imparting a charge to particles in the air as they pass through the filter and then trapping the particles with an oppositely charged plate in the unit. These devices too must be cleaned often.

Electrostatic filters have one drawback: they produce ozone, which makes asthma worse. This hazard can be reduced by the installation of a charcoal filter in conjunction with the electrostatic filter. This has been standard practice by manufacturers in the United States for some twenty years now.

There are filters that can be placed over individual outlet ducts of central heating and cooling systems. If you cannot find filters specifically designed for this use, substitute air-conditioning filters. Clean the filters once a week and replace as necessary.

Unfortunately, it is not clear that the filters available for home heating systems are fully effective. Ask for guaranteed specifications on the size of the particle that the filter will trap. Five microns or less is good. Usually, HEPA filters are best.

Any airflow tends to disturb dust. If you have an air conditioner or hot-air heating outlet in the bedroom, try to get the room fairly dust-free before turning on the air conditioner or furnace.

Some forced-air heating systems come with a humidifying element to counteract dryness. As we mentioned, this can be double trouble: dust is kicked up by the hot air, and mold may emerge from the humidifying element. The systems should come with instructions for cleaning, and the cleaning must be done on schedule. Some people have the humidifying feature removed.

Allergy sufferers find radiant-heat systems, such as electric heating and hot-water heating, preferable to forced-air systems, which blow allergens and irritants all over the place.

Air Cleaners. Room air-filtration devices, or air cleaners, are sometimes recommended for people with allergies or asthma. A 1988 report by the American Academy of Allergy, Asthma & Immunology suggested that such devices might be of some help in reducing asthma attacks, but the study's results did not reach the level of statistical significance.

Various brands of air-filtration machines using HEPA and other filters are commercially available. Other types of air-filtration devices use electrostatic precipitators and ionizers to control dust.

Electrostatic precipitators have been accused of producing ozone, but tests of filtration machines with charcoal prefilters show no apparent ozone problems. Unfortunately, the tests did not demonstrate much health benefit either, so it may be just as well to avoid the risk of ozone exposure.

A room air-filtration machine is one of the modern world's little luxuries. If you can afford it, it may be worth trying. But there is no hard evidence that such a device will really reduce allergens in the air.

All in all, a professional housecleaning and the use of exhaust fans and well-maintained air conditioners and dehumidifiers are the best proven allergen reducers.

INDOOR POLLUTION

Indoor pollution is a serious health problem. Moreover, the tighter we seal buildings to retain heat and save energy, the more acute pollution becomes.

People with allergies or asthma are often affected by small amounts of pollutants that others notice only in high doses. To give an example, some people are sensitive to tobacco smoke. Even a very little amount of it in the air makes them quite ill, giving them headaches and making it difficult to breathe. *No one should smoke, but especially not around a person who has allergies or asthma.*

Other fairly common causes of exacerbation of allergy and asthma at home are heating or cooking gas (natural or propane) and perfumed items, such as scented candles, air fresheners, and incense.

If you are sensitive to natural gas or propane, be sure that there are no leaks in your lines. For the lines that you can reach (those inside the stove and between the stove and the wall or floor), one test is to shake up detergent with a little water, wipe it on the lines, and look for small bubbles forming. The bubbles indicate leaks. But the best thing to do if you smell gas, even fleetingly, is to call the gas company.

Some people are bothered by the small amount of gas that comes from a pilot light. You can put an exhaust hood over the stove. You can turn off the pilot light and convert to an electric ignition system. But you may eventually find that you are most comfortable with an electric stove.

Space heaters that burn natural gas, kerosene, or bottled gas should be vented to the outside. These heaters produce nitrogen dioxide and carbon monoxide, neither of which is good for your breathing or general health.

Some people are bothered by fumes in a house or apartment building that is heated with oil or gas. Smoke from wood stoves and fireplaces can be troublesome, especially to asthmatics.

To reduce pollution from heating-oil fumes, clear the fumes from the basement with a vent and exhaust fan or by opening a window or a basement door to the outside every couple of days. Also, exhaust fans in the uptake lines will draw fumes into the chimney more efficiently. You can try air filters in the duct work. Have your chimneys cleaned regularly (a safety measure, in any case). Lower the thermostat setting.

If none of these measures are satisfactory, you may do better with an electric heating system, if you can afford it.

Painting and floor waxing can cause flare-ups of allergy and asthma symptoms. If this is true for you, have the job done by others at a time when you can be out of the house for several days. Working with water-based paint has less effect on asthmatics than working with oil-based paint.

Structural Pollutants

Some materials and chemicals built into home or office construction can cause allergy-like reactions.

Carpet. One suspect item used in both homes and offices is wall-to-wall carpet. No one knows at this point whether the reported illnesses associated with certain newly installed carpets are caused by the glue, the latex backings, or the carpets themselves; but the symptoms include burning eyes, nasal irritation, and breathing problems.

Insulation. If you are buying insulation, you should check the product with a reliable evaluation service and with an informed allergist. If you are buying a home, have an engineer identify the type of insulation for you and evaluate it as you would a new product.

One of the substances formerly used in insulation and still used in other structural materials, such as some plywood and wallboard, is formaldehyde. (Also, from time to time there are reports of a flawed structural product from which formaldehyde escapes in excess amounts.) The effects of formaldehyde in relation to health and allergy are the subject of considerable controversy. At high concentrations, formaldehyde is toxic, producing severe skin irritations and burning of the nasal mucosa (mucous membranes of the nose) and of the lungs. Formaldehyde is also carcinogenic.

The question is whether small amounts of formaldehyde escaping into the air in small amounts in the home or workplace are a health hazard. The answer is still not clear.

Formaldehyde, incidentally, has a fairly distinct odor. Your nose is not a bad formaldehyde detector.

Pesticides and Repellents

In recent years, the public has become much more aware of the dangers of filling homes with pesticides. More and more people, for example, are trying to control cockroaches by nontoxic means rather than with monthly visits from the exterminator.

Avoid treating house plants with pesticides and fungicides, especially during cold weather, when windows are kept closed. Try nontoxic remedies, such as washing the plants with detergent or alcohol. Throw out infested plants quickly so that they do not affect others.

Pyrethrum, a natural pesticide made from the flowers of a chrysanthemum, is related to ragweed. Pyrethrum is actually a safe, good pesticide—for everyone but certain allergy sufferers. To them it is a menace.

There have been reports of allergic and toxic reactions to heavy use of topical insect repellents containing 2,3:4,5-Bis (which has been eliminated from many products now) and even the basic DEET (*N, N*-Diethyl-*m*-toluamide). Be cautious in using these repellents. Do not spray them all over the head and body, and especially not all over a child. Use a nonspray liquid and follow the directions on the label. *Do not use products containing 2,3:4,5 Bis at all.*

Outbreaks of encephalitis are typically followed by area-spraying with the pesticide resmethrin to control mosquitoes. This substance can cause rashes and asthma.

With respect to insect repellents, cleaning substances, and similar commonly used products, use your eyes and ears to follow health news. Always read the labels before buying a product for your home, and follow the instructions for use and disposal.

For more on indoor pollution and "sick buildings," see chapters 4 and 14.

Chapter 5

ALLERGY MEDICINES

Taking the commonsense approach of avoiding troublesome allergens is, as we have said, the first and most important step in allergy treatment. Unfortunately, it is not always enough. Sometimes avoidance is impossible: children with hay fever, for example, who want to play baseball and softball aren't going to find many pollen-free ball fields. If your fiancée owns a cat and you don't feel quite secure with the ultimatum "Kitty or me!" you may need medication to treat or prevent the symptoms you experience in the company of the cat.

People with severe or chronic allergies may need immunotherapy, or desensitization (allergy shots), to tone down their sensitivity to certain allergens. But symptoms that are mild or arise only occasionally can be alleviated with drugs, such as antihistamines and decongestants. Such medicines are sometimes needed even after desensitization.

Self-medication with over-the-counter drugs is often the first treatment an allergy sufferer tries. This approach frequently is effective and usually less expensive than consulting an allergist. But self-medication may prove unsatisfactory and can be quite expensive as well, so it is best undertaken with a good understanding of the range of medicines available for allergy treatment.

TRADITIONAL MEDICINES

Certain drugs that relieve allergy and asthma symptoms have been known for centuries. The ancient Chinese used ephedrine, a stimulant that opens the airways, which is derived from a desert herb of the genus *Ephedra.*

Stramonium (jimsonweed) leaves when smoked may provide some relief from asthma. Atropine, which is found in these leaves, is the basis of the bronchodilator drug Atrovent. Unfortunately, jimsonweed can be quite toxic. When taken in large doses, it may induce unpleasant symptoms, including hallucinations; and it can be fatal.

The key breakthrough in the pharmacology of allergy treatment did not emerge from ancient remedies, however, but from modern medical research. It was the discovery of antihistamines in 1942.

ANTIHISTAMINES

Antihistamines available today provide relief from a wide range of allergic diseases, from hay fever to hives. They are not much help in directly treating asthma, their benefit in asthma being in situations where the asthma is made worse by nasal allergy; and thus, treating the nasal symptoms improves the asthma.

Since the synthesis of the first antihistamine, diphenhydramine hydrochloride (Benadryl), numerous varieties of antihistamines have been created. Unfortunately, like Benadryl, many of the older antihistamines had unwanted side effects, especially sleepiness. This was a significant drawback to the use of this type of medication. However, newer antihistamines have been developed that do not cause drowsiness, as we discuss below.

How Antihistamines Work

Antihistamines prevent histamine from acting on the cells of the capillaries (tiny blood vessels), nerve endings, and other cells that have histamine receptors. This action of histamine, working in concert with other chemicals produced by the body in response to invading allergens, causes allergy symptoms.

Recall that a double connection is needed to release histamine. The allergen molecule locks into a molecule of IgE antibody; the IgE is attached to one of the mast cells in the tissues lining the nose, lungs, or gastrointestinal tract. When the connections are made, the mast cell suddenly releases a large amount of histamine, along with other chemical substances, producing allergic symptoms. Histamine release also occurs when similar connections are made with allergen IgE and a basophil, which is a type of white blood cell. (See figure on page 4.)

Histamine makes the capillaries widen and release fluid. This may result in swelling, such as hives. In severe reactions, a significant drop in blood pressure may occur. Histamine can irritate nerve endings, causing itching. In the gastrointestinal tract, it may cause increased secretion of fluids and cramps. And it may provoke tightening of the smooth muscles in the bronchial airways.

Histamine acts upon receptors on the surface of the cells that it affects. Antihistamines have a molecular structure similar to histamine and therefore can block the histamine from reaching its normal receptors. The antihistamine connects with the cell receptors, leaving the histamine molecules with no place to latch onto, like molecular losers in a game of micro-musical chairs. When the histamine can't get to the cell receptors, the chain of occurrences that makes up the allergic reaction is interrupted.

From this, you can see why doctors and pharmacists recommend taking antihistamines before your symptoms have appeared. You want to have the antihistamine latched onto the histamine receptors before the histamine released by mast cells can get there.

Try to anticipate the need for antihistamines. For example, if you are allergic to ragweed and you hear on the morning news that ragweed counts this season are expected to reach a century-high record, take your antihistamine. Don't wait until you're a weeping, sneezing wreck.

New antihistamines, being tested for use in controlling asthma, chemically stabilize the mast cells, inhibiting their release of histamine.

Antihistamines are categorized according to the two different kinds of receptors that they act upon. There are H_1 (histamine 1) receptors and H_2 receptors. Therefore, among antihistamines, there are H_1 blockers and H_2 blockers.

The H_1 and H_2 receptors are present on many human-tissue sites, including the very-important capillaries (where H_1 receptors predominate) and the lining of the stomach (where H_2 receptors are particularly important). Therefore, H_2 antihistamines are more commonly used in treating disorders of acid secretion in the stomach, the exception being they can be helpful in hives, which is discussed later.

There are many more H_1 than H_2 antihistamines—seven classes of them, in fact. The H_1-antihistamines are particularly helpful in treating allergic rhinitis, or hay fever. But medical researchers are still studying the best way to use antihistamines in treatment. One fairly new approach is to combine H_1—antihistamines and H_2 antihistamines to treat hives. In the past, only an H_1-antihistamine was used.

ANTIHISTAMINE SIDE EFFECTS.

The most notorious side effect of some H_1-antihistamines is sleepiness. This is not always an undesirable effect. If you are suffering from severe allergic rhinitis, a soporific antihistamine may help you to get a good night's sleep; but for daytime use, the soporific effect can be a real problem.

Always check the label of an over-the-counter antihistamine or the warnings that come with a prescription antihistamine. As a general rule, be cautious about driving a car, operating dangerous machinery, or working in high places after taking such medication. It has now been shown that the newer nonsoporific (non-drowsy) antihistamines do not interfere with cognitive function in any way, whereas the other antihistamines always do, *even if they do not make you sleepy!* Your doctor can explain the circumstances under which it is safe to use any antiallergy medicine prescribed for you. Your pharmacist is another source of information, not only on prescription medicines, but on those sold over the counter as well.

A special note of caution for those who drink or take tranquilizers: many antihistamines interact with alcohol and tranquilizers to depress the central nervous system, leaving the patient really groggy.

Antihistamines tend to produce tolerance. This means that a drug that at first makes you sleepy may later not do so. This can be a plus, but another effect of this tolerance is that the drug may not work as well to relieve your symptoms. At that point, your doctor might recommend trying another class of antihistamines to see if they are more effective. If you are self-medicating and develop a tolerance, try a brand made with a different class of antihistamine.

Certain antihistamines may produce what are technically called anticholinergic effects, such as heart palpitations, retention of urine, constipation, dry mouth, and nervousness. Therefore, one should be careful about using an antihistamine described as possibly producing such effects while taking any other anticholinergic drugs—for example, dicyclomine (Bentyl), hyoscyamine (Levsin), and various combination products such as Donnatal.

Consult with a doctor before taking an antihistamine if you are taking any anticholinergic medicine, antidepressants of the MAO-inhibitor type, or if you have thyroid disease, heart disease, or high blood pressure.

NONSEDATING AND LIGHTLY SEDATING ANTIHISTAMINES

The first nonsedating antihistamine released in the United States was terfenadine (Seldane). It did not cause drowsiness and was very effective. However, in 1992 it was discovered to cause severe side effects when taken with certain other drugs or in excess doses. Terfenadine (Seldane) alters normal heart rhythm and, rarely, may cause severe arrhythmia and, even more rarely, sudden cardiac death. Obviously, these side effects, as rare as they were, were not acceptable; and terfenadine (Seldane) was pulled from the United States market in 1997. Similar side effects have been attributed to the second nonsedating antihistamine introduced in the United States, astemizole (Hismanal).

Seldane and Hismanal were found to block the potassium channels in heart muscle, which are involved in the normal generation of electrical current through heart muscle. This discovery explained the severe side effect of these two drugs. Seldane, even at normal doses, causes changes in electrocardiograms.

Loratadine (Claritin), a newer nonsedating antihistamine, was introduced in the mid-1990s. Claritin did not have this effect on heart-muscle potassium. Furthermore, even in excess doses, Claritin does not produce any changes in electrocardiograms (which measure heart-muscle electrical currents).

Because of this, loratadine (Claritin) became the nonsedating antihistamine of choice. Other so-called second-generation antihistamines were introduced recently. They are cetirizine (Zyrtec) and acrivastine (available as Semprex-D, the D meaning it is combined with pseudoephedrine, a decongestant). However, in clinical trials, cetirizine (Zyrtec) and acrivastine (Semprex-D) caused drowsiness in about 10 percent of patients compared with 5 percent of placebo-treated patients. (To keep this in perspective, the older antihistamines such as chlorpheniramine [Chlor-Trimeton] caused sedation in more than 50 percent of patients.) Therefore, cetirizine (Zyrtec) and acrivastine (Semprex-D) cannot be truly classified by the FDA as nonsedating, although they are quite close and deserve a special classification such as "less sedating." More recently, the third-generation antihistamines have been released. They are either "mirror-image molecules" (levocetirizine [Xyzal] or metabolites (desloratadine [Clarinex] and fexofenadine [Allegra]. These third-generation drugs were designed to be more effective and with less side effects than their second-generation counterparts. While fexofenadine (Allegra) does live up to this standard and has no cardiac side effects as opposed to its related terfenadine (Seldane), the others (desloratadine [Clarinex] and levocetirizine [Xyzal]) do not really have any advantage over their related (Claritin and Zyrtec).

All these new antihistamines except, at the time of publication, for Xyzal are available in combination with a decongestant (pseudoephedrine, or Sudafed: Allegra-D, Claritin-D, Clarinex-D, Zyrtec-D). Acrivastine (Semprex-D) is only available in combination with Sudafed, which is a slight disadvantage in that you cannot use the antihistamine by itself in situations where you don't have a need for a decongestant. The recommended frequency of doses of the combination products depends on the speed of the release of the decongestant.

Pseudoephedrine adds the risk of stimulant-type side effects: nervousness, insomnia, and heart palpitations. It is best, when possible, to take this medication earlier in the day, when the drug will not interfere with sleeping. Many, perhaps most, patients may do better to use the plain antihistamine and then use the pseudoephedrine when needed to relieve congestion. This is sometimes a matter of personal preference.

Keep in mind that with all the above products, it is impossible to say that one is universally better than another. One may be more effective in one patient and not very effective in another. A patient may become tolerant to one, benefit from switching to another, and then use the original product again in the future. As we've said, to determine the best drug or combination of drugs for any given patient, at any given time, is sometimes a trial-and-error process.

One of the advantages of the new antihistamines loratadine (Claritin), desloratadine (Clarinex), and fexofenadine (Allegra), which are nonsedating, is that they do not typically interact with alcohol and tranquilizers.

In general, most physicians today recommend extreme caution in taking any drugs during pregnancy. At the time of this revision, loratadine (Claritin), levocetirizine (Xyzal) and cetirizine (Zyrtec) are pregnancy category B, whereas fexofenadine (Allegra) and desloratadine (Clarinex) are category C, making loratadine, levocetirizine and cetirizine the ones deemed safest during pregnancy. See chapter 17 for details.

Here follows a list of the H_1 oral antihistamines. We list only the generic names of the drugs as there are numerous products that contain these antihistamines with and without decongestants and other medications.

Table 5.1 Oral Antihistamines

Class/Type	Generic Name	Available in
Class 1 **Ethylenediamines**		(This is a partial list of common brands, but it is important to read labels as contents change.) The brands listed often contain other ingredients such as pseudoephedrine.
	Pyrilamine maleate (AKA mepyramine maleate)	Codimal, 4-Way Fast Acting Nasal Spray; Poly-Histine products; Triaminic products
	Pyrilamine tannate	Rynatan products
	Tripelennamine hydrochloride	Pyribenzamine (PBZ) products
Class 2 **Ethanolamines** (This class of antihistamines tends to have a more marked soporific effect.)	Bromodiphenhydramine hydrochloride	Ambenyl, Amgenal, Bromanyl, Bromotuss
	Carbinoxamine maleate	Histex, Palgic, Rondec
	Clemastine fumarate	Tavist products
	Dimenhydrinate	Dramamine (used for motion sickness)
	Diphenhydramine hydrochloride	Benadryl, Nytol, Advil PM
	Doxylamine succinate	Contac Nighttime, NyQuil
	Phenyltoloxamine citrate	Atrohist, Comhist, Magsal, Naldecon, Poly-Histine
Class 3 **Alkylamines**		

(This class of antihistamines tends to be less soporific than the above.)	Brompheniramine maleate	Bromfed, Dimetapp, Dimetane, Drixoral
	Chlorpheniramine maleate	Chlor-Trimeton and numerous other products
	Chlorpheniramine tannate	Rynatan
	Dexbrompheniramine maleate	Drixoral
	Dexchlorpheniramine maleate	Polaramine
	Pheniramine maleate	Dristan Nasal, Naphcon-A eye drops, Poly-Histine, Ru-Tuss
	Tripolidine hydrochloride	Actidil, Actifed
Class 4 Piperazines		
	Acrivastine	Semprex-D* (with pseudoephedrine)
	Cyclizine	Marezine (for motion sickness)
	Hydroxyzine hydrochloride	Atarax
	Hydroxyzine pamoate	Vistaril (multiple uses: anti-itch, antinausea, mild analgesic, opiate potentiating drug)
	Meclizine hydrochloride	Antivert, Bonine, Dramamine (for nausea and motion sickness)
	Phenindamine tartrate	Nolahist, Nolamine
	Cetirizine hydrochloride	Zyrtec*

	Levocotirizine hydrochloride	Xyzal*
Class 5 Phenothiazines		
	Methdilazine hydrochloride	Tacryl
	Promethazine hydrochloride	Phenergan (multiple uses: antihistamine, sedative, antinausea)
	Trimeprazine tartrate	Temaril
Class 6 Piperadines		
	Azatadine maleate	Optimine, Rynatan, Trinalin
	Cyproheptadine hydrochloride	Periactin
Class 7 Nonsedating antihistamines		
	Fexofendadine	Allegra
	Loratadine	Alavert, Claritin
	Desloratadine	Clarinex
	Astemizole, Terfendadine	Removed from market because of cardiac toxicity

*Significantly less sedating than most antihistamines, although not nonsedating. H_2 Antihistamines

The first H_2 antihistamine, cimetidine (Tagamet), came on the market in the United States in 1982. Its primary use now is to treat stomach and duodenal ulcers. It is still used in the treatment of urticaria (hives) but has lost favor somewhat because it is a short-acting drug (frequent doses are necessary).

A newer H_2 antihistamine, ranitidine hydrochloride (Zantac), lasts longer (two doses daily are usually recommended) and is less likely than Tagamet to affect the metabolism of other medicines that a person might be taking, such as theophylline or antidepressants.

Two other H_2 antihistamines, famotidine (Pepcid) and nizatidine (Axid), complete the family for the time being.

All are used in treating stomach disorders, such as ulcers and reflux of stomach contents into the esophagus, which can trigger asthma in some people (see chapter 9).

Side effects of these drugs do not occur commonly. They include headache and confusion and, even less commonly, constipation, liver dysfunction, blood disorders, rashes, and loss of interest in sex.

The H_2 antihistamines may have the effect of increasing the rate at which alcohol is absorbed into the bloodstream from the stomach. So be careful if you are drinking, especially on an empty stomach.

Tagamet affects the metabolism of drugs and other chemical substances by the liver. If you are taking other medicines or are likely to be exposed to high concentrations of chemicals, such as pesticides, consult with your doctor if Tagamet has been prescribed for you.

TOPICAL NASAL SPRAYS

A more recent addition to allergy treatments is the topical nasal antihistamine. The first one developed was called azelastine hydrochloride (Astelin and Astepro). Recently, another one, called olopatadine (Patanase), was released. It contains the same ingredient as a previously released eyedrop (Patanol and Pataday. Olopatadine [Patanase] probably has fewer side effects in some patients, since about 10 percent of azelastine users experienced drowsiness, burning or stinging in the nose, and a bitter taste in their mouth after using azelastine; and these side effects are essentially nonexistent with olopatatdine. Both of these antihistamine nasal sprays can be used on an as-needed basis to control breakthrough symptoms of sneezing and runny and itchy nose, and they can even relieve some eye symptoms as well. [The eyes and nose are connected by the nasal-lacrimal duct; also, there is some systemic absorption of the drug.]) They can be used as an add-on to some other oral or nasal therapies, or they can be used by themselves.

Anticholinergic medications have been available for years for use with an inhaler to treat certain lung conditions and in pill form as treatment of nasal allergy. A nasal form of this medication is called ipratropium bromide (Atrovent Nasal Spray). This medication is useful in controlling rhinorrhea (runny nose). The lower strength ipratropium bromide (Atrovent Nasal Spray) (0.03 percent) is used for runny nose associated with both allergic and nonallergic rhinitis. The higher-strength ipratropium bromide (Atrovent Nasal Spray) (0.06 percent) is used for treating the rhinorrhea associated with upper respiratory infection or the common cold. Ipratropium bromide (Atrovent Nasal Spray) is relatively free of side effects, although nose bleeds and sore throat can occur in 5 to 10 percent of patients. Overall, it is very effective for the otherwise difficult to control symptom of runny nose.

NASAL CORTICOSTEROID SPRAYS

Topical corticosteroid spray medications developed in the past twenty years have become important in the treatment of seasonal and perennial (year-round) allergic rhinitis. They are available as beclomethasone dipropionate (Beconase AQ, Vancenase AQ), flunisolide (Nasalide and Nasarel), and triamcinolone acetonide (Nasacort). The *AQ* means that the medication is in an aqueous base and may provide a slight moisturizing and soothing effect as well as the anti-inflammatory effect of the steroid.

More recently, a group of high-potency nasal steroids, with decreased systemic potency (i.e., a lesser potential for systemic side effects) have been introduced. These are budesonide (Rhinocort), fluticasone (Flonase and Veramyst), mometasone (Nasonex) and ciclesonide (Omnaris). There is no meaningful evidence that one of these is better than another, although that doesn't mean that one may not work better in any given patient.

The older nasal steroids (beclomethasone [Vancenase, Beconase], triamcinolone [Nasacort], flunisolide [Nasalide]) may take up to a week to achieve maximal benefits. The newer ones (fluticasone (Flonase), mometasone (Nasonex), ciclesonide (Omnaris), and budesonide (Rhinocort) work more rapidly. Because of this rapid onset of action, a case can almost be made for as-needed use in some patients; you should speak to your specialist about this.

The new nasal steroids are best started at the first sign of symptoms or even better, right before a known allergy season. They can also work after symptoms begin but may take longer to obtain relief, especially if the inside of the nose is so swollen that the sprays don't get into the nasal cavity very well.

Most of these medications are effective when used once daily. The safety of the older nasal steroid sprays has been demonstrated in chronic-use studies for up to twelve years. Nasal ulcers can occur but are rare. To reduce the chance of ulcer formation, it may be helpful to direct the spray at different angles each time it is used. A physician should examine the nasal lining (inside the nose) periodically.

Local side effects of headache and nasal congestion are rare and often fade with continued use. Mild nasal bleeding is not common, but if it occurs, you should stop the medication and contact your physician since this may be a sign of nasal ulceration. These sprays are useful in the treatment of nasal polyps and in the prevention of their recurrence after surgery. They are also useful in rhinitis of nonallergic origin and in the management of acute and chronic sinus infections (in conjunction with other medications).

OVER-THE-COUNTER ANTIHISTAMINE AND DECONGESTANT TREATMENT

Many people manage allergy symptoms on their own, buying antihistamines and decongestants over the counter (without a prescription). In terms of cost-effectiveness as well as therapeutic effectiveness, self-treatment is a reasonable approach for short-term flare-ups of allergy symptoms. In recent years, two effective medications, formerly available only by prescription, have been made available for purchase over the counter.

The types of allergy that respond to antihistamine treatment alone, or antihistamine plus a decongestant, include mild reactions affecting the eyes, nose, and sinuses and the itch associated with some rashes caused by contact with substances to which one is allergic.

Antihistamines are not helpful with asthmatic reactions. Asthma attacks, for example, require a combination of treatments prescribed by a knowledgeable physician, typically an allergist or pulmonary specialist. Antihistamines are not going to help asthma directly, but in some patients, their use (usually along with other medications) in the control of nasal allergy can improve the asthma. (See chapter 9.) They can be useful in the initial response to treat food allergies. In severe reactions, they must be used with epinephrine injections and oral steroids. (See chapter 7.)

Most allergists do not recommend trying to treat chronic allergic disease with over-the-counter remedies or sometimes even with prescription antihistamines. By *chronic*, we mean a condition that requires you to use antihistamines for more than three months of the year, in total.

One reason for caution here is that prolonged use of over-the-counter medication, without any physician monitoring, may delay diagnosis of complications involving the sinuses, ears, or eyes. If you experience facial pain, pain above the teeth, ear pain or dizziness, or any vision problems, have your condition checked by a physician.

Even if no complications appear, if you suffer from symptoms most of the time, there are drugs other than antihistamines that might be considered. The possible benefits of trying to reduce your exposure to allergens and of immunotherapy should also be assessed.

In selecting an over-the-counter antihistamine for short-term use, we recommend starting with the least-soporific drug available. In the past several years, a nonsedating antihistamine, loratadine (Claritin) and one "less sedating" antihistamine, cetirizine (Zyrtec), have become available without a prescription. This has significantly improved the choices in over-the-counter treatments. These two medications, which come in various forms and also combined with pseudoephedrine (with the suffix *D* added to the name), should be the first choices when choosing an over-the-counter antihistamine. People's reactions to different types of antihistamine vary, so you may have to experiment to find one that works well for you. Or you might prefer to ask a physician, not necessarily an allergist, for a prescription for a different nonsoporific antihistamine.

The generic versions of the over-the-counter brands are generally cheaper and equally effective. Be aware that prolonged use of one class of antihistamine may result in a tolerance. If one antihistamine stops working, then sometimes switching to a different class may help, though this may also be a signal that the allergy has gotten worse or that there is a complication.

If you are giving a child antihistamines for allergy symptoms, keep in mind that children often react to drugs very differently than adults do. In 2008 the FDA warned against giving cold medications to infants less than two years old and was reviewing the safety of these medications in older children. It is best to consult with a pediatrician or allergist when considering any medication for a child. The same probably applies to adults over age sixty, especially if the medicine is to be taken for more than a couple of days, as older adults do not excrete medications as efficaciously as younger ones do and the medication could build up to toxic levels. Therefore, lower doses should be considered. (See chapter 16.)

DECONGESTANTS

With many kinds of allergy reactions, the patient feels a strong need for a decongestant: the sinuses are swollen, the nose is running, and so on. And there are many decongestant medicines, in both oral forms and topical sprays, available in most supermarkets and drugstores. Yet these drugs may be tricky to use. Some have a minimal or delayed effect. Some have unwelcome side effects, especially in younger children and older adults as mentioned above.

Decongestants are stimulants that work by constricting the blood vessels. They are related to epinephrine (Adrenalin) and have similar side effects. Elevated blood pressure is one possible side effect. Others may be jumpiness, anxiety, rapid heartbeat, and headaches.

Both oral and topical decongestants should be used with particular caution in young children and by people with hypertension, diabetes, heart disease, or thyroid disease and by people who are taking certain antidepressants.

Decongestants tend to counteract the sleepiness caused by antihistamines, so the two theoretically are a good team. But there are different schools of thought on whether it is a good idea to use products that combine drugs, as many over-the-counter preparations do. If you buy individually only the medicines that you are sure you need, say an antihistamine and a decongestant, you can adjust the doses to treat your symptoms precisely. On the other hand, the combined formulas are convenient to use and often effective; but since these combinations are fixed amounts, they don't have the same degree of flexibility.

Whether you buy medicines individually or in combination, be sure to read the label so that you know what you are getting and what side effects to expect. If you are taking other medicines of any sort, ask your physician or pharmacist if there is a possibility of a problem arising as a result of taking the new medicine. For example, if you are taking an anti-inflammatory containing ibuprofen (Motrin, Nuprin, etc.) or any other nonsteroidal anti-inflammatory drug (NSAID), you might want to avoid a cold or allergy product that includes aspirin. Together, ibuprofen and aspirin can create quite a case of heartburn and possibly more serious gastrointestinal problems, including bleeding or even ulcers.

In the table we list some of the more commonly used pure decongestants.

Table 5.2 Decongestants (Oral, Nasal, Ocular)

Generic Name	Common Brand Names	Comments
Oral Decongestants		
Ephedrine sulfate	Generic only	Short acting (rarely used today)
Pseudoephedrine hydrochloride	Sudafed, Novafed	Contained in many antihistamine preparations. A stimulant with side effects that may include elevated blood pressure. Check with your doctor or pharmacist if you are also taking antidepressants or other medicines.
Pseudoephedrine sulfate	Afrin tablets	Similar to above
Phenyl-propanolamine hydrochloride	Off the market	Removed from all OTC and prescription products by FDA order in 2000 because of increased stroke risk.
Topical Decongestants		For short-term use only—follow directions on label carefully.
Phenylephrine hydrochloride	Neo-Synephrine	There are oral forms, but they may not be effective.

Propylhexedrine	Benzedrex	
Naphazoline hydrochloride	Naphcon A, Clearine	Longer duration of action, also in many ocular preparations
Oxymetazoline hydrochloride	Afrin, Neo-Synephrine	Longer duration of action
	Dristan	
Tetrahydrozoline hydrochloride	Tyzine, Collyrium, Murine, Visine	Longer duration of action
Xylometazoline hydrochloride	Otrivin, Sinutab	Longer duration of action

Decongestants taken topically, in nasal sprays and drops, are more effective than oral decongestants are. They are very useful in treating the symptoms of a cold. But they are for short-term use only. It is very important to read the label and follow instructions. Topical decongestants cannot be taken for more than three to five days or more frequently than recommended without risking a rebound reaction, a more severe form of congestion (rhinitis medicamentosa).

Sometimes patients ask what medicine doctors themselves favor. No single product gets all the votes. Doctors' recommendations are based on a number of factors, including their familiarity with one product as opposed to another.

The basic similarity of many of the widely available antihistamines and decongestants is one of the reasons that the products are sold in such complicated combinations with such elaborate advertising. It becomes imperative that one reads the labels to see what ingredients are in a medication. For that reason, in this book we have used generic names with associated brand names, when appropriate.

CROMOLYN SODIUM

The drug cromolyn sodium, discovered in the 1960s, inhibits allergic reactions directly at the mast cell by reducing the release of histamine and other chemical mediators of allergic reactions. Moreover, it acts without the annoying side effects characteristic of many other medications. When it works, it can be very helpful.

How Cromolyn Works

Cromolyn works by inhibiting a mast cell's output of histamine and other chemical mediators, even when the cell is in contact with an allergen-antibody duo that would ordinarily cause histamine release and the resulting unpleasant symptoms.

Cromolyn reduces inflammation associated with allergy, and in asthma it blocks what is called the late-phase inflammatory reaction. This was the first inhaled drug to do this. Its usefulness in asthma has been superseded by the inhaled steroids, and it has recently become unavailable in the United States.

For allergic rhinitis (hay fever), there is a nasal spray called Nasalcrom. And for allergic conjunctivitis, cromolyn comes in the form of eyedrops that may help within days, sold either under the name Opticrom or Crolom.

For hay fever and other allergens. If you are interested in trying cromolyn for hay fever-type symptoms, it is best to get started well before pollen season. In perennial rhinitis, it may take several weeks before you feel a beneficial effect from cromolyn. If you put off seeing your doctor until symptoms have already developed, you may have to use the cromolyn along with some other form of treatment for a while.

Cromolyn is sometimes used to reduce symptoms from exposure to specific, known allergens. In other words, it's worth a try in the kind of situation in which you have an allergy to an animal and cannot avoid contact with the animal. But heavy exposure to allergens can overload the cromolyn mechanism, making it relatively ineffective. Cromolyn is good, but not perfect.

Topical Medications for the Eyes

Eye symptoms are common in allergies to pollen and other sorts of allergic rhinitis. Often the oral antihistamines and even some of the nasal sprays can control these symptoms adequately, but in some patients, these symptoms can be seriously troublesome.

In the late 1990s, novel nonsteroidal medications were introduced to treat these ocular symptoms. The medicines have proved very effective, allowing us to avoid using ocular steroids in most patients.

Ketorolac (Acular), an eyedrop, is the same type of drug as the nonsteroidal anti-inflammatory drugs (NSAIDS) that we commonly use in treating pain and arthritis (Motrin, Naproxen, etc.). As it became clear that allergy results in inflammation, this novel approach to reducing allergy symptoms in the eye was successfully developed. Other eyedrops in this class are diclofenac (Voltaren) and suprofen (Profenal).

Lodoxamide (Alomide), cromolyn (Crolom), nedocromil (Alocril), and pemirolast (Alamast) prevent mast cells from releasing chemicals that cause allergic inflammation.

They can be very effective but only if used properly, which means frequent and regular use. Usually they must be started before the allergy season and will not provide much benefit if used on an as-needed basis. They are not as effective as the combination antihistamine/mast cell stabilizers listed below.

Levocabastine (Livostin) and emedastine (Emadine) are potent topical antihistamines that can be used as needed and can be very effective. However, redness can result from long-term use, and other drugs may be more appropriate.

Olopatadine (Patanol or Pataday) combines the efficacy of an antihistamine with the prophylaxis of a mast cell-stabilizing agent. It can be extremely effective. Pataday is the once-daily version. The medication in the drop is identical, however. Other medications in this class have been released over the past ten years. These include azelastine (Optivar), epinastine (Elestat), and ketotifen (Zaditor, Zaditen, Zyrtec Itchy Eye Drops, Claritin Eye). The last two listed are available over the counter.

All of the above are associated with minimal side effects, mostly related to burning after the eyedrop is applied; burning is common with this type of medication.

None of these ocular medications have the potential for rebound congestion with chronic use such as that seen with the topical ocular and nasal decongestants. However, prolonged use of the topical antihistamines can result in redness but by a different mechanism.

Steroidal medications are effective but should be used sparingly. Typically, a short course will gain control of the symptoms while concurrent use of a prophylactic medication such as olopatadine (Patanol or Pataday) will maintain control when the steroid is stopped. If ocular steroids are required for more than a week, an ophthalmologist should be consulted because of the potential side effects of chronic use, especially increased intraocular pressure (glaucoma). The claim that one steroid has less potential for side effects is untrue.

ANTI-ITCH TOPICAL MEDICINES

If you've ever had a bad case of poison ivy treated the old-fashioned way, you know why today people use corticosteroid creams and ointments. Poison ivy victims used to go around for weeks painted pink with calamine lotion, which actually did little to check the spread of the rash or to relieve the itch.

Treatment with corticosteroids is much more effective for eczema and for poison ivy and other types of contact dermatitis. These disorders (see chapter 12) can occur in mild or serious forms and should not be taken too lightly. When in doubt as to the cause of a rash or when a rash continues to be troublesome for a week or more, it is best to see a doctor for diagnosis and treatment.

POISON IVY RASH

A few patches of poison ivy rash, however, are not ordinarily cause to visit the doctor. Usually, the rash can be diagnosed by anyone familiar with the effects of poison ivy and can be brought under control quickly with an over-the-counter corticosteroid cream. The same is true of an outbreak of dermatitis resulting from short-term exposure to something to which you are sensitive. The person who is allergic to chrysanthemums but includes them in the garden, the person who is sensitive to, say, flea shampoo for pets but uses it on the dog anyway, these people may develop itchy, burning rashes that need short-term treatment and may not require a physician to intervene; but it is impossible to make a generalization such as this. So when in doubt, ask your physician for help.

For preventive treatment of poison ivy, see page 198.

STRENGTH AND USAGE RECOMMENDATION

Most drugstores carry low-potency corticosteroid creams on their shelves, and there are a couple of dozen stronger varieties available through prescription.

We've used the terms *ointment* and *cream* nontechnically; but there are distinctions among ointments, creams, lotions, and gels. Ointments are the most occlusive—that is, they block the penetration of air most effectively and allow the most absorption of the steroid into the skin. Creams, lotions, and gels are, in the order listed, increasingly less occlusive and therefore more drying. So more occlusive is less drying because water is trapped, and less occlusive is more drying since water can escape.

The occlusiveness of these preparations is increased if you wrap the treated area with an airtight dressing, such as plastic food wrap. The result is more impact per dose, but with some of the stronger preparations, the dressing increases the risk of side effects, including skin thinning and infection. Never use such dressings without medical supervision.

As a rule, the fluorinated corticosteroid products are the most potent and must be used with the most care. (These products are identified in the table below.) They should not be used in sensitive areas, especially where the blood vessels are close to the surface—for example, the face, neck, or groin. Nor should they be spread over large areas or be used for prolonged periods. All topical steroids absorb through the skin. Therefore, if you are pregnant or even think you could be, do not use these medications without a physician's advice.

SIDE EFFECTS

Normally, side effects are minimal. Local side effects may include itching, dryness, or loss of skin color. Contact dermatitis sometimes results from chemicals in the medications, especially the paraben preservatives. But there are several paraben-free preparations, such as Halog, Lidex, Kenalog, and Aristocort.

TABLE 5.3 TOPICAL CORTICOSTEROID PREPARATIONS*
(in order of potency)

GROUP I (MOST POTENT)

Betamethasone dipropionate 0.05% (cream & ointment)
Clobetasol propionate 0.05% (cream & ointment)
Diflorasone diacetate 0.05% (ointment)
Halobetasol propionate 0.05% (cream & ointment)

GROUP II

Amcinonide 0.1% (ointment)
Betamethasone dipropionate 0.05% (cream & ointment)
Desoximetasone 0.25% (cream)
Desoximetasone 0.05% (gel)
Diflorasone diacetate 0.05% (ointment)
Fluocinonide 0.05% (cream, gel, ointment & solution)
Halcinonide 0.1% (cream)
Mometasone furoate 0.1% (ointment)

GROUP III

Amcinonide 0.1% (cream & lotion)
Betamethasone dipropionate 0.05% (cream)
Betamethasone valerate 0.1% (ointment)
Desoximetasone 0.05% (cream)
Diflorasone diacetate 0.05% (cream)
Fluocinonide 0.05% (cream)
Halcinonide 0.1% (ointment & solution)
Triamcinolone acetonide 0.1% (ointment)

GROUP IV

Hydrocortisone valerate 0.2% (ointment)

Flurandrenolide 0.05% (ointment)
Fluocinolone acetonide 0.025% (ointment)
Mometasone furoate 0.1% (cream)

GROUP V

Betamethasone dipropionate 0.05% (lotion)
Betamethasone valerate 0.1% (cream)
Fluticasone acetonide 0.025% (cream)
Fluticasone propionate 0.05% (cream)
Flurandrenolide 0.05% (cream)
Hydrocortisone valerate 0.2% (cream)
Prednicarbate 0.1% (cream)

GROUP VI

Alclometasone dipropionate 0.05% (cream & ointment)
Betamethasone valerate 0.05% (lotion)
Desonide 0.05% (cream)
Flucinolone acetonide 0.01% (cream & solution)
Triamcinolone acetonide 0.1% (cream)

GROUP VII (LEAST POTENT)

Hydrocortisone hydrochloride 1% (cream & ointment) Hydrocortisone hydrochloride
2.5% (cream, lotion & ointment) Hydrocortisone acetate 1 % (cream & ointment)
Hydrocortisone acetate 2.5% (cream, lotion & ointment)
Pramoxine hydrochloride 1.0% (cream, lotion & ointment) Pramoxine hydrochloride
2.5% (cream, lotion & ointment)
*Reprinted with permission of *Annals of Allergy, Asthma, & Immunology* 1997,
79:200.

The over-the-counter preparations, being less potent, are unlikely to cause side
effects. But do not use them on children under age two without checking with a
pediatrician.

ALL RASHES IN BABIES SHOULD BE MEDICALLY EVALUATED

There are many other medicines helpful in the treatment of specific allergy
complaints or in emergencies; these drugs are discussed in the appropriate chapters
ahead.

Chapter 6

IMMUNOTHERAPY (ALLERGY SHOTS)

Immunotherapy in the form of "allergy shots" is a basic weapon in the fight against allergies. The shots are not a cure, but when they work, they tend to suppress allergic reactions. This can make life much more enjoyable for those of us with allergies.

Unfortunately, some physicians prescribe series of shots that go on for years, without proper regard to whether the patient needs or is benefiting from this treatment. Fortunately, most doctors are honest.

How can you tell whether your symptoms will be diminished by allergy shots? How can you tell whether a doctor's recommendation of allergy shots is in your best interest or only in your doctor's interest?

First, you want to be sure that you actually have an allergy and that it is the sort of allergy likely to be responsive to immunotherapy. Careful testing, plus a good history, can usually lead a specialist to diagnose an allergy—or the lack of one—correctly.

However, there are mail-order laboratories and shady physicians who are not particularly interested in the correct diagnosis. They want to persuade you that you have an allergy and need treatment, whether you do or do not (see chapter 19).

Here are a few tips to help you avoid mistreatment:

1. Beware of diagnoses made exclusively on the basis of a blood test (without any physical examination or detailed history). Fraudulent or careless laboratories and doctors are apt to diagnose on the basis of a single test. As often as not, in cases of fraud or incompetence, the result of the test is quite a surprise to the patient. This is especially true of food-allergy tests. You may be told that you have an allergy to beef or tuna or wheat or some other food that you eat frequently with no apparent harm. (This was the experience of a Consumers Union investigator who mailed samples of blood to several mail-order allergy-testing labs. Nonexistent allergies were detected, while his actual sensitivities were missed.)

2. Beware of diagnoses of unusual allergies (such as an allergy to the yeast *Candida albicans*).

3. Beware of findings of multiple food allergies to be treated by neutralization techniques and dramatically restricted diets. Food allergies do not respond to immunotherapy. (However, see chapter 7 for attempts at immunotherapy for peanut allergy and tree nuts.)

4. Beware of findings that contradict your own experience. A sound allergy diagnosis usually makes sense to the patient. For example, if you test as very allergic to cats, your doctor would expect you to recall that exposure to cats makes you uncomfortable and a long vacation from cats makes you feel better. If that is definitely not true, the test result, even if genuinely positive, may not be relevant.

5. Before undertaking an expensive course of treatment, get a second opinion from a board-certified allergist. Even the best doctors will misdiagnose occasionally, and not every patient benefits from allergy shots. If allergy shots are working, the patient normally feels the benefit within a year, sometimes within six months. It is usually necessary to continue shots for a couple of years at least, but the idea is to continue only if the treatment is effective, not just in the hope that someday it may help. Fruitless treatment should not drag on for years.

IMMUNOTHERAPY: HOW IT WORKS

Frankly, medical researchers are not entirely sure how immunotherapy works, but they do have volumes of research findings that reveal some of the factors involved in successful immunotherapy.

In the late nineteenth and early twentieth century, when immune reactions were first being investigated, scientists hoped that a wide range of diseases and toxic reactions could be controlled by building up immunities or tolerances in patients. By and large, this line of research has proved enormously beneficial, eliminating scourges such as smallpox and polio through vaccinations that create antibodies to the disease.

Nevertheless, the immune system is so complex that we are still doing basic research in many areas. In studying the immune system disease AIDS, for example, investigators must search for a cure in many different directions, without knowing whether it is best to look for a vaccine against AIDS (which would be a type of immunotherapy), or to focus on inactivating the virus, or to take some other course.

Fairly early on, allergy reactions were distinguished from other immune system reactions. Unfortunately, allergy was most obvious in its most dramatic form: an animal or human in whom the researcher was hoping to build an immunity would suddenly experience a violent, sometimes life-threatening (anaphylactic) reaction upon the second exposure to the substance.

Some of these extreme sensitivities can be reduced through repeated exposure to the allergen in minute quantities—in other words, through immunotherapy leading to desensitization.

In 1909, two English doctors, L. Noon and J. Freeman, began treating hay fever with pollen extract. Hay fever responds quite well to this kind of treatment. But the first controlled scientific study of the effectiveness of immunotherapy in allergy treatment was not published until 1949. Since then, numerous studies have been done worldwide, and we have a much-better picture (although not a complete picture) of the immunotherapy process.

When the body is exposed to a particular antigen (or allergen), it may produce antibodies to that substance. As you know, the basic allergy antibody is IgE. Overproduction of this IgE antibody is typical of allergy reactions. For example, in the season when ragweed pollinates, people who are sensitive to the pollen show elevated levels of ragweed-specific IgE. (It is not known why some people produce abnormal amounts of IgE in response to allergens and others do not, but this is an exciting area of research.)

Immunotherapy in allergy medicine is done by injecting the patient with small but gradually increasing doses of an allergen to which the patient has been found to be sensitive. When this is done correctly, the patient, instead of developing allergy symptoms, gradually becomes less sensitive to the allergen.

For reasons that are not yet fully understood, some allergens in very small doses promote production of a blocking antibody. This is an IgG antibody that interacts with the invading allergen, blocking it from linking up with the IgE allergy antibody found on mast cells and basophils.

A person sensitive to ragweed who is receiving allergy shots of ragweed-pollen extract shows elevated levels of IgG-blocking antibody. During the ragweed season, that patient will not have the sharply elevated levels of IgE antibody that one would expect.

Researchers also have discovered that during immunotherapy, there is increased production of suppressor T white blood cells. It is possible that these white blood cells inhibit the production of IgE.

CANDIDATES FOR IMMUNOTHERAPY

In trying to decide whether allergy shots are likely to help a patient, a careful doctor considers the nature of the allergy, its severity, and other relevant questions, such as whether the patient can successfully avoid the allergen or whether the patient is taking medication that might interact negatively with immunotherapy, such as beta-blockers (drugs used to treat high blood pressure, angina, migraine headaches, and other conditions).

The age range in which immunotherapy is most likely to be successful is from five to about fifty. Significant success also occurs from age fifty to sixty. After age sixty, allergy immunotherapy is less successful, although there are many examples of effective treatment in this age range. In all ages, treatment plans must be individualized.

Although traditionally, allergists do not use immunotherapy with children under age five, and some of us prefer to wait until the patient is ten. Specifically, children ages two to six suffering from mite allergy have been clearly helped by allergy shots.

In general, considering patients of all ages, allergy shots work best for people with allergies to pollen, mites, and cats. Immunotherapy shows variable results in patients sensitive to mold and animals other than cats.

Recent standardization of allergen extracts used in allergy shots has improved results and reduced unwanted side effects.

ALLERGIES THAT USUALLY DO NOT RESPOND TO IMMUNOTHERAPY

- Food allergies normally do not respond to immunotherapy, although extensive work is being done in this field. For further detail, see "Food Allergies," chapter 7.
- Drug allergies are not usually treated by immunotherapy. But with certain drugs, such as penicillin and cephalosporin, desensitization is occasionally attempted when the patient urgently needs the drug. The process is tedious and somewhat dangerous. (Other drugs may also be desensitized in the appropriate individual. See chapter 8 on drug allergy.)
- Allergies to feathers and kapok are not treated by immunotherapy.
- Whether allergies to bacteria exist is a matter of debate, but in cases where they have been suspected, they have not responded to immunotherapy (that is, therapy with bacterial vaccines).
- Cockroach allergy has yet to be shown clearly to improve as a result of immunotherapy. In the United States, there is no standardized cockroach antigen available for treatment.
- Urticaria (hives) does not respond to immunotherapy. The same is generally true of eczema, except that hives and eczema associated with allergic rhinitis or asthma may clear up following allergy shots for those disorders.

ALLERGIC RHINITIS

Allergic rhinitis (caused by one or more kinds of pollen produced seasonally by trees, weeds, and grasses) responds to immunotherapy in 80 to 90 percent of cases.

Whether you would want to take shots for this sort of allergy might depend on how long the allergy season lasts for you. Six weeks of moderate sniffling might be bearable, especially with the help of a nasal antihistamine or nasal steroids (as in nasal sprays) or oral antihistamines and decongestants. But if your symptoms last three months or more or if they are very severe, then you might want to consider immunotherapy. This would be true also if, for whatever reason, you cannot tolerate or do not like the allergy medicines on the market.

Allergic rhinitis is not believed to be caused by mold spores. Immunotherapy for mold-spore sensitivity from outdoor mold does not always work as well as one would hope. The available extracts of mold allergens are not as pure and effective as the pollen extracts. (This is because the mold extracts are made from the whole mold, although only the mold spores are allergenic.)

Many people suffer from perennial rhinitis caused by dust mite allergy, which is then exacerbated by seasonal sensitivity to one or more pollens. This kind of rhinitis is a good choice for immunotherapy. Effective, pure dust mite-allergen extract is available for reducing sensitivity.

Some patients hope that by taking allergy shots, they will be able to avoid the kind of changes in their home environment as suggested in chapter 4. But unfortunately, that isn't so. Both measures are usually necessary.

ANIMAL ALLERGIES

Sensitivity to animals can sometimes be lowered by immunotherapy, but the better way is to avoid or reduce exposure to the animal (see chapter 4).

If avoidance is not possible—perhaps you are a veterinarian or you board pets for a living—immunotherapy is worth trying. A potent cat antigen is currently available and is effective.

Up to now, dog-allergen extracts have been less than optimal, but an improved product is said to be on its way.

There is little scientific data on the effectiveness of desensitization to horses, but many doctors report satisfactory results through immunotherapy. Sometimes the immunotherapy is enough if the patient also avoids grooming the horse or uses an antihistamine before riding. Be aware that an apparent horse allergy may really be a sensitivity to mold spores, which are common in stables, or even to pollen. The correct diagnosis, as always, is important.

ALLERGIC ASTHMA

When there is an allergic component to asthma, especially if it is related to pollen or dust mite allergy, the symptoms often can be reduced by immunotherapy. The same approach as in that used in cases of allergic rhinitis is appropriate: Diagnose the allergy. Limit exposure to the allergen. Desensitize the patient if possible.

There is some evidence that immunotherapy can block late-phase asthma reactions, which is a crucial step in controlling the disease.

Incidentally, there is some evidence that treating allergic rhinitis in children with immunotherapy can prevent the development of asthma.

Bees, Wasps, and Other Nasties

If you have had a severe allergic reaction (not merely local swelling) to the sting of a bee, wasp, or fire ant, it is very important, perhaps a matter of life and death, to get desensitization treatment. You should also learn how to use and always have available an EpiPen, which contains epinephrine (Adrenalin).

If you are stung, try to collect the carcass of the critter (or of one of its relatives) that got you (do not pick it up with your bare hands) and take it with you to your doctor for identification.

Allergy shots, when done properly, will usually provide complete protection against a single sting from an insect in the bee or wasp family. They also provide some protection against multiple stings. But any sensitive person who receives multiple stings should regard it as a potential emergency.

Because immunization to insect venom can be risky, the patient should be tested to determine if a venom allergy has developed. Only a small number of patients test positive in the first week after a sting. Others do not show sensitivity until later. Therefore, current practice is to test immediately for the presence of an allergy to venom. If the results are negative, a follow-up test is done five to six weeks later.

Allergy Shots: What They're Like

Allergy shots are typically started on a weekly schedule, although to speed up the process of desensitizing, one can start by giving the shots twice a week or even more frequently.

Gradually increasing doses of allergen are given with each shot until a maintenance dose is reached. The maintenance dose is a predetermined amount or the maximum dose the patient can tolerate without a reaction—whichever comes first.

While working toward the maintenance dose, one must keep to a regular schedule or else the dose must be held the same or reduced. For example, if you are getting a shot every week and miss two weeks, the dose should not be increased. If you go more than four weeks without a shot, the dose should be reduced.

Allergy shots are safe to continue during pregnancy, but it is best not to start treatment or to increase the dose at this time. The idea is to avoid a systemic reaction to the shot, which, although rare, could be harmful and possibly induce a miscarriage. After the maximum dose has been reached (which usually takes six months to a year), the shots can be administered less frequently, gradually stretching out the interval to two, three, or even four weeks.

Shots are sometimes given seasonally, either during or preceding the season in which the patient reports having suffered allergy symptoms. This approach is not recommended. The best results come when the shots are given year-round. If you are being treated for an allergy to ragweed, the dose of ragweed allergen should not be increased during the ragweed pollination period. This applies to other pollens as well.

The shots are not painful. They are given under the skin (subcutaneously and hence are referred to as subcutaneous immunotherapy, or SCIT) but not into the muscle (intramuscularly). They are usually administered by a nurse (alternatively a PA [physician's assistant] or NP [nurse practitioner] can administer the shots), but a physician must be on hand in case you experience a systemic anaphylactic reaction to the shots (with swelling of the throat, hives, difficulty breathing, and so on). If that happens, the doctor will immediately give you a shot of epinephrine (Adrenalin) and perhaps antihistamine. This will almost always take care of the problem. Very rarely, a patient may have to go to the hospital. There is an extremely slight risk that death may occur; but in the past twenty-five years, very, very few deaths from immunotherapy have been reported in the United States.

The patient should be prepared for possible reactions. Sometimes the skin around the site of the shot becomes red, itchy, and swollen, forming a raised wheal. Sometimes the whole arm begins to swell.

Even if you have experienced only minimal reactions or no reaction, you must wait in the doctor's office for a half hour after each shot to be certain that you do not develop difficulty breathing or other symptoms of anaphylaxis. Most severe reactions occur in the first thirty minutes after the shot, so it is imperative that you remain in the doctor's office during this period.

LENGTH OF TREATMENT OF SUBCUTANEOUS IMMUNOTHERAPY (SCIT)

Immunotherapy is often continued for three to seven years. Improvement should occur within a year of achieving maintenance. If this doesn't happen, it is wise to discontinue the shots.

There are certain circumstances under which a long period of treatment—a minimum of ten years—is advisable. In some cases, it may be best to continue indefinitely if the treatment results are excellent. This might be true, for example, in the case of someone with severe asthma who is much improved during immunotherapy.

Complicating conditions, such as nasal polyps or sinus or ear disease, may also dictate a prolonged course of treatment.

If it is difficult for you to get to your allergist's office, arrangements can sometimes be made to have the shots given by another doctor. Occasionally they can even be given in the home (although this is not recommended).

With home treatment, you must be scrupulous in following directions about refrigerating the allergen extract, measuring dosage carefully, and maintaining emergency medications.

Results and Costs

Allergy shots might be considered expensive, but costs should be compared to the medications used to treat them as allergy shots can reduce the amount of medications needed. It is difficult to come up with a cost estimate that is meaningful nationwide because prices vary from place to place.

The bills are covered at least in part by almost all types of medical insurance.

Among patients whose symptoms disappear or are reduced and who then stop the treatment after, say, five to seven years, a lucky one-third finds that the reduced sensitivity is a permanent condition. Another one-third experiences the return of some symptoms but remain much improved. The unfortunate other third will return to their original allergic state. This tendency to relapse is very variable; relapse may occur within a few months of discontinuing immunotherapy or even ten years later. Most relapses occur within three years of discontinuing immunotherapy.

Immunotherapy can be started again if your symptoms return, but it may not be successful the second time around.

There is no way of predicting which patients will do well on allergy shots and which will remain well if the treatment is stopped. But your odds of being helped by allergy shots are good, assuming that you are an appropriate candidate for such treatment.

Are the investment of time and money worth it for a treatment that may not yield permanent effects, even if successful? This is almost always a question that only the patient can answer. It very much depends on your circumstances. If you have limited medical insurance (perhaps hospitalization only) and are working your way through college or working to send a child to college, allergy shots may be a luxury that you have to postpone. On the other hand, some patients can manage their symptoms with medication but opt for immunotherapy, which does away with the need for sprays and pills. Although no doctor can honestly promise success in advance of treatment, all allergists have many happy stories to tell.

In the last twenty years, allergy treatment that can be administered orally has been developed, and it is called sublingual immunotherapy—SLIT to its friends. SLIT continues to be experimental but does hold promise in the future for treatment of seasonal allergies. Because of the quantity of allergens that have to be given and the possibility of some GI irritability, the extent of treatment is currently limited. The authors do not use subcutaneous immunotherapy except on patients with multiple allergies, as the process is tedious. The authors virtually never treat a patient with allergies confined to one or two seasons, as pharmacological therapy is very effective today. However, in areas of the country where the seasons are very long, such as California, this may be an effective way of treating grass and tree allergies, which have very long seasons there, whereas in the northern part of our country, the seasons are much shorter. Therefore, SCIT is much more effective than SLIT because treatment with multiple allergens can only be given effectively with SCIT.

Much work is being done on SLIT. However, studies to date have not convinced the FDA to approve this product; and therefore, SLIT is not reimbursed by insurance companies, although some practitioners affiliated with university centers do use it in accredited studies that are still evaluating it. Since it is not covered by insurance yet, this can require several thousand dollars a year of out-of-pocket expense.

SLIT is administered orally, under the tongue, and depends on absorption from that site. Unlike regular allergy shots, SCIT (subcutaneous [under the skin] immunotherapy), the optimal dose or duration of treatment required for this to be effective is not known. As mentioned, but of significant importance, the feasibility and efficacy of treating with multiple allergens in not known as well.

The advantage of SLIT is that there are less systemic reactions than with SCIT. However, SLIT can cause gastric reflux and theoretically might cause a more serious syndrome: eosinophilic esophagitis. Because the long-term efficacy and safety of SLIT are not known, the authors, at the time of publication of this book, do not recommend SLIT. However, a website associated with this book will be updated periodically, so as they used to say when we were kids, stay tuned.

Xolair technically is "an allergy shot" that is not covered in this chapter. (See chapters 5 and 9.)

Chapter 7

FOOD ALLERGIES

Lucretius observed, "What is food to one is to another bitter poison." In ancient times, a violent food allergy was a mysterious and alarming condition. Imagine a healthy guest at a Roman banquet suddenly choking and gasping then collapsing and dying. It is easy to understand why many innocent survivors were suspected of poisoning the poor victims. It is as true today as it was then that an ordinary food can kill a person who is sensitive to it.

A note from the authors about this chapter: The subject of food allergy is closely related to anaphylaxis, as you will see. Therefore, this chapter should be read in conjunction with the chapter on anaphylaxis (chapter 13).

Today we recognize a variety of food allergies. Even though significant advances have been made in recent years, food allergy is still a very difficult field in allergy medicine, both in diagnosis and management. The mechanisms are often poorly understood, there are key gaps in our knowledge, and the entire subject has been further obscured by a few physicians who practice unproven methods supported by pseudoscience about food allergy. In the allergy-medicine field, unfortunately, there is still a lot more quackery surrounding food allergy than, say, allergic rhinitis. Also, food sensitivities are very complex. There are straightforward food allergies, delayed-response allergies (which are less well understood), and intolerances that resemble allergies but do not involve the allergy immunoglobulin IgE. Adding to the confusion is the fact that the majority of patients who believe they have a food allergy do not actually have a true food allergy. Many of these persons have either a food intolerance or another unrelated condition such as lactose intolerance, irritable bowel syndrome, acne, migraines, or arthritis, to name a few conditions that have been erroneously attributed to food allergy.

Although ongoing discoveries are adding to our knowledge, a lot remains to be learned. Imagine if you were surrounded by a minefield and had to walk through it blindfolded and drunk. This is how a patient whose child almost died from peanut allergy described what it was like to avoid peanuts, as she pointed out there was inadequate labeling of foods and eating at restaurants was too risky.

Two of the most-significant advances in food allergy in the past ten years were not scientific discoveries. The first is a law passed by the U.S. Congress called Food Allergen Labeling and Consumer Protection Act (FALCPA), which became law in 2006. This law requires manufacturers of packaged foods to state on their labels if the food contains one of the eight major food allergen groups: crustacean shellfish, egg, fish, milk, peanut, soybean tree nuts, or wheat. These eight groups account for 90 percent of food allergic reactions. Food manufacturers must comply with the law by identifying *in plain English* on their product labels the food source of any ingredient that is or contains protein from one of the eight foods or food groups mentioned above. FALCPA also requires the type of tree nut (e.g., almonds, pecans, walnuts); the type of fish (e.g., bass, flounder, cod); and the type of crustacean shellfish (e.g., crab, lobster, shrimp, but does not include clams, oysters, mussels, scallops) to be declared. Manufacturers of foods packaged for sale in the United States can comply with this law in one of three ways of labeling: (1) list the item in the ingredient list (e.g., milk, egg, or soy); (2)in parentheses following the derivative food (e.g., casein [milk] or lecithin [soy];(3) near the ingredient, list in a statement that reads, "This product contains e.g. milk, wheat, crustacean shellfish (lobster)."

The only exemptions from the labeling law are for highly refined oils. Also, manufacturers may apply for exemptions for ingredients by petition to the FDA. Thus far, no exemptions have been approved by the FDA, and highly refined oils would still be labeled in most cases unless they are included in flavorings.

This law has obvious limitations. The new labeling requirements apply to retail and all food-service establishments that package, label, and offer food for human consumption. However, the law does not apply to foods that are placed in a wrapper, a carry-out box, or other containers after being ordered by a consumer. So if a pile of sandwiches is on a counter at a deli, having been prepared in advance for the day, they are subject to this labeling law. But if you order a sandwich at that same deli, and they wrap it up for you, there is no labeling requirement. The law does not apply to foods regulated by the U.S. Department of Agriculture (USDA) such as meat and poultry and their adherence is voluntary. Also missing from the law is a requirement for labeling other offending foods such as sesame seeds or other seeds, which are becoming an increasingly frequent offender. But it certainly is a good start in helping food allergic persons avoid the offending foods. In addition, warning labeling such as "May contain (e.g., milk, soy, peanut, etc.)" or "Produced in a facility that also produces milk, soy, peanut, etc.," is considered voluntary and is not covered by the law. Therefore, for example, if there is no warning on a bag of potato chips that states "May contain peanut or wheat," it does not mean that there is no risk in eating these chips for a person with those allergies.

The second major advance in the field of food allergy was the publication of the *Guidelines for the Diagnosis and Management of Food Allergy in the United States:*

Report of the NIAID-sponsored Expert Panel. These guidelines were developed by a panel of thirty-four experts to address the growing concerns about the difficulty of diagnosis of food allergies and the inconsistencies in diagnosis among various health-care providers. The link is listed at the beginning of the appendix dealing with foods (appendix C). These guidelines are unique in that they are intended for all doctors, not just allergists.

In the 1990s, the American Academy of Allergy, Asthma & Immunology formulated definitions of various food-related allergies and sensitivities. These definitions are consistent with some of the definitions included in the new federal guidelines, and we have left them in as they also include definitions of other food-related reactions not covered in the guidelines.

Here follow the academy's definitions (with the addition of a couple of subcategories):

- *Adverse reactions to a food or to food additives.*

Adverse reaction is the global term and encompasses all untoward reactions to food. These include but are not restricted to allergic reactions. An example is Chinese-restaurant syndrome—that is, the headache, tingly feeling, and other symptoms that some people develop when they ingest monosodium glutamate. This reaction is not a true allergy, as it happens, but those people who get quite sick from it should avoid monosodium glutamate.

- *Food allergy or hypersensitivity to a food.* This refers to a reaction, involving the immune system, to a given food or additive. The category includes common allergy reactions—for example, hives caused by eating shrimp. Most often, the substance in food causing an allergic reaction is a protein. Eight types of food account for over 90 percent of allergic reactions in affected persons: peanuts, tree nuts, milk, eggs, fish, shellfish, soy, and wheat. Approximately 4 percent of children under age eighteen have a food allergy in any given year. The prevalence of food allergy in this age group has grown in the past ten years by 20 percent for unknown reasons. In 2007, approximately ten thousand children were hospitalized for food allergy, compared to 2,500 in 1998. The cause of this increasing incidence could be just increased detection and public awareness, but some speculate that the contamination of processed foods with small amounts of peanut or other allergenic foods may have something to do with the rising incidence.

Another theory about the increasing incidence of food allergy relates it to deficiency of vitamin D. There is an epidemic of vitamin D deficiency in most industrialized nations related to lifestyle changes (more time spent indoors). It is estimated that 50 percent of people in these countries have insufficient levels of vitamin D and that 10 to 15 percent are actually deficient in the vitamin. Vitamin D has newly discovered roles in tolerance (tolerating and not reacting to foreign substances such as food). It also plays a role in mucosal immunity or prevention of bacteria in the gut from damaging the intestine and allowing foreign antigens, such as food, to enter the body. So a deficiency in vitamin D can reduce tolerance, making us more likely to react to and not tolerate foreign substances such as foods. And further, a deficiency of vitamin D will allow bacteria to cause damage in the intestines and allow food allergens to enter the body. Both of these theories are possible factors in the increasing incidence of food allergy and warrant further research.

- *Food anaphylaxis*. This is a serious, systemic allergic reaction that is rapid in onset and that sometimes can be fatal. It is a true allergic reaction involving the allergic immunoglobulin IgE. The symptoms, triggered by the release of histamine and other chemical mediators, can include hives, swelling of the throat, a drop in blood pressure, wheezing, and abdominal cramping. Peanuts (which are legumes), tree nuts, shellfish, fish, milk, and eggs are the most common culprits in food-induced anaphylaxis.

Note that there is a similar type of adverse reaction to food, called an anaphylactoid reaction. (The use of the term *anaphylactoid* is no longer recommended but is included here for historical significance.) This resembles anaphylaxis, except that apparently, the problem food causes release of histamine and other chemical mediators without IgE involvement. Strawberries may be an example of such a food. They can cause anaphylactic-type reactions, but no strawberry-specific IgE has been detected.

- *Food intolerance*. This is the name given to an abnormal, less-severe reaction to a food or food additive that is not mediated by the immune system. For example, people affected with lactose intolerance typically develop stomach cramps and diarrhea when they drink milk. The intolerance results from absence of the enzyme lactase, which assists in digesting lactose. The condition is common among older adults, especially African Americans, Asians, Jews, and Mediterranean peoples.

Food intolerance includes the conditions listed below.

- *Food poisoning or toxicity*. This is a reaction to bacteria (such as the salmonella bacterium often found in poultry), products of bacteria, or chemicals present in food. The symptoms can include diarrhea, nausea, fever, and occasionally, organ damage and death.
- *Pharmacologic reactions*. These are adverse reactions to some chemical in the food that acts as a drug. An example is insomnia resulting from ingesting

too much caffeine. Histamine poisoning, discussed below, also can be included in this category.

- **Metabolic food disorders**. These involve an inability to metabolize a given food. One example is lactose intolerance, mentioned above. Another example is favism, an enzyme deficiency that affects millions of people worldwide. The lacking enzyme, glucose-6-phosphate dehydrogenase, helps to protect blood cells. The disease is provoked by eating fava beans or taking certain antibiotics or other drugs. The result is severe anemia. Symptoms include headache, nausea, fever, and jaundice. Favism tends to be hereditary, especially among southern Mediterranean peoples, including African Americans and Italians.

- **Idiosyncratic food reactions**. These are adverse reactions suffered by some people that do not involve allergy mechanisms. Sulfite sensitivity is an example. Sulfite compounds, frequently used in food as preservatives, can provoke a range of allergy-like reactions, including a rapid, severe asthma reaction in asthmatics, which is discussed below.

QUESTIONABLE OR SPECULATIVE ALLERGY REACTIONS

Many substances and additives have been suspected of causing adverse idiosyncratic reactions. In some cases, the evidence against the suspect substance is rather thin.

One of the more controversial foods is sugar. There have been numerous accounts of supposedly adverse allergic or idiosyncratic reactions to sweets, especially hyperactivity and irritability in children. But there is no scientific evidence of such a sugar sensitivity. However, researchers have found that children, who eat a hearty dose of sweets, especially on an empty stomach, may experience a sharp increase of adrenaline in the blood. The mechanism is a sort of roller-coaster reaction, in which elevated blood sugar provokes an increase in insulin production, which, if excessive, causes a quick drop in blood sugar, which stimulates adrenaline production.

Children, evidently, are more likely than adults to experience this swing in hormonal reactions. The result indeed may be irritability and anxiety—and tearful birthday parties.

By and large, most Americans would do well to reduce their sugar intake for reasons of nutritional health, but not because sugar causes allergic reactions or other immune-system disorders. In fact, there appears to be little relation between food allergies and changes in behavior or mood. This is not to deny that what we eat affects how we feel, for worse and better. But there is not much scientific basis for diet fads that have been popular for years, many promoted by practitioners of marginal medical theories having no supportive scientific evidence.

Some questionable practitioners recommend dangerously restricted diets, supplemented with heavy doses of herbal extracts, whose effects have not been appropriately tested and can sometimes be dangerous.

The guiding principles of good nutrition are still to eat a balanced diet, emphasizing fruit and vegetables and de-emphasizing red meats as a protein source. It also may be prudent to seek out organic foods that are as free of pesticide residue as possible.

The issue of delayed allergy reactions to food is highly problematic because since the time until the reaction is delayed, it may be hard to recognize the association between the food and the reaction to the food. With a delayed reaction, symptoms would appear many hours or even a day after the food has been eaten, while in ordinary allergic reactions, symptoms appear quickly, usually within an hour or so.

A few delayed allergy reactions have been demonstrated. Very recently, a delayed anaphylactic reaction to beef, pork, or lamb has been discovered. (See chapter 13). Another example is milk allergy in infants, which can cause delayed reactions with gastrointestinal symptoms.

More recently, a group of disorders termed eosinophilic gastroenteritis has been discovered. Our understanding of this is evolving, but currently it is a condition that causes gastrointestinal symptoms such as pain and bloating but can also mimic reflux disease from which it needs to be distinguished. This condition can affect any part of the GI tract from the esophagus to the rectum. It is diagnosed by finding eosinophils on a biopsy. But GERD (reflux disease) can also have eosinophils, but in lower numbers. Therefore, in order to prevent confusion, some doctors recommend treating a patient for three months with anti-GERD treatment to eliminate this potential confusion. In some patients with this condition (particularly eosinophilic esophagitis), allergy tests (skin or blood) to some foods are positive; and if you eliminate these foods, they get better. Currently, studies are being done to see if patch testing for food allergies may be more reliable in this condition. But there are numerous cases of suspected delayed allergic reactions in which it is difficult to determine whether the suspect food is actually the cause of the problem and whether the reaction is an allergy or an intolerance of some sort.

A case in point would be a child who frequently eats corn cereal or cornbread in the morning and vomits or complains of nausea later in the day at school. It may not be clear whether there is a corn sensitivity present, although there are diagnostic procedures of considerable value.

Ultimately, if avoiding corn helps the child, it does not really matter whether technically it was a corn allergy that caused the nausea and vomiting. But many children have been placed on restrictive, not necessarily healthy, diets because their parents have come to believe without much evidence that their children suffer from a variety of delayed food allergies.

Incidentally, researchers theorize that in delayed reactions, the offending allergen may not be in the food itself but rather may be a substance produced in the course of digestion or possibly by interaction with a medication that the patient is taking.

How Food Allergies Work

There is a tendency to think that food allergens cause stomach upset and diarrhea, whereas airborne allergens are responsible for respiratory symptoms. But as we've mentioned, molecules of an allergenic substance can travel widely in the body and cause problems far from the original site of entry or impact. Gastrointestinal symptoms, such as nausea and diarrhea, can be present in food allergies, especially in infants. But more commonly, the skin is the target of symptoms, where the allergy reaction may appear as hives or eczema. Before the allergen even gets to the stomach, it may react with mast cells in the mucous tissues in the mouth or throat, causing symptoms such as swollen lips or itchy mouth. The sinuses and respiratory tract less commonly may be affected before or after the food allergen enters the stomach. Numerous organs are involved in systemic anaphylactic reactions, which will be discussed in chapter 13.

Some people develop migraine headaches as a result of food intolerances. The mechanisms are not always known, but it is unlikely that true food allergy plays a role. Caffeine or other chemical substances in chocolate, and amines in cheese may cause headaches. (See chapter 19.)

Food presents a complicated challenge to the body's immune system; for among the hundreds of thousands of substances that may enter the system, the body must distinguish between nutrients, wastes, and poisons. Allergic reactions are a mistake by the immune system involving, usually, a certain class of chemicals (glycoproteins) within a fairly narrow band of molecular weight. Luckily, the body is not likely to develop an allergy to just any food, or we would face a much worse problem. As it is, there are certain types of food that we know are more apt than others to cause allergy reactions. Curiously, among these problematic foods are some that are very common in the normal diet. Indeed, it is not unusual to develop an allergy to frequently ingested foods.

The onset of one kind of allergic reaction can make you more susceptible to other reactions. For example, if you are sensitive to ragweed pollen and the ragweed pollen count is high, you may become unusually sensitive both to other pollens (such as of chrysanthemum and sunflower) and to certain food allergens, in particular in melons, bananas, and chamomile tea.

Some people develop anaphylaxis when they exercise after eating certain foods. Identified culprits include celery, apples, peaches, cabbage, shellfish, chicken, and spices in the Apiaceae family (anise, caraway, coriander, cumin, celery, and parsnip).

People with this problem should not exercise until about four hours after eating and should carry injectable epinephrine (EpiPen) in case of an emergency. After the first episode, always consult a physician before exercising again.

Latex allergy, a serious problem that is increasing in frequency, is also related to food allergies, as cross-sensitivity can exist between latex allergens and a number of foods.

The following information is from the American Latex Allergy Association's website. Ranked in order of significance, these include high association or cross-reactivity with latex: banana, avocado, chestnut, and kiwi, and moderate association or cross-reactivity with latex: apple, carrot, celery, papaya, potato, tomato, melons. The list of low or indeterminate foods is very long and changing, so we refer you to the website if you are latex allergic or otherwise interested. (www.latexallergyresources.org). Foods on the above list may cross-react and cause reactions in latex-allergic individuals. Some of the foods in the list particularly in the low/indeterminate category are foods that share antigenic structures with latex and therefore are only of theoretical concern. The details of these cross-reactions are not fully known.

WHO HAS FOOD ALLERGIES?

Only about 3 to 4 percent of adults suffer from food allergies, but about 25 percent of adult Americans believe that they have food allergies. About 6 percent of children are affected, and most pediatricians are well qualified to treat childhood allergies.

Some food allergies are linked to the atopic diseases: allergic rhinitis, atopic dermatitis (eczema), and asthma, which tend to occur together in patients with a family history of these diseases. For example, there is an increased incidence of peanut allergy in children who have a relative with one of these atopic illnesses.

With certain patients suffering from one or more of the atopic diseases, food allergies definitely play a role. The younger the patient, the more likely that food is a causative agent. The likelihood that a food is provoking flare-ups of rhinitis, eczema, or the like is greater if the patient has had a sensitivity to the food from a young age.

It has been reported that food allergies in children may lead to asthma attacks. Dr. Hugh A. Sampson, who led the research, recommended that children not responding well to asthma medication should be considered for testing for food allergies.

Many food allergies occurring before age three are outgrown. This is especially true of allergies to milk, eggs, wheat, and soy. Peanut allergy was thought to be lifelong, but more recently, we are finding that up to 20 percent of young children do outgrow their peanut allergy by age five. If it is not outgrown by late adolescence, then it is likely going to be lifelong. A word of caution: persons with peanut allergy should not experiment to see if they have outgrown their allergy unless they are being guided by a physician on how to do this. And once outgrown, there can be recurrence of peanut allergy. Unfortunately, new allergies can arise as one grows older. The allergies associated with hives, angioedema (swelling), and sometimes anaphylaxis often appear in late childhood or young adulthood; but they can appear at any age.

While most food allergies are acquired by age two, food allergies can even arise in old age, and they may well be misdiagnosed at that time because the general health picture is complex.

PROBLEM FOODS AND ADDITIVES

Certain foods and additives are more likely than others to cause adverse reactions. But there are no hard-and-fast rules. You may thrive on one of the foods mentioned here and react badly to some normally innocent substance.

In infants and children the most common foods to cause allergic reactions are cow's milk (2.5 percent), egg (1.3 percent), peanut (0.8 percent), wheat (0.4 percent), soy (0.4 percent), tree nuts (0.2 percent), fish (0.1 percent), and shellfish (0.1 percent). The allergies to milk, egg, soy, and wheat usually disappear by the time the child starts school; the other allergies tend to persist for a lifetime.

Many infants and toddlers, approximately 25 percent, are intolerant of orange juice and other fruit foods and may get diarrhea or develop a rash around the mouth. These symptoms do not suggest an allergy and are not usually cause for any concern, although you should notify your pediatrician of such symptoms. You can try a different fruit or dilute the juice.

Given that milk, egg, soy, and wheat allergies are often outgrown, the adult list of most-common foods causing allergic reactions consists of shellfish (shrimp, lobster, crab, crayfish, 2 percent), peanut (0.6 percent), tree nuts (0.5 percent), and fish (0.4 percent). If an older child or adult has a reaction to one of these foods, that sensitivity tends to persist. Reactions to fruits and vegetables are common (5 percent) but not as severe. Allergy to seeds such as sesame seed is an increasing problem. Of course, almost any food is capable of causing an allergic reaction.

In the following sections, we review the major food-allergy groups that are covered by the Food Allergen Labeling and Consumer Protection Act of 2006. This information is not intended to be all-inclusive and will change over time. ***It is of utmost importance to read all food-product labels carefully***. Also, ingredients may change from time to time, so labels need to be checked every time you shop. If in doubt, call the manufacturer. Always take extra precaution when dining in restaurants or eating foods prepared by others. If you are ever in doubt about any product or dish, don't eat it. An excellent resource in writing this book and for persons with food allergy is the Food Allergy Initiative website (www.faiusa.org).

MILK

The federal Food Allergen Labeling and Consumer Protection Act (FALCPA) requires that any packaged food that contains milk as an ingredient must list the word *milk* on the label as described in the labeling requirements.

As cow's milk is usually the first foreign protein introduced into an infant's diet, it follows that cow's milk allergy is the most common food allergy in infants and young children. It occurs more commonly in infants who are fed cow's milk formula as opposed to infants breast-fed or fed a less-allergenic formula. This allergy is usually outgrown. Milk allergy can be manifested by eczema and gastrointestinal symptoms. Less-common symptoms are asthma and rhinitis. Symptoms can include difficult to control asthma, rashes, nasal congestion, poor growth, lethargy, throwing up (dietary-protein enterocolitis syndrome), bloody stools (dietary protein proctitis), pulmonary bleeding (hemosiderosis), and anaphylaxis. Obviously, every parent should be alert for signs of milk allergy (see chapter 16).

There are twenty or more proteins in milk that may produce an allergic reaction. They are divided into two groups, whey and casein proteins. The caseins give the milk its milky appearance. The whey proteins include the lactoglobulin, lactalbumin, and others. Most of these allergenic proteins are heat resistant, so boiling the milk will not help in most cases, but it may be worth a try for those patients who are allergic to heat-labile proteins. However, some of the proteins can even become more allergenic after boiling.

People who must avoid milk because of allergies should be sure to get adequate calcium and vitamin D in their diets. Vitamin D helps in the absorption of calcium. Sometimes, though rarely, a milk-sensitive person can tolerate yogurt or certain cheeses, such as goat's cheese. A vitamin-mineral supplement is also helpful in maintaining adequate calcium intake. A pediatrician should routinely be certain that plenty of calcium and vitamin D are included in the formula or in vitamin drops if a child has milk allergies. An adult who eats a balanced diet ordinarily has nothing to worry about with respect to calcium, but a milk-allergic woman should consult with a physician on the best way to supplement calcium, especially after menopause.

The following ingredients indicate the presence of milk: artificial butter flavor, butterfat, and butter oil; casein and caseinates (in all forms); cheese flavor; curds; ghee; hydrolysates (casein, milk protein, protein, whey, whey protein); lactalbumin; lactalbumin phosphate; lactoglobulin; lactoferrin; lactulose; nougat; rennet; rennet casein; Recaldent (used in tooth-whitening chewing gums); Simplesse (a whey protein-based fat substitute used in low-calorie foods); whey (in all forms).

Cow's milk may be found in the following foods: nondairy products, processed milk products, such as powdered or evaporated milk; breads, frozen and refrigerated soy products (which are often manufactured on dairy equipment and contaminated with milk), cakes, cereals, cookies, crackers and pastries, butter and margarine, except margarine made with soybean oil; caramels; chocolates and other candies; cheese; chewing gum, cream sauces and soups; ice cream, sherbet, puddings; pastas; various canned and processed meats, cold cuts, luncheon meats and hot dogs; certain nondairy milk substitutes containing caseinate; pies with cream filling or made with butter; yogurt. Even shellfish can be a problem as it is sometimes dipped in milk to reduce the fishy odor, so you must ask this when purchasing it.

There is often confusion regarding kosher terminology in food labeling. A D or the word *dairy* near the circled letter K or U means the product contains milk. A product labeled pareve is considered milk-free by the supervising rabbinical organization.

However, a food may be considered pareve even if it contains traces of milk protein. Therefore, you cannot assume that pareve is safe if you have milk allergy.

There are some food ingredients that may sound suspicious, but these are considered safe in milk-allergic individuals: cocoa butter, coconut milk, calcium lactate, calcium stearoyl lactylate, oleoresein, cream of tartar, sodium stearoyl lactylate, and lactic acid (although lactic acid starter culture may contain milk).

Sheep's milk and goat's milk are not safe for persons with cow's milk allergy since most cow's-milk-allergic individuals are also allergic to these milk.

Egg

Egg allergy also can be quite dangerous in children. It is the white, which is more allergenic, that causes the problem; and raw white is more likely than cooked white to provoke symptoms. But even cooked whites may be potent allergens, and an egg-sensitive person must avoid the yolks, since they can be contaminated with whites. In one study, half of egg-allergic children will tolerate small amounts of egg protein in extensively heated (baked) products such as breads, cakes, and cookies. Egg-sensitive children are rarely allergic to chicken and other poultry.

Reactions can include hives and angioedema, flare-ups of atopic dermatitis, nausea, vomiting, and anaphylaxis.

Youngsters usually outgrow the allergy to egg by age five, but this allergy occasionally continues into adulthood. Vaccines produced in eggs (influenza, measles/mumps/rubella [MMR], rabies, and yellow fever) may also cause a reaction, but the culprit in vaccine reactions may also be gelatin used in the vaccines. However, the MMR vaccine has been shown to be safe in egg-allergic individuals; and the current recommendation is that persons with egg allergy may receive the MMR vaccine without testing. The most-recent recommendations are that persons with egg allergy should be skin-tested to the influenza vaccine before administration. However, as this book was being finished, new data suggests that this may be unnecessary and that egg-allergic persons can safely receive the vaccine when administered by doctors knowledgeable in egg allergy.

The federal Food Allergen Labeling and Consumer Protection Act (FALCPA) requires that any packaged food that contains egg as an ingredient must list the word *egg* on the label, as described in the labeling requirements. Very sensitive people may even have to avoid preparing foods with egg whites. A food that contains any of these ingredients must be avoided as it contains egg protein: albumin, apovitellin, dried egg, powdered egg, egg solids, egg substitutes (e.g., Egg Beaters), eggnog, fat substitutes, globulin, lecithin (which is obtained from either soy or egg, but often, one cannot be sure which), Livetin, lysozyme, mayonnaise, meringue, ovalbumin, ovoglobulin, ovomucin, ovomucoid, ovotransferrin, ovovitelia, ovovitellin, silici albuminate, Simplesse, vitellin.

The following may contain egg protein: artificial flavoring, natural flavoring, nougat. Eggs act as an emulsifier in cooking, which means they help ingredients to mix smoothly. Instead, you might want to buy a commercial egg replacer, which may be made from ingredients like potato starch or tapioca. Applesauce also works as an emulsifier. Half a cup of applesauce can replace one egg in most recipes. Two other egg replacements in recipes are (1) one teaspoon baking powder, one tablespoon water, and one tablespoon vinegar and (2) one teaspoon yeast dissolved in one-fourth cup warm water.

Numerous other products may contain egg protein, such as baked goods, breaded foods, cream fillings, custards, candies, canned soups, casseroles, frostings, ice creams, lollipops, marshmallows, marzipan, pastas, salad dressings, and meat-based dishes, such as meatballs or meat loaf. Egg whites and shells also may be used as a clarifying agent in soup stocks, consommés, wine, and alcohol-based and coffee drinks.

Legumes: Peanut

Soy or peanut allergies are fairly common in both children and adults. Both foods are legumes. We will discuss peanut first. The federal Food Allergen Labeling and Consumer Protection Act (FALCPA) requires that any packaged food that contains peanut as an ingredient must list the word *peanut* on the label as described in the labeling requirements.

Often, the oil of these legumes (and of nuts) is safe for allergic individuals. Refined peanut oil is subjected to steps that remove or break down the allergenic proteins and are considered safe for peanut-allergic individuals. In fact, refined peanut oil is exempt from allergen-labeling laws. However, since it is difficult to determine the degree of refinement of commercial peanut oil, it is probably better to avoid it altogether especially in highly sensitive persons. Moreover, cold-pressed, expelled, or extruded oils, which are often called gourmet oils, are typically cold-pressed at 149 to 203°F, which leaves the allergenic protein intact. The oil is delicious but allergenic. The decision as to which oils are safe must be left to your own physician.

One of the most potent of all allergens is the protein in peanuts. As far as is known, it has been responsible for more food-allergy deaths than any other allergen, killing about one hundred persons every year in the United States. The sensitive person must scrupulously avoid raw and roasted peanuts and any form of cooked peanuts.

One must constantly be alert to the possibility that peanuts may have been added to a recipe. For instance, a Brown University student died suddenly a few years ago after eating in a fast-food restaurant where the chili had been thickened with peanut butter. Spaghetti sauce can also be thickened with peanut butter. In a similarly accidental fashion, a teenage boy suffered an anaphylactic reaction and nearly died after eating a doughnut that was described as almond coated but was actually coated with sliced peanuts. Nu-Nuts and other artificial flavored nuts contain peanut protein.

It is considered too risky for a person with peanut allergy to eat at ethnic restaurants (such as African, Chinese, Indonesian, Thai, and Vietnamese), bakeries, and ice-cream parlors due to the common use of peanut and the risk of cross-contamination—even if you order a peanut-free item. Many candies and chocolates contain peanut or can be accidentally contaminated with peanut protein during manufacture.

Lupin(e) is a legume that may cause a reaction in someone with peanut allergy. Lupine is used in many gluten-free and high-protein products. In many European countries, particularly Italy and France, lupine flour and/or peanut flour may be mixed with wheat flour in baked goods. Tree nuts are usually processed in the same facility on the same machinery with peanuts and therefore may contain trace amounts of peanut protein.

A peanut-allergic person must always carry an epinephrine autoinjector (EpiPen), wear a MedicAlert bracelet, and never hesitate to call (after self-administering the EpiPen) for emergency transport to a hospital at the first experience of any symptom. (See chapter 13.)

For unknown reasons, there has been a striking increase in peanut allergy in the past twenty years, and children are increasingly at risk. Of interest is that this is not the case in China, where there is a larger per capita consumption of peanuts. This may be because in China, peanut is largely boiled, but in the United States, it is largely roasted. Something about roasting may make the peanut more allergenic (or boiling may make it less allergenic). One theory about why peanut allergy is increasing in the United States suggests that it is the minute amounts of peanut often present in foods processed in factories that process multiple kinds of food that cause children to develop allergies. This is consistent with the science of immunology as we know it, whereby miniscule amounts of a food ingested are more likely to cause the development of allergy to that substance whereas ingestion of larger amounts lead to "tolerance" of the food, which means the immune system tolerates it without a problem. Our consumption of processed foods has been rising exponentially over the last several decades, leading to this rise in peanut allergy because of exposure to minute amounts of peanut allergen in this processed food. Another theory, in accordance with the cleanliness hypothesis discussed elsewhere, implies that the recommendation to avoid peanuts early in life is backfiring and increasing the incidence of peanut allergy. In the late 1990s, it was felt that feeding peanuts or peanut butter to children under age three who were at risk for peanut allergy (because one or both parents had allergies of some sort) increased their chances of developing a sensitivity to peanuts. More recently, data analysis has shown the opposite may be true, that avoiding peanuts early in infancy will greatly increase the chances of developing a peanut allergy; and the American Academy of Pediatrics changed their opinion about early avoidance, and this opinion also applies to the pregnant or breast-feeding mother. Therefore, until further analysis is available, the current recommendation is that after four to six months, kids at risk for development of peanut allergy (and other toddlers as well) can eat peanut-containing foods.

A peanut-allergic person should beware of hydrolyzed vegetable protein (HVP) in some food products. Peanuts are sometimes used in Europe to produce this. Labeling laws should prevent this from happening in the United States; but imported products, even though they must comply with the allergy-labeling laws, might fall through the cracks.

Patients allergic to peanuts do not necessarily have to avoid tree nuts and vice versa. However, packaged or processed tree nuts can be contaminated with peanut material; and recently, it has been found that up to 50 percent of peanut-allergic individuals are also allergic to a tree nut.

Since peanuts are in the legume family, a person who is allergic to peanut may also be allergic to other legumes. Watch out for peas, beans, acacia, black-eyed peas, chickpeas (garbanzos), lentils, licorice, senna, soybeans, and tragacanth. But before you avoid these other good sources of protein in your diet you should discuss this with your allergist.

LEGUMES: SOY

The federal Food Allergen Labeling and Consumer Protection Act (FALCPA) requires that any packaged food that contains soy as an ingredient must list the word *soy* on the label as described in the labeling requirements. Soy protein may be present in bread, cake, crackers, candy, high-energy bars or snacks, cereals, ice cream, lecithin, margarine, infant formulas, canned or processed meats and sausages, canned fish, salad dressings, sauces, shortening (including Crisco), soups, broths, soybean noodles and pasta (of course), Chinese food, and even peanut butter.

With respect to children's allergies, soy formulas are the best substitute for a milk formula for bottle-fed babies. If your infant does not seem to do better on soy, it may be that she or he has an allergy to that too. Your pediatrician will recommend a substitute diet. It is too risky for a person with soy allergy to eat at Asian restaurants, not only because soy is such a common ingredient, but also because of the risk of cross-contamination.

These names indicate the presence of soy: edamame, miso, natto, shoyu sauce, soy (concentrate, fiber, isolate, milk, protein, sauce, etc.), tamari, tempeh, textured vegetable protein, and tofu.

Studies have shown that most people with soy allergy will tolerate soy oil and soy lecithin. As a matter of fact, soy oil is exempt from the labeling law.

TREE NUTS

Allergies to tree nuts are most commonly manifested by hives and anaphylaxis. Occasionally, gastrointestinal complaints may occur. This allergy is usually lifelong, although one study showed that 10 percent of persons outgrew it. Persons are usually allergic to more than one nut, so the recommendation by allergists is that all nuts be avoided if there is a problem with one.

Nuts are very difficult to avoid because they are used so widely. However, here are the worst offenders. (In parentheses is the approximate incidence of that nut causing problems amongst tree-nut-allergic individuals, showing that walnuts are the most allergy provoking.) There are six families, and cross-reactivity may occur within a family (in other words, if you are allergic to one kind of nut, you may be allergic to its relatives): *family 1*, Brazil nuts(less than 5 percent); *family 2*, cashews (20 percent) and pistachios (related to the mango,7 percent); *family 3* macadamia nuts(< 5 percent); *family 4*, English and black walnuts(34 percent), hickory nuts, and pecans(9 percent); *family 5* (nuts and fruits of the plum group), almonds(15 percent), apricots, cherries, plums, nectarines, peaches; *family 6*, filberts and hazelnuts(< 5 percent).

The federal Food Allergen Labeling and Consumer Protection Act (FALCPA) requires that any packaged food that contains tree nut as an ingredient must list the "specific tree nut" on the label as described in the labeling requirements. The following common nuts are considered tree nuts under this law: almond, Brazil nut, cashew, chestnut, filbert/hazelnut, macadamia nut, pecan, pine nut (pignolia nut), pistachio, walnut. In addition to these common nuts, the following uncommon additional tree nuts also require disclosure by this law. However, the risk of an allergic reaction to these nuts is unknown: beechnut, ginkgo, shea nut, butternut, hickory, chinquapin, lychee nut, coconut, pili nut.

Patients allergic to tree nuts do not necessarily have to avoid peanuts and vice versa. However, packaged or processed peanuts can be contaminated with tree-nut material; and recently, it has been found that up to 50 percent of peanut-allergic individuals are also allergic to a tree nut.

Tree-nut proteins can be found in cereal, crackers, cookies, candy, chocolates, energy bars, flavored coffee, frozen desserts, marinades, salad dressings, chicken breading, barbeque sauces, and some cold cuts, such as mortadella, which can have pistachios. Other unexpected exposures to tree nut can occur when eating pancakes, meat-free burgers, pasta, honey, fish dishes, and pie crust. Mandelonas are peanuts soaked in almond flavoring.

Ethnic restaurants (e.g., African, Chinese, Indian, Thai, and Vietnamese), ice-cream parlors, and bakeries are considered too risky for people with tree-nut allergy due to the common use of nuts and the possibility of cross contamination, even if you order a tree-nut-free item. They should probably be avoided.

Tree-nut protein is found in foods such as marzipan (almond paste), nougat, Nu-Nuts artificial nuts, pesto, and nut meal.

Tree-nut oils may contain nut protein and should be avoided.

Avoid natural extracts, such as pure almond extract and natural wintergreen extract (for the filbert/hazelnut allergy). Imitation or artificially flavored extracts usually are safe.

The following are not considered nuts: nutmeg, water chestnuts, and butternut squash. Tree-nut oils are sometimes used in lotions and soaps. Shea nut, although not usually found in food products except in Africa, is often used in lotions.

Certain alcoholic beverages may contain nut flavoring and should be avoided. These beverages are not currently regulated by the FALCPA (Food Allergen Labeling Act), and you may have to call the manufacturer in order to determine the safety of ingredients such as natural flavoring.

SHELLFISH (CRUSTACEANS AND MOLLUSKS)

There are two groups or varieties of shellfish: crustaceans and mollusks. If you are sensitive to one variety of shellfish, beware of other shellfish in the same group. For example, if you are allergic to oysters, be careful with clams and scallops; but there is no reason to think that tuna will be a problem. In this example of an oyster (mollusk) allergy, you might be able to tolerate crustaceans, but there can be cross-reactivity with that group also. You need to discuss this with your allergist first.

The two "shellfish" groups with this risk of cross-reactivity are (1) mollusks (abalone, clams, cockle, mussel, octopus, oyster, quahog, scallops, snail, and squid) and (2) crustaceans (crab, crayfish, lobster, prawn, shrimp). There is a high degree of cross-reactivity within the two groups but less so between the two groups. In other words, if you are allergic to crab, you need to avoid crayfish, lobster, prawn, and shrimp; but you might be able to tolerate octopus. Again you should not play around with these facts and try things on your own, as these reactions can be deadly. If you have been diagnosed with a shellfish allergy, never eat any kind of shellfish without consulting your doctor first.

It has recently been discovered that most shellfish-allergic children have sensitivity to dust mite and cockroach allergens, which might say more about evolution than allergy.

The federal Food Allergen Labeling and Consumer Protection Act (FALCPA) requires that any packaged food that contains crustacean shellfish as an ingredient must list the "specific crustacean shellfish" on the label as described in the labeling requirements. But note this applies to crustacean shellfish only and not to the mollusk group. Remember, this law only intended to include the eight most common food allergens. Some comfort might be found in the fact that crustacean allergy tends to produce particularly severe reactions compared to mollusk allergy.

Seafood restaurants pose a problem if you have a shellfish allergy, even if you don't order the food you are allergic to. There is often cross-contamination and even reactions to vapors in the air. The same applies to ethnic restaurants (Chinese, African, Indonesian, Thai, and Vietnamese), and they should all probably be avoided. When eating out, people with shellfish allergies should always check with the chef to make sure that shellfish are not cooked on the same skillet or in the same oil as other food are. You also should make sure that your dishes are not prepared with the same utensils or on the same work surfaces as shellfish. Restaurants with steam tables that patrons sit around should probably be avoided because of the risk of exposure to fumes and of cross-contamination.

If you are shellfish allergic, you have to be careful with the following ingredients on labels: bouillabaisse, fish-stock flavoring, seafood flavoring, and surimi.

Fish (Finned)

If you are allergic to one kind of finned fish, you may be allergic to other kinds or even to all finned fish. There is a common antigen in all of them. However, as mentioned above, there is no reason to avoid shellfish, unless you are allergic to shellfish as well. More than half of all people who are allergic to one type of fish are allergic to others, so our recommendation to someone allergic to fish is to avoid all fish. The finned fish include anchovies, bass, catfish, cod, flounder, grouper, haddock, hake, herring, mahimahi, perch, pike, Pollock, salmon, scrod, sole, snapper, swordfish, tilapia, trout, and tuna as well as less-common varieties.

Fish allergen can cause atopic dermatitis, hives (urticaria), and angioedema. It is rarely associated with asthma, but a very fish-sensitive person may get an asthma reaction from the odor of fish cooking. Fish allergen's greatest danger is that it can cause anaphylaxis. This allergy is rarely outgrown.

The federal Food Allergen Labeling and Consumer Protection Act (FALCPA) requires that any packaged food that contains fish as an ingredient must list the "name of the specific fish" on the label as described in the labeling requirements. A fish-allergic person must be very careful when eating foods prepared by others (parties and restaurants). Fish-allergic persons must avoid fish-oil vitamin supplements as they are likely contaminated with fish proteins. Seafood restaurants pose a problem if you have fish allergy, even if you don't order the food you are allergic to. There is often cross-contamination and even reactions to vapors in the air. Also you can assume that worcestershire sauce, caesar salad, and caesar dressing are not safe if you are fish allergic, as they usually contain fish ingredients (anchovies). While hardly used anymore, fish glue can pose a problem. In fishing communities, fish allergen can be found in house dust. Carrageen is used as a thickener in ice cream and other foods. It is a marine plant and is safe to eat.

Fish-allergic people also have to stay away from imitation crabmeat, which frequently is made with surimi, a processed fish product. Surimi is also used in certain meatless food products such as meatless hot dogs and pizza toppings.

Fish allergens are more susceptible to manipulation by cooking or processing than other food substances are. For example, most persons allergic to fresh-cooked salmon or tuna can eat canned tuna or salmon without having a reaction. However, if you are fish allergic, we are not recommending you order a tuna melt while reading this book without getting your allergist's approval first.

Wheat

Wheat allergy can cause atopic dermatitis and, sometimes, asthma and urticaria and, rarely, exercise-induced anaphylaxis. Wheat allergy should not be confused with celiac disease (gluten enteropathy or nontropical sprue), which is a sensitivity to the gluten in wheat and other grains. People with celiac disease have to avoid barley, rye, and oat as well. Wheat contains four allergens: albumin, globulin, gliadin, and wheat gluten. About one of five people with wheat allergy is allergic to one or more other grains as well. This allergy is often outgrown by age three and rarely persists into adulthood.

People with wheat allergy must follow restricted diets because wheat is so widely used. The federal Food Allergen Labeling and Consumer Protection Act (FALCPA) requires that any packaged food that contains wheat as an ingredient must list the word *wheat* on the label as described in the labeling requirements. It is ordinarily found in bread, cookies, crackers, and other baked goods; many beverages, including ale, beer and malted milk; breakfast foods, bran and cereals; candy; ice-cream products; canned baked beans; chili; couscous; any flours; gluten; pasta; breaded foods; batter-fried foods; meat products such as burgers, meat loaf, hot dogs, and sausage; seitan; semolina; and some soy sauces and other sauces, salad dressings, gravies, surimi(shell fish substitute), and soups.

Less commonly known sources of wheat are bulgur, starch, durum, emmer, einkorn, farina, gelatinized starch, hydrolyzed vegetable protein, kamut, natural flavoring, soybean paste, hoisin sauce, spelt, triticale, vegetable gum, and whole-wheat berries.

There are flour substitutes for people with wheat allergy. These include amaranth, arrowroot, buckwheat, corn, flax seed meal, wheat-free millet, oat, potato, quinoa flour, rice, soybean, tapioca, and chia seed flour. Triticeae gluten-free oats (free of wheat, rye or barley) is a safe source of cereal fiber.

Spelt and kamut are grains closely related to common wheat, and are not usually tolerated by wheat allergic people.

Sesame Seed

"Open sesame" from the *Arabian Nights* stories refers to the unique feature of sesame pods that burst open when they ripen. The increased consumption of these seeds has opened up another can of worms in Western countries. The incidence of sesame-seed allergy has been rising in recent years. This is likely due to the increasing use of these seeds in foods sold in the United States. Europe and Canada have added sesame seed to their food-allergy-labeling laws. The United States has not yet followed suit. The more common an allergenic food is consumed in a country, the higher the incidence of allergies to that food. Therefore, it is not surprising that the incidence of sesame allergy is very high in the Middle East. In Israeli children, it is the third most-common allergen behind milk and egg. If you are allergic to sesame seed, you do not necessarily have to avoid other seeds (e.g., poppy, pumpkin, rapeseed, sunflower, and flaxseed [linseed]).

The following names indicate the presence of sesame-seed protein in a food: benn, benniseed, gomasio (sesame salt), halvah, hummus, seeds, sesame oil (AKA gingelly or til oil), sesamol, sesamolina, sesamum indicum, simsim, tahini, vegetable oil.

Given the widespread use of sesame in baking and ethnic cooking of all varieties, it is not wise to eat at bakeries or ethnic restaurant (e.g. African, Asian, Indian, Middle Eastern, etc) if you have an allergy to sesame. Even if you don't order a dish with sesame, there is a high risk of cross-contamination. Let's not forget that many rolls at fast-food restaurants are covered with sesame seeds.

Many snack foods such as candy, protein or granola bars, pretzels, pita or bagel chips, rice cakes, trail mix, may contain sesame seeds. Sesame seeds may be found in a wide variety of other foods, including margarine, sauces, dips, soups, salad dressing, processed meats, and vegetarian burgers.

Some Ayurvedic drugs used in alternative medicine may contain sesame oil. Sesame oil is used in the manufacture of some pickles.

ADDITIVES AND CONTAMINANTS

Food additives can cause a variety of adverse reactions. Most are not allergens themselves; but they may exacerbate asthma, urticaria, or cause gastrointestinal symptoms.

The subject of adverse reactions to food additives is much too large to cover in this book. A recent online review of food additives turns up an astounding number of potential culprits. Among food additives there are at least 2 color fixers, 70 edible thickening agents, 58 excipients, 8 fat substitutes, 128 flavors, 15 food-acidity regulators, 28 food antioxidants, 66 food colorings, 230 food emulsifiers, 36 preservatives, 39 sequestrants. In addition, there are various anticaking agents, antifoaming agents, color-retention agents, humectants, stabilizers, and thickeners to name a few. Indeed, the Food and Drug Administration (FDA) publishes a small volume commonly known by the acronym *EAFUS* (*Everything Added to Food in the United States*), which lists 2,922 substances allowed for addition to foods in the United States. This is not to say that everything added to food can cause problems. But individual case reports abound, and many have not been verified; so we will attempt to cover some of the more common problematic additives, including only those that cause reactions that mimic allergic diseases.

How many people are affected by food additive sensitivity? Several studies mostly in Europe have attempted to answer this question and have come up with very low numbers, less than 1 per one thousand individuals.

Sometimes a food such as milk may be contaminated with small amounts of a drug, such as penicillin, to which a person is allergic. Food contaminants make up another category that is too broad to cover adequately in this book. Contaminants include agrochemicals (pesticides, hormones, antibiotics, veterinary drugs, fertilizers, etc), and environmental contaminants (chemicals that are present in the environment in which the food is grown, harvested, transported, stored, packaged, processed, and consumed).

Synthetic Food Colorants (Dyes) There have been recent reports from a medical journal in the United Kingdom of a link between six food colorings and hyperactivity in children, but this has not been widely confirmed. However, the European Union has enacted warning labels and a voluntary ban, hoping to phase out products containing these six artificial colorings by 2010. These include sunset yellow (FD&C Yellow No. 6), carmoisine (red coloring in jellies), tartrazine (FD&C Yellow No. 5), Ponceau 4R (red coloring), Quinoline Yellow, Allura red AC (FD&C Red No. 40). We will discuss the coloring first.

TARTRAZINE (YELLOW DYE NO. 5)

Several food dyes have come under scrutiny in the past as potential health risks. Tartrazine (FD&C Yellow No.5), a coal-tar derivative, had been linked to bronchospasm in asthmatics and to hives and angioedema. Further evaluation has led to the conclusion that tartrazine-induced asthma does not occur even in aspirin-sensitive asthmatics as was once believed. And after more investigation, it is felt that tartrazine is rarely, if ever, a cause of hives and angioedema. Therefore, we will continue to include it in this book.

The problem with tartrazine sensitivity is that it is not always listed on food-product labels as an ingredient. It is now used less than in the past; but it may be present in flavored drinks, candies, sherbet, pudding, frosting, dry cereals, and even medicines. Any food product or medicine colored yellow or green may contain tartrazine.

SUNSET YELLOW (YELLOW DYE # 6)

Sunset yellow also known as FD&C No. 6 has been much less commonly linked to asthma and urticaria than tartrazine is. There have been isolated cases of gastrointestinal illness confirmed by challenges that were "blinded." There is a lack of evidence to prove an association of this coloring with asthma or urticaria.

OTHER SYNTHETIC COLORANTS

Several other synthetic food colors have been implicated in urticaria, angioedema, asthma, and atopic dermatitis. These include amaranth (FD&C Red No. 2), erythrosine (FD&C Red No. 3), brilliant blue (FD&C Blue No. 1), Ponceau 4R, carmoisine, quinoline yellow, patent blue, azorubin, new coccine, indigo carmine (FD&C Blue No. 2), brilliant black BN, and fast green (FD&C Green No. 3). However, just as with the first two synthetic colorants listed above, there is no compelling evidence for these colors in exacerbating urticaria, angioedema, asthma, or atopic dermatitis.

NATURAL FOOD COLORANTS

Many natural colorants are added to food, perhaps making them "unnatural" in a sense. They include annatto, carmine, carotene, turmeric, paprika, beet extract, and grape-skin extract. Several medical studies have shown that challenges of mixtures of these colorants can cause asthma, hives, and eczema and GI cramping and vomiting.

ANNATTO

Annatto is an extract from the seeds of the fruit of the Central and South American achiote tree. It is a red coloring with a slightly sweet and peppery taste. This extract has been shown to cause asthma and angioedema. The incidence of this sensitivity is probably extremely low in the range of one per ten thousand people.

CARMINE

Carmine and cochineal extract are derived from small insects that live on the prickly pear cactus. It is a deep-red colorant. It is used widely in cosmetics without many reports of allergic reactions. There is a report of a soldier who experienced anaphylaxis after being smeared with a carmine-containing makeup stick to simulate burns in a fire drill. There have been a number of reports of carmine-induced asthma and anaphylaxis. Some of the anaphylaxis has been delayed, several occurring hours after exposure. Because of the increasing incidence of this problem as of January 2011, products in the United States containing carmine or cochineal extract will have to be clearly labeled.

CHEMICAL FOOD ADDITIVES

MONOSODIUM GLUTAMATE (MSG)

Monosodium glutamate, which is naturally present in some foods, such as Camembert cheese, is widely used as a flavor enhancer by cooks in restaurants and in commercially prepared food. MSG, routinely used in many Chinese restaurants, is famous for producing the Chinese-restaurant syndrome that afflicts some people after eating Chinese food. The symptoms include a burning sensation in the back of the neck, headache and general aches and pains, facial or chest tightness or pain, sweating, and nausea. It can also produce upper-body tingling, numbness, weakness, drowsiness, and palpitations. It will produce hives in some patients and sometimes provokes a flare-up of asthma, which can be delayed up to twelve hours. Recently, MSG has been linked to persistent rhinitis in some patients; so if someone has persistent nasal symptoms without any known cause, then we might want to eliminate MSG in the diet and see if the nasal symptoms improve. As mentioned above, this is not an allergy. Indeed, everyone will experience at least some of these symptoms if they ingest a large amount of MSG. Particularly susceptible people should avoid the substance. (Unfortunately, food manufacturers often do not list monosodium glutamate specifically on labels.) Many Chinese restaurants will eliminate MSG if the customer so requests.

SULFITES

Sodium bisulfite and other sulfite compounds are effective, cheap, and tasteless food preservatives added mostly to prevent browning of foods. Unfortunately, sulfites can cause a range of allergy-like reactions, from rhinitis and asthma to anaphylaxis. Anyone who has ever suffered an unexplained episode of anaphylaxis should consult an allergist to determine whether sulfite sensitivity might be the cause. The incidence of sulfite sensitivity is unknown; however, it is known that about one in twenty-five asthmatics will react to sulfites.

Sulfites also can cause severe, even devastating, asthma attacks in asthmatics. The cause of these attacks was a mystery for many years because such a wide range of food was involved and sometimes patients would react to a particular food and sometimes not. It took scientists quite a while to figure out that it was the preservative, not the food, which was causing the asthma attacks and other reactions.

Fresh vegetables caused trouble because they were often sprinkled with sulfites to keep them colorful and crisp (it is no longer legal in the United States to use sulfites in a salad bar or on fruits and vegetables elsewhere).

The amount of sulfites required to cause a reaction varies from person to person. Almost all sensitive people will react to one hundred parts per million or more. It is safe to say that foods with less than ten parts per million are safe even for sulfite-sensitive persons. Foods and beverages containing more than ten parts per million must be labeled as sulfite containing. Therefore, persons with sulfite allergy should be able to avoid sulfites by reading labels. Keep in mind that the terms *sulfur dioxide, sodium* or *potassium bisulfite, sodium* or *potassium metabisulfite,* and *sodium sulfite* carry the same meaning as sulfites or sulfiting agents. Avoidance of sulfites in restaurants is more difficult. The FDA ban on the use of sulfites on fruits and vegetables (except potatoes) has helped, but there are still other foods that may contain sulfites.

Here is a partial list of common foods and their sulfite content.

Highest levels (> one hundred parts per million parts per million): dried fruit (excluding dark raisins and prunes), lemon juice (nonfrozen), lime juice (nonfrozen), wine, molasses, sauerkraut juice, grape juice (white, white sparkling, pink sparkling, red sparkling), and pickled cocktail onions.

Medium/high levels (fifty to one hundred parts per million): dried potatoes, white vinegar, gravies, sauces, fruit toppings, maraschino cherries.

Medium levels (ten to fifty parts per million): pectin, shrimp (fresh), corn syrup, sauerkraut, pickled peppers, pickles/relishes, corn starch, hominy, frozen potatoes, maple syrup, imported jams and jellies, and fresh mushrooms.

Low levels (< 10): Packaged foods with less than ten parts per million, which is considered a safe level, do not have to have sulfites listed on their content labels. These include malt vinegar, canned potatoes, beer, dry soup mix, soft drinks, instant tea, pizza dough (frozen), pie dough, sugar (especially beet sugar), gelatin, coconut, fresh fruit salad, domestic jams and jellies, crackers, cookies, grapes, and high-fructose corn syrup.

Sulfites may be present in various pharmaceuticals particularly in liquids and aerosols. If possible, they should be avoided by switching to similar non-sulfite-containing products. There are no laws covering sulfites in pharmaceuticals, but drug companies have moved in the direction of removing sulfites from medications used for the treatment of asthma. One exception is injectable epinephrine, which contains sulfites and is a lifesaving treatment in severe asthma attacks and anaphylaxis. It has been shown to be safe in sulfite-sensitive individuals and should never be withheld for that reason.

BENZOATES/PARABENS

The benzoates and, to a lesser extent, the chemically related parabens are used as preservatives and antimicrobials in foods. The parabens are used extensively in cosmetics. One of the benzoates (p-Hydroxybenzoic acid AKA salicylic acid) resembles aspirin in its chemical structure and can cause reactions similar to aspirin allergy in aspirin-sensitive people. Parabens are more known for their role in contact dermatitis and will be discussed in the skin-allergy chapter. The benzoates have been shown to be possible though very uncommon causes or exacerbating factors in hives (both acute and chronic), asthma, eczema, pruritus, and persistent rhinitis (in the study described under MSG). One case of hives around a child's mouth after he rubbed food on it was attributed to benzoic acid.

NATURALLY OCCURRING TOXINS

Various types of food poisoning result from toxins produced by bacteria and other organisms. Some types, especially botulism, can be fatal.

Some toxic reactions resemble allergic reactions; and one, produced by a fish toxin, mimics allergy almost exactly because it is caused by histamine. But the histamine, rather than being released by the victim's own immune system, is produced instead by bacteria in the fish. The fish involved are of the scombroid family and include tuna, bonito, mackerel, swordfish, sailfish, marlin, sardines; but nonscombroid species, such as mahimahi, anchovies, and herring, can also cause the problem.

The poisoning occurs when the fish have been inadequately refrigerated. But cooking or refrigerating fish once they have been affected does not destroy the toxin. The fish smells normal. Symptoms occur fifteen minutes to several hours after ingestion and usually last for several hours but on occasion can persist for several days. Typically, the patient suffers nausea and other gastrointestinal problems, as well as hives, headache, and flushing of the face. The most common symptom of all is flushing of the face and neck, which is accompanied by a sensation of heat and discomfort. The rash most frequently takes the appearance of a sunburn rather than urticaria. The full-blown reaction can be confused with anaphylaxis. An allergic reaction to fish, however, usually involves one person, whereas a toxic reaction will involve everyone who eats the fish.

ADDITIVES OF LESS OR NO SIGNIFICANCE

Aspartame is a sweetener that has enjoyed considerable popularity recently. Numerous anecdotal reports of adverse reactions, including hives and angioedema, to aspartame have been made. Evaluation of individuals with self-reported aspartame sensitivity failed to prove any of these cases. Another study showed it is not a cause of chronic hives.

SORBATE/SORBIC ACID

Sorbic acid and sorbate are widely used for the prevention of mold growth on food products. Sorbic acid can also cause contact urticaria around the mouth, especially in children who smear sorbate-containing foods around their face. Sorbic acid has caused contact dermatitis on rare occasion.

BUTYLATED HYDROXYANISOLE (BHA)/BUTYLATED HYDROXYTOLUENE (BHT)

BHA and BHT are popular antioxidants used in a wide variety of foods. It has not been shown to trigger hives or eczema, but in one study, 2 of forty-five asthmatics experienced a worsening of their asthma when given a large amount.

NITRATES/NITRITES

Sodium nitrate and sodium nitrite are used as curing agents in meat products. They have not been shown to trigger hives. One case of anaphylaxis has been reported and was confirmed when the person was given them again in a hospital setting. Another person with generalized itching was made worse when given nitrates.

FLAVORS

Numerous flavoring substances are used in foods and drugs. Many flavorings contain hundreds of different chemical compounds.

Few reports of allergic reactions to flavors exist. Flavorings do not usually contain allergenic proteins, but they can on rare occasions.

There was a recent report of four milk-allergic patients who had reactions to meats: two cases involved consumption of hot dogs and two cases involved consumption of bologna. The culprit was traces of a milk protein (hydrolyzed sodium caseinate) that made up part of the natural flavoring in the products. Another recent case was of an individual who suffered life-threatening anaphylaxis after eating a soup mix. The soup contained peanut flour part of the natural flavoring.

The only examples that have been reported involve milk and peanuts; but the possibility exists that similar reactions might occur to soybeans, eggs, seafood, and other allergenic materials used occasionally in the formulation of certain flavorings.

Flavorings can also cause contact dermatitis in the oral cavity on rare occasions. Most of these involve products that are in prolonged contact with the mouth, such as chewing gum, toothpaste, hard candy, cigarettes, or denture products. Some of the possible culprits are anethole, anise oil, cinnamon and cinnamic compounds, eugenol, menthol, peppermint oil, and spearmint oil. These substances have more potential to be a problem at higher concentrations.

LECITHIN

Lecithin is used as an emulsifier in both foods and drugs. The primary source of lecithin is soybeans, although lecithin may also be made from eggs, rice, sunflower seeds, and rapeseed. Soy lecithin can contain soy allergen. Despite the widespread use of lecithin as a food ingredient, allergic reactions to soy lecithin have been described on only a few occasions probably because the level of residue protein is very small and below the threshold necessary to cause a reaction in most sensitive persons. Remember, also, that lecithin itself is used in small amounts.

PAPAIN

Papain is an enzyme used primarily as a meat tenderizer. There have been rare case reports of anaphylaxis caused by it. In one study, five of five hundred pollen-allergy patients with no history of food-allergy reactions had positive skin tests to and positive reactions when challenged with papain. No firm conclusions can be drawn from this study, however.

GUMS

Many different types of gums are used in foods and drugs. The major gums are guar, tragacanth, xanthan, carrageenan, acacia, locust bean, and alginate. Several of these gums are legumes, including guar, tragacanth, locust bean, and acacia. Remember that peanut, also a legume, is very allergenic, and there is cross-reactivity in some people with peanut allergy with other legumes.

Gums, particularly guar gum, can cause occupational asthma. There are several case reports of anaphylaxis resulting from eating foods or beverages containing guar gum. There is one case report of anaphylaxis resulting from the ingestion of guar gum in several foods and beverages.

Gum tragacanth was implicated in one case of anaphylaxis, as was gum arabic (acacia gum), and carrageenan may have caused anaphylaxis resulting from its use in a barium enema. Thyroid tablets containing acacia gum caused worsening of chronic urticaria.

LACTOSE

Lactose is a sugar present in cow's milk. Commercially produced lactose can contain residues of milk proteins. Lactose is present in many prescription and OTC pills and is also a common food ingredient. No confirmed cases of allergic reactions of milk-allergic individuals to lactose have been described. Lactose intolerance, which is not an allergy, is discussed elsewhere.

GELATIN

Gelatin is most commonly derived from beef or pork and therefore has a low allergenic potential. Kosher gelatin is made from fish skins from several species of fish including cod and thus is potentially allergenic in fish-allergic people. However, the allergens in fish are located in the edible muscle tissue whereas gelatin is obtained from the fish skins, but minute fragments of muscle tissue are likely to adhere to the skin. The gelatin-making process involves rather significant processing; and as we pointed out in the section on fish allergy, fish proteins are very susceptible to processing, often rendering the final product as safe in fish-allergic persons (e.g., canned tuna). In one recent study, thirty codfish allergic persons were given large amounts of commercial fish gelatin (blinded challenge—no one knew what they were getting), and none of them had reactions.

Beef and pork gelatins are often used in vaccines, and allergic reactions to the gelatin-containing vaccines have been reported. However, allergic reactions to gelatin used as a food ingredient are rarely reported. One researcher studied twenty-six children with allergic reactions to vaccines. Seven of the twenty-six had allergic reactions (two had reactions before vaccination and five had reactions after vaccination).

INULIN

Inulin is a sugar found in many different types of plants including chicory, artichoke, salsify, and jerusalem artichoke. Inulin is frequently injected to check kidney function, and there have not been any allergic reactions in this situation. Inulin is also used more these days as a food ingredient because it can stimulate beneficial bacterial growth in the intestines. Recently, there have been reports of people having anaphylaxis to inulin after ingestion of salsify, artichokes, and several inulin-containing foods. This was proven with positive blood and skin tests to the foods and rechallenging the people with the foods in a blinded fashion.

WHEAT STARCH

Starch is used a lot in various foods, but the starch is mostly made from corn, which is not very allergenic. However, starch is occasionally made from wheat. To date, there have been no reported cases of wheat starch causing allergic reactions, but caution may be warranted in extremely wheat-sensitive people.

EDIBLE OILS

Edible oils are derived from allergenic foods such as peanut, soybean, and sunflower seed, although they may also come from less commonly allergic foods such as corn, olive, or safflower seed. Allergens are proteins, and highly purified oils do not usually have detectable protein in them. Therefore, peanut oil, soybean oil, and sunflower seed oil can be safely ingested by people allergic to these foods. However, oils that are not highly refined, gourmet, and cold-pressed oils can contain allergenic proteins and may cause allergic reactions in allergic people.

OTHER DRUG ADDITIVES

Benzalkonium chloride (BAC) is a preservative used in asthma nebulizer solutions (albuterol and metaproterenol). Up to 60 percent of asthmatics may react to BAC and get closing of their airways from it (paradoxical bronchoconstriction). Beware of the symptoms of this reaction, which are cough and a burning sensation and sometimes facial flushing and itching. Drug companies have reduced the amounts of BAC, and this is not as much of a problem anymore; but if you experience such a reaction, tell your doctor about it as there are ways to prevent it. Other medications may contain BAC, including nasal saline, nasal steroids, and nasal-decongestant solutions.

Benzyl alcohol is commonly used as a preservative in many drug solutions and injectables. This has rarely caused contact dermatitis and angioedema.

Propylene glycol is used in various creams, ointments, gels, and oral and injectable medications. While it can be toxic to infants in high doses, the reason we mention it is that it can cause contact dermatitis.

Diagnosis and Treatment

The diagnosis of possible food allergies is aimed at determining whether allergy or some other disorder is causing the troubling symptoms. The next step is to pinpoint the exact food or family of foods that is responsible. Many times, patients themselves figure out which food caused the problem; but it is best to confirm an informal diagnosis, as many times, patients have ideas about food allergies that are not correct. Indeed, surveys show that as many as 25 percent of people think they have food allergies when in fact only 3 to 4 percent actually do.

For example, some children who seem intolerant of certain foods actually are suffering from reflux or stomach ulcers or other gastrointestinal illnesses. Many people, children and adults, contract moderately serious intestinal infections or infestations that cause gastrointestinal symptoms, fatigue, and apparent food intolerances. For example, there is a parasitic disease, giardiasis, caused by giardia, a common parasite in drinking water. The parasites frequently are spread by beavers in rural water supplies, and they exist in city water sources as well. Day-care workers who have to change numerous diapers are often infected. The disease can also be spread by sexual contact. There is a test for giardiasis, and antibiotic treatment is effective.

The doctor taking the patient's history through extensive questioning is important in trying to narrow the field of possibly allergenic foods. Your physician might ask you to keep a food diary, which is a written record and timetable of what food you have eaten at what times, and what symptoms you have experienced. You can save time by starting such a diary yourself before consulting a doctor.

If a certain food or family of foods appears to be the culprit, then you may be asked to eliminate that food from the diet to see if the symptoms subside.

If no particular food stands out as suspect, then the patient may be put on an elimination diet. All common allergens are eliminated from the diet and then introduced one at a time to see if they provoke symptoms. Common nonallergenic foods are rice, bananas, applesauce, and lamb.

To test for sensitivity to food additives, there is a liquid nutritional diet, available by prescription, that contains no additives. The patient may be asked to limit food intake to this liquid for several days to see if the symptoms subside. This is not much fun for the patient.

Skin tests can be used in diagnosis. A negative skin test is reliable in ruling out a food allergy. But skin tests for food allergies yield a high percentage of false positives—that is, the patient has a positive reaction to the food during the skin test but really isn't allergic to it. So in general, what you can say from a positive test is that you may be allergic to it, unless of course the history confirms it as a true positive. A skin test alone should not be the basis for diagnosing food allergy.

The RAST (blood test) is more expensive and is less sensitive to food allergies than skin testing is. There is a form of RAST called ImmunoCAP that is the preferred

RAST test, and studies suggest it may be as good as or better than skin testing. RAST is useful if the patient's skin is already irritated by eczema or if the patient seems to have suffered a life-threatening reaction to the food in question.

A food-challenge test, in which the patient actually ingests the suspect food in small, increasing amounts, can be quite conclusive. But this kind of test should be done only in a hospital or a well-equipped allergist's office in case a dangerous adverse systemic reaction is provoked. A challenge test is usually ill-advised for any food to which you have shown a systemic reaction in the past, although sometimes it is important to find out if there is still sensitivity, as in the case of children as they grow older and often lose their sensitivities to many of the common food allergens; then a challenge might be done.

The means of giving the test food vary, but one way is to use a gelatin capsule containing the food in powdered form. If no symptoms appear, the dose may be upped on subsequent tests.

Typically, the test is done in a single-blind or double-blind form. In the single-blind, the patient does not know if a food or a placebo is being administered, but the doctor does know; in the double-blind, neither patient nor doctor knows.

Among the types of test not recommended are cytotoxic testing (a type of blood test discussed in chapter 19), sublingual testing (the food is put under one's tongue), and intradermal testing. The American Academy of Allergy, Asthma & Immunology has determined that cytotoxic and sublingual tests are not effective. Intradermal tests, as already mentioned, are risky and potentially life threatening.

TREATMENT

Treatment, alas, is avoidance. For certain food allergies, your doctor may prescribe auto-injectable epinephrine (EpiPen). Anyone who has experienced an anaphylactic reaction should have auto-injectable epinephrine (EpiPen) always available. It buys time to get to an emergency room. (See chapter 13.) and it now comes in a double pack which protects you if the reaction re-occurs after 20 minutes, as many do. If you have any sort of immediate allergic reaction to a food that is a component of anaphylaxis you should carry auto-injectable epinephrine (EpiPen) in case a future exposure causes a worse reaction. If you have asthma and symptoms suggestive of food allergy you also should carry autoinjectable epinephrine (EpiPen), and the same applies to those with an allergy to foods typically associated with severe reactions (e.g., peanut, tree nuts, fish, shellfish). We are making generalizations here about who needs to carry and when to use epinephrine (EpiPen). This is an important decision that should ultimately only be made with your physician, who knows your individual circumstances best. People with food allergies should always consult an allergist and should have a treatment plan in place before a reaction occurs. And if indicated, EpiPen should be carried at all times; but if you were to experience a reaction and not have the EpiPen, then call 911 immediately.

National Jewish Health (formerly National Jewish Medical and Research Center) in Denver first reported successful desensitization to peanuts in patients with a history of serious allergic reaction to them. Unfortunately, the treatment is risky because it requires injections of peanut allergen. In fact, the study was stopped because of a serious reaction in one of the study patients. One avenue of research is going on now to find a "modified antigen" that can be injected to confer immunity to peanuts without endangering the patient.

Similarly, the allergens in shrimp and in many other foods have been isolated and genetically sequenced, and we expect that it will be possible to use immunization techniques to help many food-allergic patients through allergy shots. But beware of a doctor now who claims he can give you shots to help your food allergies—that would be quackery.

Another approach being investigated is to use anti-IgE (Xolair) an injectable drug that is currently indicated to treat more-severe asthma patients. It lowers the IgE in the blood and could in theory reduce a patient's sensitivity to a food allergen. Keep in mind that the initial goal is not to get to the point where the person can eat the food freely. Our goal right now is to reduce their sensitivity so they tolerate accidental exposures, as this is what causes the most problem in these persons. The initial results of these studies demonstrate improvement in some patients, but some patients do not respond at all.

There has recently been a study that shows promise of a well-tolerated Chinese herbal medicine that may reduce allergic sensitivity to peanut. Over the past couple of years, there have been reports of studies using oral desensitization (a safer route than injection) to help egg—and milk-allergic subjects tolerate small amounts of these foods as would happen in an accidental exposure. Most recently, this has been done with peanut and hazelnut. After the patients have become desensitized, they have to have daily "doses" of the food in order to maintain their desensitization. If they stop these daily doses for a few days and then restart, severe reactions have occurred. And since you may be tempted to try this yourself, we must again warn again you that **this cannot be done without medical supervision in case the person has a severe life threatening reaction to the food.**

Recently, successful desensitization to fish has been accomplished at a Scandinavian medical center.

But technology, which brings us cures, also brings worries. The use of genetic engineering to "improve" foods may transfer allergenic proteins from one type of plant to another or perhaps create new ones. For example, scientists at the University of Nebraska have found that soybeans modified with genes from Brazil nuts will provoke a strong, potentially fatal allergic reaction in people allergic to Brazil nuts but not to soybeans.

As mentioned above, if you are allergic to a food, you may be allergic to others in a related food group. A list of related food groups is provided in the appendix, and helpful food allergy resources on the Internet are included there as well.

Chapter 8

DRUG ALLERGIES

In 1900, the official U.S. government pharmacopeia, which lists all existing drugs, was a skinny little book of a dozen pages covering a hundred drugs.

Today, *The Complete Drug Reference,* compiled by the United States Pharmacopeial Convention Inc., a nonprofit organization that sets standards of strength, quality, purchasing, and labeling for medical products in the United States, lists over 5,500 prescription and over-the-counter drugs. An adult patient receives an average of eight to ten drugs during a hospital stay. Seventy-five million adults take two or more drugs per day on a regular basis. More than fifteen million Americans take aspirin regularly.

Thanks in part to these many medicines, we are now able to overcome most of the diseases that afflicted humankind and our domestic animals for most of our history. We live longer, and daily life is more comfortable with the relief of normal aches and pains. But for every step of progress, there is a price.

One price is that many important drugs can cause troublesome, even dangerous, allergic reactions in some people. These sensitive people form only a small percentage of the total population, probably about 5 percent. The chance of any given individual having an allergic reaction to a drug is only about 1 percent to 3 percent, because even if you are among the 5 percent that may develop a sensitivity, certain drugs are much less likely than others to trigger it.

Drug allergies, thus, are infrequent. But like food allergies, they can be quite severe, even fatal, when they do occur. The most notorious allergen among drugs is penicillin, which accounts for about 75 percent of deaths from anaphylaxis in the United States. Ironically, penicillin is also the greatest lifesaver of the past sixty years. Many other drugs, especially other antibiotics, are occasionally allergenic.

Adverse Drug Reactions

Drugs, like foods, can cause various kinds of adverse reactions: allergies, intolerances, toxic reactions, and so on. An adverse reaction to a drug is any untoward reaction or nontherapeutic effect of that drug. A newer classification system of adverse drug reactions has been introduced recently. Type A is dose dependent and predictable, such as an overdose. Type B is not dose dependent and is unpredictable.

Side effects too are numbered among adverse reactions; they are not as universal and predictable as overdose effects, but they tend to affect significant numbers of those who take any given drug. Many older antihistamines, for example, have the side effect of making most people drowsy. Pseudoephedrine, often used to treat nasal congestion and sinusitis, may make your heart race. Antibiotics often cause diarrhea.

A side effect that is categorized as common may appear almost invariably or may affect only one in twenty people. A side effect that is rare may affect one in ten thousand or occur with even less frequency than that.

A drug intolerance is an exaggerated response to a drug. For example, people who are extremely sensitive to aspirin may get a ringing in the ears and feel nauseated after taking just one tablet. The average person would experience these unpleasant effects only after taking many aspirin.

There are also so-called idiosyncratic reactions to drugs. These vary according to the individual and often are not well understood. It is believed that in some cases, enzyme deficiencies or other genetic predisposing factors may be involved. (An example of an idiosyncratic reaction is the bone marrow failure that occurs, rarely, after use of chloramphenicol, an antibiotic. This occurs in approximately one in thirty thousand uses.)

Finally, of course, there are allergic reactions to drugs.

About 15 percent of patients treated with drugs experience adverse reactions, and very often these people wrongly say that they are "allergic" to the drug that caused the problem. But as we mentioned, only a fraction of such adverse reactions are due to allergy. By definition, a drug allergy must involve the immune system: either the antibody arm (more-immediate reactions) or the cellular arm (more-delayed reactions) of the immune system.

It is important to know the difference between an allergy and intolerance because if you mistakenly report having an allergy to a drug, a doctor may be forced to give you a less-effective medication to avoid setting off an allergic reaction, whereas with an intolerance, you may be able to take a drug again or with continued use you may begin to tolerate it. This is especially important if there are few or no alternatives to the drug.

Often patients think that if a drug gives them diarrhea, they are allergic to it. But diarrhea is a common side effect of antibiotics and other drugs, caused by changes in the bacterial environment in the intestines.

On the other hand, if you are truly allergic to a drug, the doctor must know this because that drug or another in its family could cause you life-threatening difficulty.

TRUE DRUG ALLERGIES

The key to identifying a drug allergy is that it resembles other kinds of allergy. For instance, you will not get an allergic reaction the first time you take that drug. A sensitivity must build up. But that buildup can occur quickly, with the result that allergy symptoms can appear during the initial course of therapy, even though everything went well for the first couple of doses. Moreover, some people are exposed to drugs inadvertently or without realizing it because some drugs are present in food we eat. A baby may be exposed to penicillin through breast milk. Penicillin and other drugs may also be present in cow's milk or in meat from farm animals. (One is not supposed to milk or slaughter an animal being treated with penicillin, but it happens anyway.) In these cases, someone will have built up a sensitivity to the drug without realizing it.

Assuming a normal exposure to drugs, drug allergies often appear in early adulthood, but there are no age limits. Some children have allergic reactions to drugs. Some elderly people develop drug allergies even after having taken a drug many times.

OCCURRENCE

Frequently, an allergic reaction to a drug occurs within minutes to one hour after taking the drug. If you are very allergic, even a minuscule dose will produce symptoms. There are also delayed reactions that take hours to two to three days to appear. Rarely, there are reactions that are even more delayed. For example, hives resulting from a sensitivity to penicillin can occur several weeks after taking the drug and last up to four months. As a rule, the more rapidly the symptoms appear, the more dangerous the reaction. Symptoms arising within an hour of taking the drug are potentially life threatening. The delayed symptoms are normally less serious but still require evaluation by a physician.

MAJOR ADVERSE REACTIONS TO DRUGS

A drug reaction in the first few minutes to an hour (and even up to a day or more in the case of omalizumab [Xolair]) after exposure that includes the following symptoms requires immediate, expert medical attention: swelling (sometimes with hives), difficulty breathing or swallowing, vomiting or stomach cramps, itching, choking, weakness, and a sense of impending doom. These are signs of a dangerous reaction—anaphylaxis. Choking and difficulty breathing are caused by swelling in the throat that is closing off the windpipe. This sounds serious, and it is. That sense of impending doom is appropriate. You might die.

If you experience any swelling of the lips, tongue, eyes, fingers, or hands—even without choking or wheezing—call your doctor or an ambulance immediately. Do not take the next dose of the drug.

Typical symptoms of a drug allergy are itching associated with hives or a rash, angioedema (swelling), and sometimes a fever.

Itching is so characteristic of drug allergy that there is a medical adage, "Without itching, doubt drug allergy." The itching is often related to hives, which is the next most-common manifestation of drug allergy.

If you are taking a drug and develop hives or itching, do not take another dose. Contact your doctor immediately. Your doctor will have to assess whether to try to continue the drug or use another.

Another occasional sign of an allergy reaction is a cyanotic, or bluish, tinge to the skin; in dark-skinned people, this can be seen in the lips, nail beds, palms of the hands, and soles of the feet.

Joint aches and fever may also occur. If you develop rash or any of the symptoms mentioned above, report this promptly to your doctor.

Incidentally, one sign of drug allergy is that the symptoms usually clear up or begin to improve within several days after the drug is discontinued. Of the drug-induced adverse reactions described in the discussion that follows, some are allergic in nature or include at least some involvement of the immunological system. Others exacerbate allergic conditions or can be confused with allergy.

HIVES AND RASHES

Acute hives can be a sign of a dangerous drug allergy and should be treated as a medical emergency, especially following an injection of a drug.

A sensitivity to nonsteroidal anti-inflammatory drugs may cause hives and in some cases be associated with chronic hives as well as with asthma attacks (see the section below on respiratory manifestations). This sensitivity is sometimes linked to a sensitivity to the food additive tartrazine, a yellow dye. Unfortunately, the anti-inflammatories involved include some of the most widely used medicines for aches and pains: aspirin and ibuprofen. If you are sensitive to these medicines, your doctor may recommend a substitute, such as choline magnesium trisalicylate (Trilisate).

Rashes are a frequent manifestation of drug allergy. Commonly, they are morbilliform; that is, they resemble a measles rash, with multiple tiny red dots all over the body. The rash is itchy but not severely so.

A morbilliform rash can be the result of a drug allergy or of a number of viral diseases. There is a distinguishing sign between the two, however; an allergic rash may cover your body, but it will not affect your palms and soles. A viral rash usually does not spare the palms or soles.

Sometimes an allergic rash progresses to become thick and very red and itchy.

Occasionally, when it is difficult to determine whether a rash is caused by the illness being treated or by the drug used to treat the illness, diagnosis requires a biopsy of the rash.

Most rashes are relatively harmless, but they may develop into exfoliative dermatitis. This is a condition in which the rash spreads over the entire body and the skin begins to shed. This is similar to what happens as the result of a burn, and as with burn victims, there is great danger of infection. Some patients afflicted with exfoliative dermatitis, chiefly among the elderly, do not survive.

Exfoliative dermatitis can also result as a complication of eczema (atopic dermatitis) or psoriasis.

Almost any drug can cause a rash; but the drugs that most commonly do so include sulfa drugs, amoxicillin, synthetic penicillin (such as dicloxacillin sodium and methicillin sodium), penicillin, cephalosporins (which are chemical cousins of penicillin), and hydantoin. Patients with mononucleosis have a 9-in-10 chance of developing a measleslike rash from amoxicillin and certain other antibiotics in the penicillin family. Certain leukemias also tend to make one susceptible to developing a rash when taking amoxicillin. By and large, this kind of allergy is not terribly serious, which is a small favor when one is so sick already.

The rashes that follow treatment with penicillin and the cephalosporins are notable for their longevity. They may last up to four months after treatment is stopped.

PHOTOSENSITIVITY

Photosensitivity reactions occur when a drug that is present in skin reacts with light. Usually the light must be sunlight, but artificial light is sometimes sufficient. Diagnosis is usually simplified by the fact that the reaction is limited to areas of skin exposed to light.

Photoallergic reactions resemble contact dermatitis but can recur months after the drug is stopped, if the skin is exposed to light. Among many drugs that can cause these reactions, the most commonly implicated are sulfa drugs and salicylamides (used in medicated soaps and acne medications).

Phototoxic reactions, which are not allergic in nature, may be caused by coal-tar derivatives and other substances, including the antibiotics doxycycline and ciprofloxacin as well as the newer floroquinolone drugs such as Levaquin and Avelox. A phototoxic reaction may give rise to an exaggerated sunburnlike rash that can blister.

Skin reactions caused by drugs applied to the skin, or by handling drugs or chemicals, are discussed in the chapter on atopic dermatitis, chapter 12.

SERUM SICKNESS

Serum sickness is caused most commonly by penicillin but also by many other types of drugs, including cephalosporins, sulfa drugs and other antibiotics, phenytoin (used for epilepsy), and propylthiouracil (used to treat hyperthyroid conditions). Serum sickness is so named because it was originally associated with vaccines made from animal serums. These symptoms may be mild or severe and last several days to several weeks. Usually, recovery is complete; but in rare cases, there is permanent neurological damage or involvement of internal organs, including the heart, kidney, liver, pancreas, and adrenal glands.

Treatment includes stopping the offending drug and taking antihistamines and oral cortisone, depending on the severity of the symptoms.

DRUG FEVER

Most drugs are able to cause fever in susceptible persons. Certain anticancer drugs, for example, ordinarily result in fever. Also, the injection of a drug can cause local inflammation in the area where the shot was given, and the inflammation can cause a rise in temperature. But in some cases, the fever is part of an allergic reaction.

Fever associated with allergy can be confusing to both physician and patient, especially when an antibiotic is being used to treat an infection that produces fever. If after five days of treatment the patient is free of fever and then the fever flares up, what is going on? Is the original infection recurring as the bacteria become resistant? Is there a new infection? Or is this drug fever?

If there are accompanying signs of allergy, such as a rash, the answer may be obvious. But sometimes, such signs are missing. To reach a diagnosis, the physician should try to find out if there has been a history of drug allergy in the patient's past. One can also try stopping the drug, and if allergy is the cause of the problem, the fever will usually subside quickly.

The drugs most commonly implicated in drug fever are penicillin and the cephalosporins, sulfa drugs, certain drugs used to treat high blood pressure (typically, methyldopa), and procainamide and quinidine used to treat heart-rhythm irregularities.

It is important to identify and treat the cause of the fever because more serious manifestations may follow, including hepatitis (liver inflammation), vasculitis (inflammation of the blood vessels), and severe rashes.

DRUG-INDUCED LUPUS

Lupus (systemic lupus erythematosus) is a disease in which the body makes antibodies against its own tissues. These antibodies (autoantibodies) can seriously damage the kidneys, brain, blood vessels, liver, and heart. Certain drugs can produce similar effects, causing the production of antibodies, although no underlying disease is present.

The most commonly implicated drugs are hydralazine (used to treat high blood pressure), procainamide (for heart-rhythm irregularities), and isoniazid (an antituberculosis drug). Other drugs that may cause lupus are methyldopa (for high blood pressure), phenytoin (for epilepsy), and even birth-control pills.

In drug-induced lupus, the patient is likely to develop fevers, joint pains, and rashes—and these may occur months to years after the patient has started to take the offending drug. Usually, the symptoms fade rapidly when the drug is stopped, but the autoantibodies may remain in the body for years.

VASCULITIS

Vasculitis, or inflammation of the blood vessels, caused by drugs is usually associated with rashes, as the blood vessels of the skin are involved. But often the vasculitis shows itself in black-and-blue marks, especially on the legs. Other parts of the body, including the kidneys and joints, can be involved. The drugs that most commonly cause allergic vasculitis are penicillin, sulfa drugs, hydantoin (used to treat seizures), and allopurinol (used for gout). A rare form of vasculitis may very occasionally be associated with the asthma medications Accolate and Singulair. (See chapter 9.)

RESPIRATORY MANIFESTATIONS

Asthma can be exacerbated by a number of drugs, especially aspirin and beta-blockers, the latter even when applied topically, as in the case of eyedrops for glaucoma. Recently, it has been shown that some asthmatic patients can tolerate the newer and very highly selective beta-blockers. Whether you can tolerate these medications would be a decision made by your own physician.

About one in ten asthma patients are sensitive to aspirin, ibuprofen (Motrin, Nuprin), indomethacin, and related nonsteroidal anti-inflammatory drugs (NSAIDs). You may be able to substitute Trilisate. Acetaminophen (Tylenol) is not usually a problem.

In cases where a patient is sensitive to aspirin or an NSAID, a procedure to desensitize that patient to aspirin and NSAIDs can be done—usually in a special facility with intensive-care capability. This would only be done when aspirin and/or an NSAID must be used for arthritis or another condition for which there is no other safe alternative. This is an uncommon situation, and the need for decision to desensitize a patient should be made by an allergist and a rheumatologist.

In rare cases, the asthmatic with nasal polyps who takes aspirin or another NSAID may experience a life-threatening asthma attack. This sensitivity is not a true allergy, but it can aggravate asthma and in varying degrees. It is rather difficult to diagnose and does not show up with skin testing.

As noted previously, people who are sensitive to the yellow dye tartrazine (FD&C No. 5) or to sulfites should read labels on over-the-counter medicines and question their pharmacists about prescription drugs. Both of these are very rare sensitivities.

The lungs can be affected by reactions to drugs. Among the problem medications are penicillin, sulfa drugs, and even, although rarely, cromolyn, which is used to prevent asthma symptoms. In cases involving the lungs, patients develop a cough seven to ten days after starting the drug treatment. A chest X-ray shows a picture that resembles that of pneumonia. The blood count reveals increased numbers of eosinophils, a type of white blood cell often involved in allergic reactions.

Nitrofurantoin, an antibiotic used to treat bladder infections, has a number of side effects to watch out for, including fever, chills, coughing, and chest pain. These symptoms appear in approximately one of five hundred patients who take the drug, and they usually disappear one or two days after the treatment is stopped. Methotrexate can cause similar problems. It is an anticancer drug; it is prescribed for some kinds of arthritis. Recently it has been used as a steroid-sparing agent (to reduce the need for steroids) in severe asthma.

Coughing is a common side effect of a class of drugs called angiotensin-converting enzyme inhibitors (such as captopril, enalapril, and lisinopril), which are used to treat high blood pressure. Coughing clears up after the drug is stopped. These same drugs can cause idiopathic angioedema, which can be serious and even life-threatening as it can involve the throat. If you are taking any of these drugs and have any form of angioedema (swelling of the lips, under the skin, etc.), contact your doctor immediately to decide whether it is related to the drug and whether or not you should stop the drug.

BLOOD, LIVER, AND KIDNEY REACTIONS

Allergic and toxic reactions to drugs can cause changes in the blood, including a reduction in platelets and a risk of abnormal bleeding; a decrease in the number of red blood cells (anemia); and a decrease in the number of white blood cells. These disorders are generally noticed only when a blood count is done, either routinely or because the patient is feeling sick.

An increase in eosinophils is often associated with allergy, and is discussed below under "Diagnosis and Treatment." Because the liver metabolizes drugs, it may become involved in adverse drug reactions. The symptoms of liver damage are often subtle or nonexistent. They may include stomachaches, nausea, or yellowing of the skin (jaundice). But in blood testing, one can run various tests for liver function. The drugs most often associated with liver damage include isoniazid (used for tuberculosis), certain antidepressants and other mood-altering drugs, birth-control pills, and some antibiotics.

The kidneys, because of their general excretory function, also may be affected by drugs in the bloodstream, including penicillin and the related cephalosporins, sulfa drugs, diuretics (water pills), hydantoin drugs (used for seizures), and NSAIDs.

PENICILLIN

As you may have gathered from the frequency with which penicillin has been mentioned here, it is the major villain in the story of adverse drug reactions. The first reported death from penicillin was in 1949, and today it causes some four hundred to eight hundred deaths per year. Put another way, about one in every ten thousand doses of penicillin leads to anaphylaxis. About one in every one hundred thousand doses results in death.

The age group most at risk is adults twenty to forty-nine years old. The more seriously ill the patient, the greater the risk of a serious reaction. Penicillin makes no distinction between male and female or among ethnic groups; all are equally liable to become allergic.

Over a period of years, one may mature out of a penicillin allergy. If you have experienced only a rash, especially a delayed rash, the chances are that if it were necessary, you could use penicillin again if your skin tests to penicillin were negative. If you have developed hives and other signs of an anaphylactic reaction, you may never be able to use penicillin. Future tests for penicillin sensitivity should probably be done only in the well-equipped allergist's office or hospital. Recently a test for penicillin allergy (Pre-Pen) was recently put back on the market after being unavailable for a number of years. Desensitization is even trickier, although it can be attempted in critical cases where the infection is life threatening and there are no alternative antibiotics that would be effective.

Variants of penicillin taken orally, such as amoxicillin, almost always cause reactions in people sensitive to penicillin. The symptoms may be delayed days or even weeks.

Cephalosporins, which are chemically related to penicillin, contain allergenic factors similar to those in the penicillin molecule. But cephalosporins are not usually as potently allergenic as penicillin itself. The oral cephalosporins include Ceclor, Keflex, Ceftin, Suprax, and Velosef.

People who are truly allergic to penicillin have about a 5 percent to 16 percent chance of reacting to a cephalosporin. Typically, if penicillin causes a delayed, mild reaction, such as a rash, then it would be medically acceptable to try treating the patient with a cephalosporin in a case in which the drug is needed and there are no good alternatives. The best procedure is to give the first dose in the doctor's office a little at a time over several hours.

ANESTHETICS AND INSULIN

Painkillers and various anesthetics cause allergic and toxic reactions fairly frequently. Some opiates, for example, may cause direct histamine release. If you have ever developed a rash or any kind of adverse reaction to a painkiller, sedative, or anesthetic, you should report this to your doctor. Possibly you should avoid drugs of the same type that caused you a problem. Often, another class of drugs can be substituted.

Symptoms such as weakness, changes in heartbeat, and fainting when local anesthetics are injected are not usually due to allergy but rather to the stress of the experience. But if there is doubt as to the cause and you want to know if you are in any danger using local anesthetics, skin testing can indicate whether an allergy exists. If the skin tests are negative, then gradually increasing doses of the drug are injected to be certain that tolerance is good.

Anaphylaxis and other severe allergic reactions can occur during the administration of general anesthesia. This is manifested during surgery by a sudden, calamitous drop in blood pressure and even cardiac arrest. Other allergic stigmata such as hives and rash are not always present. This type of reaction can be confused with many other nonallergic reactions during surgery. It is essential to establish when an allergic reaction has occurred because it will occur again and can be prevented by appropriate premedication. This is a very important point, and patients who have had this type of reaction during general anesthesia should discuss it with their own physicians. In some cases, the reaction may be due to latex allergy, and it is important to identify the cause. (See p. 184.)

Insulin allergy can be highly problematic to diabetic patients who need this substance to maintain health. There are various methods of coping, which should be reviewed with a physician specializing in diabetes.

CHYMOPAPAIN AND STREPTOKINASE

Papain and chymopapain, derived from the papaya tree, are enzymes used in a variety of products from meat tenderizer to toothpaste. Chymopapain was used in treating herniated disks. Unfortunately, it also caused anaphylaxis in about one of every one hundred persons treated. It is believed that exposure to meat tenderizer and certain grass pollen may predispose people to react badly to chymopapain, and it is rarely used today.

Typically, patients are tested for chymopapain sensitivity by both an in vitro (laboratory) blood test and a skin test before the chymopapain is injected into the disk, but these tests are not always reliable.

Streptokinase, another enzyme, dissolves blood clots and is used to treat circulatory-system disorders, such as heart attacks and phlebitis. Unfortunately, many people are allergic to it and develop anaphylaxis.

X-RAY DYES

X-ray dyes, more appropriately called radiographic contrast media, are often used prior to certain CAT scans, myelograms, angiography, kidney X-rays, and so on. The dye helps the radiologist see the organ being studied. But the intravenous injection results in allergy-like reactions (termed anaphylactoid) in one of fifteen cases, in dangerous reactions in one of fifty cases, and in death in one in forty thousand.

If you have ever had an allergy-like reaction to an X-ray dye, this must be noted in your medical records. Be sure to mention the reaction to any doctor contemplating such diagnostic testing. There are new dyes to which you may be less sensitive but which are not used routinely because they are expensive. One of these newer dyes, however, should be used if you have had any previous reaction, no matter how mild, to X-ray contrast media.

Also, pretreatment with antihistamines and corticosteroids is very helpful in preventing or damping a reaction.

Severe reactions are less common when, as in a myelogram or barium enema, the dye is not injected into a vein.

It was formerly thought that a history of shellfish allergy was a predictor of reactivity to these dyes, but this is absolutely not so. However, a history of hay fever or asthma does increase the risk slightly and may justify the use of the newer dyes in these patients. Latex allergy can also play a role in allergic reactions occurring during invasive radiological procedures (such as dye injection).

PREVENTION OF DANGEROUS DRUG REACTIONS

Other antibiotics and painkillers too may cause anaphylactic reactions. Chymopapain, as just discussed, can be dangerous.

The single most important thing that you can do to prevent an overwhelming anaphylactic drug reaction is to stay within reach of medical help for a half hour to forty-five minutes after having an injection of a drug, especially penicillin.

Oral doses of a drug are much less likely to cause a severe reaction than injected doses do. Delayed reactions are usually milder than those that arise in the first half hour or so. But this does not mean that you should ignore symptoms associated with an oral dose of medicine, whether they occur soon after the medicine is ingested or are delayed.

Anytime that you have taken a medicine and develop any swelling or itching, go directly to the nearest emergency room or doctor's office. If you start to feel worse en route, call 911 for emergency medical help.

If you have found that you have a drug allergy, it is important that you mention this to your doctor before trying a new medication. *It is wise to learn which other common drugs belong to the family of drugs to which you are allergic. You should avoid that whole family of drugs.*

When a doctor prescribes a new drug, always remind her or him of your allergy. Unfortunately, a doctor may have forgotten your allergy or, worse, failed to have taken your earlier report seriously. Another prudent safeguard is to check with your pharmacist as to whether a prescribed drug is related to the drug or class of drug that previously caused you difficulty.

To avoid delayed but nevertheless serious manifestations of drug allergy, it is important to notice and remember any and all reactions that you may have had to a drug in the past. A remembered rash or fever that cleared up suddenly when you stopped taking the drug may be helpful in diagnosing a troublesome reaction in the present. Alert your doctor to any possible sensitivity before starting a course of treatment. Ask that the information be included in your medical records.

DIAGNOSIS AND TREATMENT OF DRUG ALLERGY

Diagnosis of drug allergy is often uncertain, and treatment is usually simple avoidance.

This avoidance, by the way, can also be helpful in the diagnosis. If the drug is withdrawn and the symptoms disappear relatively promptly, the chances are that the cause of the trouble was some sort of allergy.

Elevated levels of eosinophils in the blood, together with other signs of allergy, such as a rash, indicate that an allergic process is present. But an increased number of eosinophils by itself is rarely enough reason to diagnose drug allergy.

Skin tests for drug allergy are imprecise and can be dangerous. Nevertheless, they may be undertaken, always under a physician's supervision, when it is important to determine whether an allergy really is present. This situation arises most often in the case of patients who need treatment for certain infections, such as staph infections, or for some other condition for which there is really only one drug of choice.

Skin testing for penicillin sensitivity, while risky, is of value in that it reveals the sensitivity in most (but not all) instances in which a sensitivity does exist. Skin testing involves testing with several components of penicillin as well as the whole drug. At the time of writing this chapter, it is not possible to test accurately for penicillin allergy as a very important test (minor determinant), which predicts anaphylaxis is not available for testing. Skin testing is also fairly reliable for sensitivity to insulin, chymopapain, and local anesthetics. Some centers are doing research on other drug-allergy testing.

RAST (a laboratory blood test) is not recommended for diagnosing drug allergy at present. However, penicillin is the only drug for which a RAST is available. When the RAST is done if the result is positive, then it is likely that the patient is allergic to penicillin. A negative test is not sensitive enough to indicate whether or not it is safe to give penicillin.

If a drug-sensitive patient must have the drug in question, a program of desensitization may be undertaken under controlled conditions (preferably in an intensive care unit). Penicillin and insulin are the drugs for which desensitization is most often attempted, frequently with good results. There are frequent reports of successful desensitization with many other drugs as well; however, successful desensitization in just one patient (as in a case report) is not a guarantee that in a second patient it might not be successful or even cause a severe reaction.

The treatment of symptoms of drug allergy is usually with antihistamines and corticosteroids, if necessary. Often, just stopping the drug is sufficient.

Chapter 9

ASTHMA

Asthma, one of our most common diseases, afflicts about 6 to 7 percent of adults in the United States and about 8 to 9 percent of children. About 11 percent of Americans (32.6 million persons as of 2006) experience asthma symptoms at some point in their lives. Deaths from asthma number over five thousand annually.

Simply described, asthma is reversible obstruction of the airways, caused by muscle spasm or mucus blocking or both. In chronic asthma, the airways may become structurally narrowed by scarring. As we discuss below, prevention of this "remodeling" of the airways is a major goal of the new approach to asthma treatment.

The most characteristic (but not universal) asthma symptom is wheezing, which is a musical sound like a faint whistle, produced usually while one is exhaling. Lack (or shortness) of breath, coughing, bringing up mucus, and a feeling of tightness in the chest are also common symptoms.

The airways of the lungs are similar to the branches on an upside-down tree. Air moves through the main trunk of the tree (the trachea, or windpipe) into two main branches (the left and the right bronchi) to the lungs. The bronchi, which are relatively large tubes, subdivide into smaller and smaller branches. The smallest, the bronchioles, lead into clusters of tiny sacs in the lungs, called alveoli. There are millions of alveoli, and it is here that air is exchanged with the blood. Oxygen enters the blood; carbon dioxide is removed and exhaled.

In a typical asthma reaction, lung-muscle tissue surrounding the small breathing tubes tightens, mucus production in the cells lining the airways increases, and the bronchial walls swell and become inflamed (caused by an influx of various types of cells from the blood as well as leakage of fluid and proteins from the blood). Sometimes the mucus forms small plugs that clog the airways and take the shape of the air passages. When these mucus plugs are coughed up, they resemble bits of string or rope, ranging in size from about the diameter of a piece of spaghetti to the diameter of a pencil.

With all this happening, normal airflow is reduced; and in particular, exhalation is incomplete. This results in a feeling of dyspnea, or shortness of breath, and sometimes a feeling that one cannot breathe at all (the term *asthma* derives from a Greek word meaning "panting," or "breathlessness"). Asthma can flare up anytime of the day or night, and many asthmatics wake up in the early morning hours with difficulty breathing because asthma worsens in the early morning hours, as do many other diseases.

The mechanisms and physiology underlying an asthma reaction are not entirely understood; but studies indicate that in the person predisposed to asthma, the mucous membrane cells lining the lungs may not be as tightly packed as is normal, allowing allergens and other molecules to get below the membrane to where the mast cells are. The mast cells may then release chemical mediators, causing asthma symptoms.

One theory about the cause of asthma holds that people prone to this disease are affected by a dysfunction of one part of the nervous system. In the autonomic nervous system (which governs our body organs), there are two opposing subsystems: the sympathetic and the parasympathetic systems. They have opposing actions and should balance each other. One slows the heart, and one quickens it; one opens airways, and one closes them, and so on.

In the sympathetic nervous system, there are so-called beta-adrenergic receptors, which respond to epinephrine (adrenaline) stimulation by relaxing the airways and by increasing CAMP levels in the lungs. It is believed that in an asthmatic, these beta-adrenergic receptors may not function properly, allowing the contrary reaction of the parasympathetic nervous system—constriction of the airways—to take place unchecked, unopposed.

ASTHMA: AN INFLAMMATORY DISEASE

There may actually be no single underlying cause of asthma. The mechanism may vary from patient to patient (which would explain the variety of asthma patterns). Hopefully, our understanding of genetics will allow us to identify these subsets of asthma patients. This will surely improve our ability to take care of these patients in a more-individualized way. In the 1990s, researchers clearly identified the key characteristic of asthma: chronic inflammation in the airways. Prior to this, asthma had just been thought of as a disease causing spasm of the smooth muscle surrounding the airways.

Control of the inflammation is essential to controlling the disease.

Inflammation is a normal physical reaction to trauma, a reaction that usually is curative but sometimes causes severe problems. Familiar types of inflammation include the swelling, redness, and pain that follow, say, a knife cut on the hand or overexposure to the sun. The inflammation can be quite painful for a day or two, but it is part of the healing process.

When the skin tissue is injured, certain cells release chemicals that recruit inflammatory cells to rush to the area to begin healing. This healing involves new tissue growth, often with scarring.

Inflammation in the airways, as in asthma, is not a desirable type of inflammation. The process causes thickening of the airway wall, excess mucus production, and sloughing off of the cells lining the airways. Collagen, a substance produced by the body for scar formation (among other purposes), is deposited along the outside of the airways (beneath what is called the basement membrane). Edema (swelling) causes narrowing of the airways.

The cells responsible for these reactions include mast cells, which, as we have said, play a major role in allergic immune system activity, and various other white blood cells. Among the white blood cells are neutrophils (especially in severe asthma), eosinophils (involved in allergic and related reactions), and TH2-type lymphocytes.

Asthma is not the only disease related to inflammation. Another example is the inflammation of the joints in rheumatoid arthritis. So many other illnesses are caused by inflammation that it is a recurring theme in most diseases throughout the body.

With asthma, inflammation of the airways makes them hypersensitive to any irritation and liable to constrict and pinch off the flow of air. Swelling and mucus production also reduce airflow. Perhaps most important, scarring can actually remodel the structure of the airways for the worse so that they become fixed or irreversibly obstructed.

The first two editions of this book speculated that maybe controlling airway inflammation can prevent airway remodeling later in life. We are now happy to report that it can. Recently, evidence from biopsy studies is confirming that inhaled corticosteroids can reduce remodeling of the airways. Now, one of the most important areas of current asthma research is

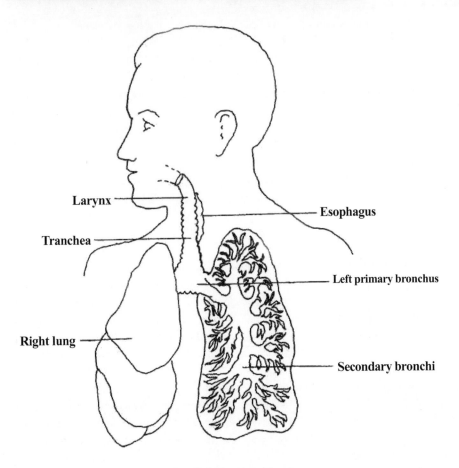

The Respiratory Tract

the question of how much can treatment with anti-inflammatory medications prevent the undesirable scarring and remodeling of the airways. Parallels with the treatment of other inflammatory diseases, such as rheumatoid arthritis, suggest that the answer is remodeling and can be prevented to a significant degree. The question is significant in that it dictates how aggressively we should use inhaled corticosteroids in younger asthmatics. The next edition of this book may have an answer.

CAUSES OF ATTACK

Although this book focuses on asthma that is triggered by allergy, not all asthma is related to allergy. Asthma attacks can be brought on by exercise, cold air, aspirin or other nonsteroidal anti-inflammatory drugs, environmental pollutants, odors or irritants, smoking or exposure to cigarette smoke, infection, and laughing. It can also be related to gastroesophageal reflux, a fairly common problem, especially among older people. Acidic fluid from the stomach moves upward into the esophagus, which in some instances causes asthma to worsen.

One clue to diagnosing the kind of asthma resulting from gastroesophageal reflux is that the attacks come mostly at night and usually affect older people. When one is lying down, the stomach contents can more easily flow into the esophagus—gravity isn't helping to keep the fluid in the stomach. But another even more common cause of nocturnal asthma is a natural reduction in pulmonary function. This occurs in all people at night and in the early morning but is exaggerated in asthmatics. A rule of thumb is that reflux should be considered in any patient with difficult to control asthma and in others as well. An antireflux medication trial of sixty to ninety days is indicated to rule it out.

EXERCISE

In the past, many asthmatics were invalids from childhood on. An example is Martin Scorsese, the film director. His asthma kept him indoors mainly focused on watching old movies on TV. This was very influential in his choice of careers, and thus he was one of the luckier asthmatics of that older generation. Through advances in medication and a better understanding of the disease, most people with asthma can now lead full lives without any limitations. In fact, they can lead highly athletic lives. Among the world-class sports stars who have asthma are the Olympic gold medalists Jackie Joyner-Kersee (in track) and Nancy Hogshead (in swimming).

Vigorous physical activity can improve lung function, reducing the impact of an asthmatic reaction. An aerobic exercise program can help asthmatics but should be undertaken in consultation with a doctor and should be done systematically, gradually building up aerobic capacity.

Most athletes with asthma need to keep inhalers with medication on hand, to be used as prescribed, usually fifteen minutes before beginning to exercise. But youngsters will sometimes resist carrying an inhaler. It helps if the coach accepts asthma treatment as a matter of routine and if he or she treats the inhaler like any other piece of equipment. A physician or parent may have to explain to the coach that the youngster is physically fit.

ASTHMA TRENDS

The first two editions of this book did not have much good news about asthma trends. This has changed for the better now. The worldwide incidence of asthma had been increasing over the past forty years. Unfortunately, it is still increasing, and we mention possible causes below. Also, mortality from asthma had been increasing until the late 1990s. Figures vary; but according to the American Academy of Allergy, Asthma & Immunology, the incidence of asthma rose about 75 percent in the past thirty years and continues to rise worldwide. The suspected reasons are multifactorial:

The obesity epidemic that we are experiencing is a likely factor here in the United States. Obesity, because of mechanical reasons, contributes to the development of asthma and makes asthma worse in existing asthma patients. Our change in lifestyle has resulted in vitamin D deficiency as well. It is estimated that 15 to 20 percent of children are now vitamin D deficient and up to 50 percent have inadequate levels, though not actually deficient. This is probably because we spend more time indoors and use more sunblock because of our increasing awareness of the sun causing skin cancers. Sunlight is needed to produce vitamin D in the body. This vitamin D deficiency can lead to immune changes resulting in more allergies (including food allergies). Recently, a relationship between low levels of vitamin D and asthma severity has been reported. Further research on this is ongoing.

In the late 1970s, doctors started recommending the use of nonaspirin treatment of fever in children because of the discovery that it can lead to Reye's syndrome. Therefore, children were all abruptly switched to acetaminophen (Tylenol). Acetaminophen can block chemicals in the lung (glutathione), and this may lead to lung inflammation because of loss of protection from free oxygen radicals. Indeed, graphs of acetaminophen use in the United States line up with the rising incidence of asthma. Other possible factors for this increasing incidence of asthma are increasing incidence of allergies, increasing air pollution, poor air circulation in newer buildings, and perhaps even an increase in the diagnosis of asthma by physicians due to improved methods. Asthma-related death rates, which were dropping until the late 1970s, began rising in the 1980s. This resulted in targeted interventions by many national-government health departments to update the way asthma was being treated by physicians, both specialists and nonspecialists. Physicians had not been widely incorporating the use of new treatments in their treatment of asthma, particularly inhaled corticosteroids. These interventions seem to have paid off, as the mortality rate in most countries has gone down significantly in the past ten to fifteen years. However, there are still, worldwide, approximately 250,000 deaths annually from asthma.

The severity of asthma (as with many other diseases) is disproportionately high among impoverished African Americans and Hispanics living in inner cities. The causes of this disturbing situation probably include high exposure to allergens and polluted air as well as less access to medical care and education. African Americans also seem to be genetically more severely atopic as well.

Recently, we have learned that cockroach allergen is a major inner-city hazard. Urban and suburban air often have high levels of ozone, which interferes with respiratory function. Polluted air also typically has high levels of sulfur dioxide, hydrocarbons, and particulate matter.

Over the past fifty years, many dwellings and workplaces were sealed and insulated to save energy, with a corresponding rise in indoor contaminants and allergens. This may be exacerbating some respiratory ailments.

All in all, the picture is not entirely clear. For example, some studies demonstrate that on days with high levels of air pollution, hospitalizations for asthma increase and in general asthma symptoms get worse. But the findings are not all consistent; and in some instances, other factors, such as viral infections or allergen levels, may be involved.

Asthma epidemics have occurred in Japan and New Orleans. In Japan, air pollution seemed to be the cause; but in New Orleans, the cause is believed to have been *Alternaria* mold spores.

In Australia, asthma mortality rates doubled in the 1980s. In that country, a weed was given some of the blame. *Parietaria judaica* pellitory, also called sticky weed and pellitory, is a prolific pollen producer during much of the year. It has caused so much allergic rhinitis and asthma that the government has classified it as noxious, which means you have to destroy it if you find it growing on your property.

STRESS

Stress used to be listed as one of the causes of asthma, but now our understanding is that although stress may aggravate asthma, it does not cause it. Keep in mind that stress can aggravate most other illnesses as well. Asthma attacks can be precipitated by rapid air movement in and out of the lungs, which occurs in exercise and also in laughing and crying. As a result, in the past, asthma had been mislabeled an emotional disease.

In children, depression and asthma together seem to be a potentially lethal combination, although it is not clear exactly how the two are linked. A study of children who have died of asthma indicates that a distressed home life and depression put the children at greater risk.

Dr. Bruce Miller, a psychiatrist at the National Jewish Medical and Research Center in Denver, suggests that there may be an underlying physiological explanation for the role of stress. Stress at first stimulates the sympathetic nervous system (which would be helpful to asthmatics). But if the stress is not relieved—for example, if the stress is caused by the death or absence of a parent—this can lead to depression, in which the parasympathetic nervous system becomes dominant. As described above, the parasympathetic nervous system tends to close the airways.

If this theory of the relationship between depression and asthma is correct, adults as well as children are more at risk if they suffer from both asthma and depression; and indeed, the mortality of asthma is increased in patients with depression.

LATE-PHASE, OR INFLAMMATORY, REACTION

In several types of allergy, especially allergies to food and drugs, doctors are especially worried about the immediate reaction, which tends to be the most dangerous. In asthma, however, a delayed reaction, called the late-phase, or inflammatory, reaction, can be highly troublesome, even life threatening. For simplicity of understanding, we divide the allergic reaction into an early and late-phase reaction. In reality, there is a continuous flow of these two reactions into and overlapping each other.

The immediate, or early-phase, reaction in asthma begins within minutes of exposure to an allergen or some other causative factor; peaks in about a half hour; and resolves within two hours. This reaction is caused by the release from mast cells of preformed chemical mediators, such as histamine and certain leukotrienes. These mediators dilate the blood vessels (from which fluid then leaks into the tissues); they cause smooth-muscle contraction (leading to bronchoconstriction) and attract inflammatory white blood cells. The early reaction responds well to Adrenalin-type drugs (also called beta$_2$-agonists—see under "Treatment," p. 128). In a controlled experimental environment, the late-phase reaction begins in about three to four hours after exposure to an allergen or other trigger and may subside in a day or so. This is what one might expect from a laboratory study of a patient allergic to, say, cats, who is exposed experimentally to cat allergen.

In real life, however, the lungs of the asthmatic person may be chronically inflamed due to ongoing exposure to multiple triggers. The inflammation brings the lungs into a condition of hypersensitivity and hyper-reactivity (irritability). That is why it is so important to control the inflammation.

The late-phase inflammatory reaction is caused both by the chemical mediators released initially and by newly formed chemical mediators, which are created as part of the immune system reaction. The newly formed mediators include other leukotrienes, prostaglandins, thromboxanes, and platelet activating factor. The effects of these substances include bronchoconstriction, inflammation, and excess mucus production.

The inflammatory reaction does not respond to Adrenalin-type drugs, but there are four kinds of treatment that do help. Cromolyn and nedocromil (mast cell stabilizers), both of which have been discontinued, reduce both the short-term and long-term inflammatory reaction in asthma. Leukotriene inhibitors perform a similar function, as explained in chapter 5. Allergy shots reduce sensitivity to allergens and can prevent the late reaction from developing. Corticosteroids, preferably inhaled, prevent and reduce inflammation.

DIAGNOSIS

The symptoms of asthma may be confused with ordinary bronchitis or a cold or hay fever. The authors have seen numerous patients with a history of having had "bronchitis" every fall for many years when in reality, this was asthma. In the case of asthma that is caused by exercise, you may think that you are extremely out of shape. Unfortunately, the experience of an asthma attack during or following physical activity is likely to discourage further efforts toward physical conditioning.

Any of the following symptoms should prompt you to call a doctor:

- Shortness of breath, whether following exercise, in the morning, in the middle of the night, or indeed at any time
- Wheezing

- Coughing up phlegm, especially if it is discolored or bloody
- Persistent cough
- Chest tightness or pain

In taking a medical history, the doctor should ask you about similar respiratory episodes in the past. Often, patients report a history of frequent "bronchitis" when growing up.

Through a physical exam, chest X-ray or CT scan, and tests, the doctor will focus on determining whether the breathing difficulties are the result of asthma, heart disease, emphysema, lung tumor, cystic fibrosis (in young children), hypersensitivity pneumonitis (a dangerous, progressive condition affecting the lungs in some cases of untreated allergy), infection, or some other cause. Other uncommon but important conditions to be alert for are alpha-1 antitrypsin (AAT) deficiency and lymphangioleiomyomatosis (LAM). The former is diagnosed by a blood test; and the latter, which affects women in their thirties and forties, requires a lung biopsy. It is important to differentiate both illnesses from asthma as preventative care is helpful in both diseases, and in AAT, replacement therapy may be available.

A disease sometimes associated with asthma is allergic bronchopulmonary aspergillosis, which can sometimes be detected by chest X-ray or blood tests and often shows a fever accompanying the asthma attacks. This disease, caused by a fungus, requires a somewhat different approach to treatment.

In the physical examination, especially with children, one sees at times a distension of the chest resulting from asthma. The distension is caused by the asthmatic's reduced ability to exhale air from the lungs. The physician may also hear wheezing when listening to the chest. Examination of the nose may reveal nasal polyps or evidence of allergic rhinitis.

The pulmonary-function test (see chapter 3) is often the key to making the diagnosis. The test will usually detect difficulty in exhaling air from the lungs. The diagnosis of asthma will become almost certain if the difficulty in exhaling is diminished after treatment with a bronchodilator (patients with emphysema are not helped much by a bronchodilator).

If the diagnosis is still unclear, a mecholyl-challenge test may be recommended. This test involves inhaling increasing concentrations of methacholine while changes in pulmonary function are monitored. Below a certain concentration, the nonasthmatic will not show any reaction; but a person with asthma and certain other conditions, such as hay fever, will begin to wheeze and show a decrease in pulmonary function.

ALLERGENS

If asthma is diagnosed, the next step is to determine what triggers the attacks. If the asthma is related to an allergy, this is often apparent in the patient's history and can be confirmed by skin tests or RAST, a blood test (see chapter 3).

In children under age three, as compared with older children and adults, pollen allergy is less commonly the cause of asthma. In most of the country, the pollen season is relatively short and sensitization is relatively slow to develop, so this form of allergy rarely appears in toddlers. But in places like Southern California, where the pollen seasons last up to eight months, asthma associated with pollen sensitivity can be a problem as early as age two.

Allergies triggered by nonseasonal factors, such as dust mite or animal dander in the home, can become a problem and lead to asthma at an early age, even among toddlers.

In patients aged five to fifty, allergy of some sort often plays a significant role in causing their asthma. After age fifty, allergy is less likely to be involved. But this is not a hard and fast rule. There are people who develop allergic asthma in their seventies, and there are young children whose asthma is not allergic.

The patient's history often reveals what is causing the asthma. Your doctor will ask if allergies run in your family. Are your asthma attacks more likely to occur in some places than others? at the office? at home? Are the attacks seasonal? Are they set off by odors or fumes? exercise? aspirin? certain foods? And so on.

Sometimes the probable cause is fairly obvious. The patient reports spending a weekend at a house with a cat and getting an attack of asthma. Or the patient's asthma flares up after eating Chinese food, suggesting sensitivity to monosodium glutamate or sulfites.

In children under age three, food allergies tend to be as important as allergies to inhalants, such as dust mite allergen, cat dander, and pollen. From age three until adulthood, inhalants are much more likely culprits.

FOOD ALLERGIES

When foods are associated with childhood asthma, the foods most often at fault are milk, wheat, corn, and eggs.

Among adults, foods are uncommonly the cause of asthma, but the possibility cannot be ignored. Sometimes the relationship between asthma and food allergy is difficult to pinpoint. For example, in one patient who seemed to have asthma all year round, no matter what she ate, food allergy did not seem a likely cause. But then the patient mentioned to her doctor that the only time of the year when she felt well was during the Jewish holiday of Passover—when she ate unleavened bread! The patient, it turned out, was sensitive to yeast.

A sensitivity to aspirin and other nonsteroidal anti-inflammatory (NSAID) medicines often causes problems for asthmatics. It is felt that up to 10 percent of asthma patients may be sensitive to these medications. If you have nasal polyps, you are even at higher risk of being sensitive to aspirin and other NSAIDs. Another uncommon cause of asthma attacks among adults is a sensitivity to food additives, including FD&C Yellow No. 5 (tartrazine) and sulfites, used as coloring and preservatives in a wide range of foods, such as salad dressing, beer, cider, potato chips, and so on. (See chapter 7.)

OTHER TRIGGERS

You should be aware that your asthma may be caused by some substance that you use in your work or hobby. There is a phenomenon called baker's asthma, caused by sensitivity to flour. And one patient suffered weekly attacks of asthma, which she and her doctor finally realized always occurred a few hours after she had dried the family laundry. She was extremely sensitive to the fabric softener. The family settled for less-soft laundry, and the patient had no more attacks.

Some medications may make asthma worse; so your doctor should be aware, as always, of any medicine that you take at all frequently. The most-frequent offenders are beta-blockers (both oral and ophthalmic) and aspirin, which is discussed above. The oral beta-blockers are used mainly to treat high blood pressure, and the ophthalmic beta-blockers are used for glaucoma. There are claims that some newer beta-blockers are completely safe for asthmatics; but this is not the case, as they all can cause worsening of asthma, both gradually and suddenly. A better description would be that some are "safer" and that the newer ones are safer and might be tolerated in some patients. This is a call by your physician, and of course, alternative medication is always preferable. However, if you are on a beta-blocker and at any point in time your asthma worsens, the use of the beta-blocker should be revisited and discontinued if necessary.

ASPERGILLUS

Asthma can be seriously complicated by infection with the *Aspergillus* fungus. This occurs in about 1 to 2 percent of asthmatics. *Aspergillus* proliferates in unclean humidifying systems, causing a type of chronic inflammation of the lungs called hypersensitivity pneumonitis. It is a very common environmental mold and is one of the molds responsible for the "molding" of bread as well as being a major component of "mildew."

Aspergillus infections usually affect only patients already weakened—for example, those with abnormal immune systems or cancer. These infections are treated with fungicidal drugs. Allergic bronchopulmonary aspergillosis (ABPA) can turn moderate asthma into a fatal illness even in the absence of other serious problems.

Essentially, ABPA is an allergic reaction to *Aspergillus* fungi growing in the bronchial tubes. When this happens, the asthma patient suddenly begins to require more frequent doses of steroids to prevent breathing distress and begins to suffer from fever and at times coughs up brown plugs of mucus. A chest X-ray is likely to show signs of pneumonia.

If a timely diagnosis is not made, the disease may progress to the point that the lungs become fibrotic (scarred). Steroids no longer relieve the asthmatic symptoms.

The patient suffers chronic breathing problems similar to emphysema and may eventually succumb to the disease.

Diagnosis is made on the basis of the clinical history of the disease; a positive result in skin testing for sensitivity to *Aspergillus fumigatus;* a high level of the allergy antibody, IgE, in the blood, as well as an elevated eosinophil count and the presence of precipitating antibodies to *Aspergillus.* Finally, a CAT scan may reveal a widening of portions of the air passages.

The treatment of ABPA is with a long period of steroid medication (prednisone). Sometimes, antifungal antibiotics are used. Immunotherapy is contraindicated because it sometimes makes the disease worse. ABPA cannot be prevented. This mold is present everywhere, and it seems some asthmatics are susceptible to having it grow in their airways.

TREATMENT

Often, people postpone treating asthma, hoping it will go away. This is unwise. Although asthma may go into remission, over time, delaying treatment can be fatal.

Children with asthma have the greatest chance of getting better: 33 percent improve. Unfortunately, 33 percent get worse, and 33 percent remain the same. If asthma starts in early childhood and does not improve by adolescence, the person will probably have it for life. Many teenagers find their asthma disappears, only to have it reappear later in life.

Asthma that begins in adulthood usually continues indefinitely. An exception may be asthma that develops following a flu or pneumonia—sometimes this kind of asthma will recede in about a year.

In allergic asthma it is important to do all that one can to reduce exposure to any relevant allergens (see chapter 4). But in some cases, immunotherapy (allergy shots) may also be recommended to decrease sensitivity to these allergens. Immunotherapy can be especially beneficial for people with allergic asthma who are inclined to suffer late-phase reactions, leaving them sick for days or weeks.

The decision to try immunotherapy is reasonable in the following situations:

- The asthma is seasonal but so severe that it requires significant medication, and skin tests or RASTs show a pollen sensitivity.
- The patient suffers from asthma all year, and tests show a sensitivity to one of the common perennial allergens, especially dust mite allergen.
- The asthma is difficult to control with medication, or use of the medication doesn't fit with the patient's lifestyle.
- The asthma is caused by sensitivity to an animal, and the patient cannot (or will not) avoid the animal.
- The asthma is associated with rhinitis and the symptoms are difficult to control, with the patient feeling sick much of the time.

- And more recently, a European study shed light on how we might prevent the development of asthma in children with seasonal allergies. This study found that children with seasonal pollen allergies (birch tree or grass pollen) who are treated with immunotherapy are less likely to develop asthma in the future. The protective effect remains after the allergy shots are stopped.

ADRENALIN-TYPE DRUGS (BETA2-AGONISTS, SYMPATHOMIMETIC DRUGS)

There are many useful drugs in the treatment of asthma, and among the most important are the sympathomimetic drugs or beta$_2$-agonists; they are in the Adrenalin-epinephrine drug family. They increase the production of CAMP in the body. They should be available for use by essentially all asthma patients as the rescue inhaler. Rescue inhaler is the inhaler used to treat symptoms and to prevent exercise-induced symptoms. Asthma medications are divided into two general categories, rescue medications and controller medications, which we discuss later.

The term *beta agonist* refers to a substance that interacts with the beta-adrenergic receptors of the sympathetic nervous system. Therefore, beta agonists have a sympathomimetic effect, meaning that they imitate the effects of the sympathetic nervous system: they relax airways but can also stimulate the heart.

Epinephrine (Adrenalin) is the strongest of these drugs. It is administered by injection in life-threatening emergencies, when the patient is suffering from allergic shock (anaphylaxis) or an acute asthma attack. It is available in inhaled form without a prescription (Primatene), but this over-the-counter drug is both less safe (because of side effects) and less effective than prescription inhalant medicines.

The prescription sympathomimetic drugs (beta$_2$-agonists) are usually taken by means of inhalers. These drugs are frequently taken preventively, especially before exercise.

Basically, these beta$_2$-agonists come in two forms: short acting and long acting. The former is used as rescue, or reliever, medication. From now on we will refer to them as the rescue inhaler. They relieve acute symptoms and can also be used to prevent exercise-induced asthma. Keep in mind though that these drugs are bronchodilators. Therefore, if the trigger in question is an inhaled allergen, such as cat allergen, do not use the inhaler before exposure to a cat.

What can happen is this: exposure to cats provokes an asthma attack; therefore, you (unwisely) use your inhaler before visiting a friend who has a cat. After arriving on the premises with the cat, you sneeze several times but do not feel much in the way of chest tightness. After four hours with the cat, however, you feel the need to use your inhaler. Two hours later, you need the inhaler again, but this time, it does not work well. You end up in the hospital with asthma exacerbation.

By using your inhaler, you opened your airways to cat allergen. Had you not used your rescue inhaler inappropriately before going there, in all likelihood when you started sneezing, you also would have noticed some chest tightness or coughing.

Although in general, use of anti-inflammatory medication may work as a preventive, we advise exiting the cat premises at the first appearance of any asthma symptom.

Do discuss with your doctor when and when not to use your rescue inhaler.

The most commonly prescribed rescue inhalers (beta$_2$-agonists) are albuterol HFA (ProAir HFA, Proventil HFA, and Ventolin HFA), pirbuterol (Maxair), and Xopenex HFA.

There are specific techniques for getting good results from an inhaler or nebulizer (an electric pump propels air through a solution of the drug, and the vapor is inhaled through a mouthpiece). Pay close attention to your doctor's instructions. If the patient is a child, check from time to time to see if he or she is continuing to inhale the drug in the right way.

Instructions for use of a metered-dose inhaler are given in the appendix. Children and older adults may benefit from a holding chamber, or spacer, which helps in using the device correctly. Breath-actuated inhalers are also on the market. One beta$_2$-agonist is available in a breath-actuated device, the Maxair Autohaler, but may be discontinued at the end of 2013 because it contains the older non-HFA propellants, which can damage the ozone.

The first long-acting beta$_2$-agonist (LABA) released was salmeterol xinafoate (Serevent). It comes in a standard "press and breathe" inhaler and in a dry powder inhaler device (Serevent Diskus), which keeps track of the number of sprays used and warns you (with red numbers) when the medication is running low. More recently, a second LABA was introduced called formoterol (available in the United States as nebulizer solution [Perforomist] and a dry-powdered inhaler device [Foradil]). *These LABAs should **never be used alone** without an accompanying anti-inflammatory medication as recent studies suggest that when used alone, they may result in life-threatening asthma exacerbations.*

Salmeterol and formoterol act to keep the airways open for twelve hours or more. They are useful, therefore, at night for controlling nocturnal symptoms but are often used both morning and night to improve asthma control. It takes about thirty to sixty minutes for salmeterol to take effect, and then it will last until evening. Formoterol begins working in several minutes, which in some patients may make it more appealing. However, if you are using formoterol, because of this rapid onset of action, you should not confuse it as your rescue medication, which it is not.

Words of caution are in order. **Serevent or Foradil is never to be used for acute symptoms or exacerbated asthma and should be used in conjunction with an anti-inflammatory.** Some patients feel so good taking these LABAs that they stop their anti-inflammatory medication; this can lead to a disaster. Second, remember to keep on hand a rescue inhaler (short-acting beta$_2$-agonist) in case symptoms flare up despite the Serevent.

The rescue inhaler is generally used on an as-needed basis. But it is important not to use the beta$_2$-agonists more frequently than recommended. The previous two statements may sound conflicting. Excessive use of the rescue inhaler is a sign that the asthma is out of control and that a physician should be consulted unless you have an asthma plan that tells you what to do in this situation.

Side effects of all of these sympathomimetic drugs include shakiness in the limbs, heart palpitations, headaches, and rebound bronchospasm. These drugs must be used cautiously by people with heart disease, hyperthyroidism, or diabetes.

Cromolyn (Intal) and nedocromil (Tilade) are mast cell stabilizers. They prevent the allergic reaction from occurring by inhibiting release of histamine and other chemical mediators from mast cells. They are being mentioned here because of their historical significance, but at the time this book was being written, they had been discontinued because of issues of manufacturing them with an allowed (HFA) propellant. In the past they were useful as anti-inflammatory or controller medications. Over the years, steroid inhalers have been shown to be safe and more and more children and adults were switched to the more potent inhaled steroids. Also, the leukotriene inhibitors were preferable in other patients who were on Intal and Tilade. The reduction in sales coupled with the expense of switching to an HFA-like propellant (ozone layer safe) is the factor that has contributed to the decision of the manufacturer to discontinue Intal and Tilade inhalers.

LEUKOTRIENE MODIFIERS

Leukotrienes are one of the numerous chemicals, also including histamine, released by mast cells and other cells during immune system reactions. Leukotrienes are lipids, normally present in white blood cells. In immune system reactions, they can cause muscle contraction that constricts bronchial airways; and they increase the permeability of the small blood vessels, which leads to edema, or swelling. They also stimulate mucus production and inflammation. Their effects are relatively long lasting. Our understanding of these chemicals and the receptors on cells that they attach to has mushroomed in recent years; four of these receptors have actually been cloned, giving us very detailed information about them.

There are three leukotriene modifiers currently on the US market.

These medicines are zafirlukast (Accolate), zileuton (Zyflo), and montelukast (Singulair). A fourth (pranlukast [Onon])is available around the world but not yet in the United States. They are useful in some patients in treating mild to moderate asthma. They may be considered as an alternative for inhaled corticosteroids in more-mild asthmatics. They appear to reduce the need for corticosteroids in some cases of mild to moderate asthma.

Accolate and Singulair have already been used successfully in some patients as a replacement for oral corticosteroid medication. Initially it was thought that a rare side effect of these medications was a form of vasculitis (inflammation of the blood vessels). It turned out that a preexisting vasculitis surfaced as oral steroids were reduced after a small minority of patients was begun on these agents.

A side effect associated with Zyflo has been reversible liver damage in some 10 percent of patients. Therefore, liver function must be monitored in patients taking this medicine. Because of this, Zyflo is not commonly used.

Singulair has the advantage of being available in a once-daily pill for adults and, in a lower dose, in a chewable pill and in granules for children.

The role of these medications is managing asthma with lower doses of inhaled corticosteroids in a subset of patients. They are also useful in treating allergic rhinitis symptoms in some patients, and this is discussed in chapter 5.

There is evidence that the leukotriene modifiers are helpful in severe asthma as steroid-sparing medications, and the authors of this book have used them successfully in severe asthma, but always in combination with inhaled steroids and other medications.

CORTICOSTEROIDS

Corticosteroids are invaluable in reducing symptoms in patients with chronic, moderate-to-severe asthma. The main corticosteroids are methylprednisone (Medrol) and prednisone. There are also corticosteroid inhalers for asthma, including budesonide (Pulmicort), ciclesonide (Alvesco), fluticasone (Flovent), mometasone (Asmanex), beclomethasone dipropionate (Beclovent, Qvar, and Vanceril). Because of the regulation of ozone-damaging propellants in aerosol medications, triamcinolone acetonide (Azmacort) and flunisolide (Aerobid) will cease to exist in the next year or two. The inhaled steroids have fewer side effects compared to oral steroids. Of the inhaled steroids listed above, all (except Qvar, Azmacort, and Aerobid) are dry powder inhalers (DPI). DPIs are preferred because there even fewer side effects because of the improved delivery of the medicine to the lungs with less deposited in the back of the throat. Qvar, while not being DPI, may be more useful in certain patients because of the size of the particles in the aerosol—they are more easily deposited in the small inflamed airways in the lungs.

Corticosteroids stimulate the production of CAMP, increase receptors for the sympathomimetic drugs so that they work better, stabilize the mast cells so that they do not release histamine and other chemical mediators of the allergic response, and decrease inflammation overall (including inflammation in the airways). While these statements and others are the result of scientific experiments, the most truthful statement is that we don't really know how they work. But without them, we would be lost in our treatment of asthma, allergies, and other diseases as well.

Corticosteroids can provide dramatic relief from asthma. Unfortunately, when taken orally, they have a variety of serious side effects, including the suppression of the body's normal secretion of adrenal hormones, which are vital to the correct function of many organs of the body and to an effective physiological response to stress. They also cause fluid retention and sometimes weight gain, giving patients an undesirable moon-faced appearance. In long-term use, one must watch out for osteoporosis (bone weakening), diabetes, high blood pressure, the development of cataracts and glaucoma, stomach ulcers, and loss of potassium (this can be without symptoms or can be signaled by a feeling of weakness, muscle cramping, and eventually heart arrhythmia) to name a few side effects.

Even the inhaled steroid sprays have some side effects. Cough and hoarseness occur occasionally. The cough is a result of irritation of the airways from the spray, and the hoarseness is reversible usually by just lowering the dose. The sprays may also sometimes cause a fungal infection of the throat (thrush or yeast), which can usually be prevented by rinsing the back of the mouth with water after using the spray. The risk of thrush with Qvar can be reduced by using an extender device, or spacer (Aerochamber, InspirEase), to deliver the medication more directly into the airways. Beclomethasone (Qvar) is a metered-dose inhaler device that produces an aerosol spray with particles that are small enough, so a spacer is not needed. The newer dry powder inhalers are less likely to cause this side effect because less drug is deposited in the back of the mouth and throat. They should never be used with a spacer.

It is prudent to use the lowest effective dose of inhaled corticosteroids. In some cases, that dose can be reduced by adding a long-acting beta$_2$-agonist (LABA) such as salmeterol (Serevent) or formoterol (Foradil, Perforomist) to the treatment program. These combination inhalers are called Advair (salmeterol plus fluticasone), Dulera (formoterol plus mometasone), and Symbicort (formoterol plus budesonide). A word of caution is in order here. We have been using LABA medications for ten years, and most specialists feel they have revolutionized our ability to control asthma. Recent studies have suggested that there might be some safety concerns with these LABAs and that they "may have resulted in excess mortality." Therefore, it may be prudent to maintain the higher doses of inhaled corticosteroids and forego the addition of the LABA. Unfortunately, as this book goes to press, the jury is out on this issue.

Children using the inhaled corticosteroids should have their growth monitored. While there may be some slowing of growth seen in children on higher doses, it is encouraging that studies have shown these children end up reaching their expected adult height; it just takes them longer to get there. Postmenopausal women, who are at risk for osteoporosis, should discuss with their physicians appropriate calcium and vitamin D supplements, the possibility of hormone replacement therapy, and even treatment with biphosphonates, which is for those on higher doses of inhaled steroids. Annual eye exams should be performed in patients on higher doses or in patients with a family history of glaucoma.

Naturally, given the side effects of oral corticosteroids, both patients and their doctors are usually eager to reduce or stop their use as soon as it is safe to do so. This may be possible when the asthma becomes stable, or perhaps through the use of other medication, such as inhaled corticosteroids. But the correct way to stop is slowly, through a weaning process.

If you are taking oral corticosteroids, do not try to discontinue use all at once. This can be dangerous, even fatal.

Your doctor should give you very detailed instructions on how to reduce your steroid dosages. In general, if oral steroids cannot be stopped entirely, they are given every other day, when possible, to avoid entirely suppressing adrenal gland function and reducing other side effects.

If you are on high daily doses of oral corticosteroids, there are steroid-sparing drugs that may make it possible to taper off the basic steroid medication. These drugs include the leukotriene antagonists discussed above and omalizumab (Xolair), which is discussed below. As mentioned, with our cautionary note, adding a LABA to an inhaled steroid will, in general, allow lower doses of inhaled steroids to be used. Other drugs that have been tried in the past with variable success are troleandomycin (Tao), which is an antibiotic; methotrexate, an anticancer drug that is also an anti-inflammatory; and oral gold, which is also an anti-inflammatory. But these drugs have certain toxicities and should be administered only by physicians experienced in their use.

If you are on regular doses of oral corticosteroids or high doses of inhaled steroids or have been on either in the past year, you should wear a MedicAlert bracelet because in an emergency or during surgery, you may need additional corticosteroids to supplement your weakened adrenal glands. The suppression of the adrenal glands can last up to eighteen months after you have stopped taking these drugs.

THEOPHYLLINE

Theophylline is not used often today to treat asthma. It has become a third-line therapy for patients who are poorly controlled on all other medications. We mention it because for many years it was a mainstay of therapy and is still used extensively around the world.

Theophylline opens the bronchial passages. It may work in part by interfering with the action of an enzyme (phosphodiesterase) that breaks down CAMP—that helpful chemical that counteracts bronchoconstriction. Asthmatics need more CAMP than they have, and they definitely do not need to have it broken down.

In some patients, theophylline acts as a stimulant, interacting with numerous other drugs; so there should be good, regular communication between doctor and patient to make certain the drug is being used appropriately. It can be prescribed in a long-acting form or shorter-acting forms, depending on individual needs. For example, long-acting theophylline, when taken in the evening, sometimes helps to control nocturnal symptoms.

The purpose of theophylline is to prevent an asthma attack from taking place and to maintain good pulmonary function throughout the day. It must reach a certain level in the bloodstream to be effective. That level, called the therapeutic level is pretty close to the level at which side effects occur. For this reason, it is a difficult drug to use safely. This narrow therapeutic window is further complicated by the fact that various environmental and dietary factors affect the theophylline level and can cause toxicity to develop. These are listed below.

A patient should not self-medicate with larger or smaller doses of the drug. Too much in a person's system can be dangerous, as can too little. The average range in which patients do better is ten to twenty micrograms per milliliter of blood; over twenty is too high. There is some evidence that theophylline, at lower levels, functions as an anti-inflammatory medication, thus providing a new use for this medication. A doctor should test blood levels of theophylline periodically (at least once a year) if the patient is being maintained on the drug, and especially if the patient's condition changes.

The elimination of theophylline from one's system is slowed down by certain medications (erythromycin, cimetidine, and others); by high-carbohydrate, low-protein diets; and by diseases such as viral infections and liver and heart disease. Even flu shots may have this effect. If you continue your regular doses of theophylline while it is being eliminated less effectively by your blood, levels of the drug will rise.

Conversely, high-protein, low-carbohydrate diets, charcoal-broiled meats, cigarette smoking, and certain medications like phenobarbital and phenytoin may cause theophylline levels to fall. When this happens, asthma that has been stabilized may get worse. Therefore, you and your doctor should maintain good communication about what is going on in your life to be sure that theophylline medication is achieving the blood levels that work best for you.

Because of the narrow therapeutic to toxicity ratio and because better and safer medications have been introduced, theophylline has been discontinued in most asthma patients over the past twenty years. It is now considered a third-line medication and is started in patients who are not controlled after all other medications have been added.

OMALIZUMAB (XOLAIR)

One of the more novel treatments to be introduced for asthma in the past fifty years is omalizumab (Xolair). This injection is a monoclonal antibody. A monoclonal antibody is a monospecific antibody, meaning they all attach to the same antigen. In this case, the antigen is the IgE antibody. And monoclonal means they are made by cells that are all cloned from the same parent cell and are therefore identical.

Omalizumab is only given to more-severe asthmatics that are poorly controlled even on high doses of inhaled steroids or on chronic oral steroids. The patients must have an elevated IgE and evidence of an allergy to a perennial allergen (mite, cat, cockroach, etc.) in order to be eligible to take this drug. Even then, not all patients respond. The injections are given every two or four weeks; and a response, if it is to occur, will be noticed usually after several months, but sometimes it will take up to six months. The effects may not be dramatic but might include reduced numbers of exacerbations and hospitalizations, reductions in inhaled-steroid doses, and decreased rescue-inhaler use.

There are two major issues with its use. First, it has caused anaphylaxis in about 1/1,000 injections. More concerning is that while most of these anaphylactic episodes have occurred in the first two hours after injection, some have occurred later. So patients are encouraged to wait in the office for a couple of hours after an injection and must carry an EpiPen for the next twenty-four hours. Since patients who are eligible for omalizumab (Xolair) are on the severe end of the spectrum of asthma, this side effect of anaphylaxis is potentially more risky for them.

The other issue is with cost. The annual cost runs from $10,000 to $30,000. These injections, if they work must be given for a long time, perhaps even for the lifetime of the asthmatic. Cost is a major factor these days given the concern of rising health-care costs and its effect on our nation's economy. Remember, however, that it is used for the most severe of asthmatics and this group of asthmatics is by nature the most costly, with frequent hospitalizations and emergency room visits. So if one considers the potential savings related to omalizumab (Xolair) use in reducing asthma exacerbations, it doesn't look as expensive. Omalizumab (Xolair) is approved for use in patients aged twelve and over. However, recent studies have demonstrated that it works and is safe in children ages six to twelve. While we are waiting for official FDA approval for this younger age group, it is considered appropriate to now use it in this age group as physicians are allowed to vary away from this type of age restriction in what is called an off-label use.

NEW UNDERSTANDING OF ASTHMA

Significant advances in the understanding of asthma as a disease of inflammation in the airways took place in the late 1980s. Gradually, the management has shifted toward much-earlier use of anti-inflammatory drugs. In the 1990s, the National Heart, Lung, and Blood Institute (a branch of the National Institutes of Health) developed two new programs to address the need for updating our physicians in the treatment of asthma. The unstated goal of these programs was to address the rising death rate from asthma in the United States and elsewhere. The first program was made up of U.S. experts and called the National Asthma Education and Prevention Program (NAEPP). The second program was made up of international experts and was called the Global Initiative for Asthma (GINA). Both of these panels of experts issued guidelines incorporating recent changes in our understanding of asthma that were directed to all physicians in order to update their understanding and management of asthma.

If you have asthma, select a doctor who is aware of new methods being introduced. Most board-certified specialists in allergy or pulmonology would be appropriate choices. A specialist associated with a teaching hospital usually will be up-to-date. Calling the National Jewish Health's Lung Line can help you find a board certified specialist in your area (800-222-5864). Educating yourself by following medical news from a reliable source is also an important protection against continuing to be treated with outdated methods; however, one must be careful when surfing the Internet, as there is as much information as there is misinformation.

Self-monitoring

With asthma, it can sometimes be very difficult to figure out whether symptoms you are feeling are serious or not. Feelings of anxiety, rapid heartbeat, breathlessness, or nervousness can be due to lack of oxygen because of the asthma or to the effects of certain medications or to anxiety or to all three causes.

Acute Attacks

Asthma attacks vary from person to person and time to time. An acute attack can begin suddenly, peaking in minutes, or develop more gradually over hours or days. Death can occur if a patient neglects their symptoms.

The earlier you are aware that you may be in trouble, the better you will be able to manage the attack. You should also have a plan worked out with your physician on how to handle emergencies and who will cover if the physician is not available. Your doctor may advise you to keep a peak flow meter at home to test respiratory function yourself. A drop in peak flow may be a warning that an attack is approaching and that an adjustment in medication is needed. Detailed instructions for the use of the peak flow meter are given in appendix B.

You should know what medicines to take or increase in bad times and should always be able to reach your doctor to discuss changes in medication and if a trip to an emergency room may be in order.

You should discuss with your physician what signs to look for that may indicate that your asthma is getting worse. The following general rules were formulated in 1997 and updated in 2007 by the National Institutes of Health in *Guidelines for the Diagnosis and Management of Asthma*. The publication is part of the NIH National Asthma Education and Prevention Program. See appendix E for how to access this valuable document on the Internet.

- You begin to use your short-acting $beta_2$-agonist inhaler after not having needed it for a while, or you start to use it more frequently than is typical for you.
- You finish a canister of a short-acting $beta_2$-agonist inhaler in a month.
- The short-acting $beta_2$-agonist inhaler does not provide you with the relief it used to.
- You awaken in the morning needing to use your short-acting $beta_2$-agonist inhaler because of chest tightness, or you begin to awaken at night to use it.
- Everyday activities leave you winded or breathless.

- You start coughing, wheezing, or having shortness of breath or begin producing sputum.
- Your peak-flow number goes down.

If you experience any of these changes, do not wait until there is a crisis—call your doctor.

Health-care providers assign considerable importance to the categories of asthma severity, ranging from "mild intermittent" to "severe persistent." While you may use the terms loosely, in the medical community they signify specific symptoms for which specific therapy is indicated. Here we use the terminology suggested by the NIH's *Guidelines for the Diagnosis and Management of Asthma.*

The NIH emphasizes that all asthma patients, no matter how mild or severe their asthma, will benefit from education in the character of the disease and how best to manage their individual conditions. We agree and feel that it is part of a physician's responsibility to provide education personally and, when possible, to help patients educate themselves outside the doctor's office. In fact, the reason we have written this book is to provide a source of information for asthma and allergy patients.

Your doctor should help you create a self-management plan and an action plan tailored to your level of need. In almost all communities, there are opportunities for further education through lectures or group programs at local hospitals for adults and teenagers. Asthma camps can be found nationwide and serve young children and teenagers. There are a variety of support groups for parents of children with asthma.

See appendix D for how to access such resources.

INTERMITTENT ASTHMA

You have intermittent asthma if you experience symptoms no more than twice per week, with normal breathing otherwise. The flare-ups of symptoms are brief (hours to a few days) with varying intensity. Nocturnal symptoms occur no more than twice a month. (You may call these flare-ups asthma attacks; your doctor may call them exacerbations.)

For this level of asthma, no long-term medications are needed; in other words, no inhaled corticosteroids, mast cell stabilizers, or long-acting bronchodilators. Quick-relief measures are appropriate, that is, inhaled beta$_2$-agonists used no more than twice a week.

Your doctor should help you to learn how to manage your asthma, avoid allergens and irritants, and deal with any unexpectedly severe asthma attack.

MILD PERSISTENT ASTHMA

You have mild persistent asthma if your symptoms occur more than twice a week but not every day. Flare-ups may interfere with your normal activities. Nocturnal symptoms appear three to four times per month.

For this level of asthma, you should be taking one long-term control medication that is used daily. The preferred controller is low doses of an inhaled corticosteroid. An alternative might be a leukotriene modifier.

You should have a quick-relief medication, that is, a short-acting beta$_2$-agonist, which you can use as needed. As explained above, if you are turning more and frequently to the quick relief, you may need instead an additional long-term medication.

You should learn how to use a peak flow meter as part of your general management plan for the asthma.

MODERATE PERSISTENT ASTHMA

You have moderate persistent asthma if the disease limits your physical activity and asthma attacks, or exacerbations, are frequent (two or more times per week), bothering you at night as well as during the day.

Long-term control should be provided by either medium-dose inhaled corticosteroids or a somewhat lower dose combined with a long-acting bronchodilator (salmeterol [Serevent] or formoterol [Foradil]). (If needed, the dose of corticosteroids can be boosted.) Please see the discussion of these choices earlier in this chapter. As before, quick relief can be provided by inhaled beta$_2$-agonists; but if they are used on a daily basis or with increasing frequency, more long-term control is indicated. Leukotriene modifiers may also be recommended.

SEVERE PERSISTENT ASTHMA

You have severe persistent asthma if you have continual symptoms that limit physical activity; and flare-ups, or exacerbations, occur frequently. Nocturnal symptoms are also frequent. Tests of pulmonary function indicate that the disease is severe.

For long-term control, you may be prescribed a high dose of inhaled corticosteroids and a long-acting bronchodilator and oral corticosteroids. Theophylline might be added, and if you are allergic, omalizumab (Xolair) might be tried. Your doctor should encourage a controlled reduction in the use of oral corticosteroids whenever possible. This weaning process can be abandoned when necessary, and then started over. You can use the beta$_2$-agonists for quick relief, keeping in mind that increased use indicates that a change is needed in long-term control. Your doctor may also recommend leukotriene modifiers.

You should use a peak flow meter to monitor pulmonary function.

RESULTS

You know that your asthma treatments are working well when your symptoms (breathlessness, coughing) subside in frequency and severity; you have fewer attacks, or exacerbations, and fewer visits to the hospital; you can carry on normal activity, including sports and other physical activities; you are experiencing minimal side effects from your medications; your doctor tells you that your pulmonary function has improved; and above all, you feel better and are more satisfied with your state of health.

Today, more so than ever in the past, most asthma sufferers—even those with severe asthma—can lead full, productive lives if they receive proper medical attention.

Chapter 10

Hay Fever And
Other Forms Of Rhinitis

Adolescence is when many teenagers develop the characteristic symptoms of allergic rhinitis—runny nose, itchy eyes, and a tendency to sneeze repeatedly. Indeed, teenagers are more prone than any other age group to develop rhinitis; about 30 percent of adolescents suffer from allergic and nonallergic rhinitis, compared with 10 to 15 percent of the total population.

At whatever age it first strikes, rhinitis can be seasonal or perennial, allergic or nonallergic in nature. Allergic rhinitis affects some 10 to 15 percent of the population, which means that 30 to 45 million peole in the United States are affected. At this prevalence, that would mean that 677 million to 1 billion are affected worldwide; but the prevalence is actually somewhat lower in less-developed countries because of the "cleanliness hypothesis," which is discussed elsewhere. The disease frequently disrupts normal life, causing loss of sleep, poor concentration, fatigue, and even depression. Some $3 billion is spent in the United States annually on treatment.

According to some medical historians, allergic rhinitis was much less common before the Industrial Revolution. This is also consistent with the cleanliness hypothesis, which is discussed elsewhere.

As the name suggests, perennial allergic rhinitis is a year-round problem, caused by a sensitivity to dust mite allergen, pets, or other allergens to which you may be exposed no matter the season. It is often aggravated by seasonal allergies.

Seasonal allergic rhinitis is caused by a sensitivity to the pollen of grasses, ragweed, weeds and trees. It is popularly known as hay fever, although there is no fever. Typically, so-called hay fever is a reaction to ragweed pollen and occurs late in summer. It was named hay fever because it occurs when hay was often harvested, but it has nothing to do with hay and it causes no fever unless there is a sinus infection complicating it. In the Eastern United States, approximately 75 percent of seasonal rhinitis is associated with allergy to ragweed. A sensitivity to grass pollen affects about 50 percent of those with seasonal rhinitis, and a sensitivity to tree pollen is present in about 10 percent. The reason the figures add up to more than 100 percent is that sensitivities overlap, with a few people (about 5 percent to 10 percent) allergic to all three kinds of pollen. About 25 percent are allergic to both ragweed and grass pollen.

When seasonal rhinitis occurs in late spring or early summer, it is sometimes called rose fever, another misnomer. Because roses are highly visible at just the time of year when grasses are pollinating, people naturally associate roses with summertime rhinitis. Actually, the pollen of colorful flowers—the much-maligned goldenrod as well as the rose—tends to be heavy and sticky and is not easily transported by air. These plants are pollinated by insects, with the pollen designed to go from the flower to the insect. It is the virtually invisible pollen spread by the wind that most easily enters the nose and mouth, causing annoying respiratory symptoms.

On dry, windy days, pollen may fill the air and travel great distances. (Ragweed pollen can travel up to five hundred miles!) Keep your home and car windows closed on such days, and use an air conditioner if possible.

Speaking of travel, exposure to diesel fuel is likely to stimulate allergic reactions to pollen. Diesel exhaust contains chemicals (polyaromatic hydrocarbons) that stimulate IgE production in the upper respiratory mucosa. Diesel extracts have been demonstrated to produce a response to ragweed pollen sixteenfold greater than the response to the ragweed allergen alone.

If your hay fever is worse on rainy or damp days than on dry, sunny days, then you are more likely allergic to mold spores than to plant pollen. In general, seasonal mold allergies in the United States tend to be more common in the grain-growing states of the Midwest, for molds thrive on these plants. But allergenic molds are common in humid areas wherever there are trees and lawns, for mold grows well on dead leaves and grass cuttings. The allergic teenager who hates raking leaves or mowing lawns may not just be lazy—the jobs may leave him feeling sick. Another chore may be more appropriate for this youngster.

In the United States, the most-important outdoor molds are *Alternaria, Cladosporium* (also called *Hormodendrum*), and *Aspergillus*. Their spores, which appear in early spring, reach their highest levels on warm, humid summer days. The spores almost disappear with the first frost, but unless there is snow on the ground, there may still be mold spores in the air.

THE NATURAL HISTORY OF ALLERGIC RHINITIS

Most people who develop allergic rhinitis do so before age twenty, often between ages twelve and fifteen. The course of the disease for any given patient cannot be predicted because of the many variables involved, including pollen levels where the patient lives and works, general health of the patient, and so on. Typically, however, the disease persists for many years, with perennial rhinitis showing more staying power than the seasonal kinds. With seasonal rhinitis, one study has shown that, in a four-year period, about one in twenty women and one in ten men recover and have no further symptoms.

Allergic rhinitis is often associated with asthma, and in some cases, the asthma appears first. Rhinitis and asthma are in the triad of allergic atopic diseases, the third being eczema, or atopic dermatitis. Although patients often have two of the diseases, it is unusual to have all three. In the United States, allergic rhinitis is the most common of the atopic diseases.

RHINITIS SIGNS AND SYMPTOMS

As you can tell from its name, rhinitis (which means "inflammation of the nose") typically affects the nose. But in some patients, eye symptoms may dominate, or the inflammation may move into the sinuses or ears.

In allergic rhinitis, nasal itching and serial sneezes (five or more sneezes in a row) are common. A watery secretion from the nose, with postnasal drip, is characteristic. An obstructed, stuffy nose is commonly reported. The nasal discharge can become quite copious, irritating the skin of the outer nose and upper lip. The patient tends to rub the nose and upper lip with a swiping gesture known as the allergic salute.

Nasal obstruction, if it is more or less constant, can interfere with drainage of the paranasal sinuses, causing headache. The ache results from air pressure outside the sinuses as the absorption of air within the sinuses creates a negative pressure, or vacuum. If nasal congestion blocks the Eustachian tube, you may get earaches, and your hearing will be muffled. Nasal congestion leads to loss of the senses of smell and taste.

Some patients report only itching and burning of the eyes and sometimes a marked sensitivity to light. The sclera and conjunctiva, which form the lining of the eye, can become red and swollen (see chapter 11).

In chronic cases of rhinitis, especially in young children, the area around the eyes may be puffy and dark, as if the patient has two black eyes. These are called allergic shiners.

Itching of the throat, palate, and ears may provoke a patient to try to scratch the palate or throat with the tongue, which produces a clicking sound. One distinguished medical professor, ordinarily a very polite person, used to surprise students by putting his fingers in his mouth to scratch his throat—although only at the height of the allergy season.

The allergy may affect your mood, causing you to feel weak, sick, depressed, irritable, and tired. You may lose your appetite. Since these symptoms closely resemble those of clinical depression, the patient may end up in a psychotherapist's office or be treated with antidepressant medication. The diagnosis is especially difficult in the rare cases in which depression is virtually the only symptom. To discover the real culprit, the physician must look for a seasonal pattern or other environmental factor.

Some people with seasonal rhinitis suffer only at mid-pollen season. Others are so sensitive that they are reliable harbingers of spring. No sooner are the first grains of pollen in the air than they are on the phone to their allergists.

Some patients recover quickly as soon as the pollen season passes, but others suffer for several weeks longer. The nasal mucosa is primed so that it will react to many different nonspecific stimuli, such as smoke or odors.

PERENNIAL ALLERGIC RHINITIS

The symptoms of perennial rhinitis tend to be less dramatic than those of seasonal rhinitis, except that obstruction by congestion is a far more prominent feature. Symptoms associated with such obstruction—including sinus headaches, chronic ear problems (especially in children), chronic sore throat caused by mouth breathing and postnasal drip, and itchiness of the nose and throat—are an important part of the picture.

Most often, the person suffering from perennial rhinitis is allergic to one or more common substances in the environment—dust, mite, or animal dander—the substances that in chapter 4 we advise you to clean out of your home. Occasionally, a food is the cause. And in places like Southern California, where the pollen season lasts most of the year, so does the rhinitis.

The patient with perennial rhinitis develops very sensitive nasal mucosa, which may react to all sorts of nonspecific irritants, even changes in temperature. When pollen season comes around, the additional assault on the nasal tissues can make the symptoms much worse.

DIAGNOSIS

In taking your history, in examining you, and in deciding what tests to run, the doctor will try to determine whether allergy is the main problem and what it is that you are allergic to. He or she will want to know if you have a family history of hay fever, eczema, or asthma. Expect a lot of questions relating to exactly when your symptoms appear and when they are at their worst, so if possible, bring some notes on this subject (see chapter 3).

The doctor must be sure that no nonallergic condition, such as nasal polyps or a sinus infection unrelated to allergy, is responsible for your symptoms. He or she will try to find out if there is an asthmatic component to your illness and will ask about medicines you may be taking that may cause or worsen your symptoms.

Recurrent infections (colds) resemble allergic rhinitis, but usually, the pattern of occurrence is different in that allergies tend to arise or get worse in the spring or summer and to last longer than colds do. Also, with colds there is less itching and less repetitive sneezing; there is often fever; and the inside of the nose looks different from that of patients with allergies.

Occasionally, especially with children, the physician will find something stuck up the nose; and removal of the foreign object provides a prompt happy ending.

Hypothyroidism (low levels of thyroid hormone) can produce nasal stuffiness. Hypothyroidism can be detected by a blood test. It is typically associated with fatigue and sometimes with hair loss. Pregnancy is often accompanied by nasal stuffiness. This is normal.

Overuse of topical nasal decongestants causes chronic nasal congestion (rhinitis medicamentosa). A number of other drugs—including reserpine, alpha-methyldopa, and beta-blockers—can cause nasal congestion. Cocaine and some other illegal drugs cause a nasal condition similar to rhinitis medicamentosa.

Vasomotor rhinitis is very similar to perennial allergic rhinitis, but the cause is unknown. Symptoms are typically made worse by eating spicy food, by strong odors, or by sudden changes in temperature. Allergy tests (skin tests and RAST) will be negative (see chapter 3).

Another condition that tests negative for specific allergens is NARES (nonallergic rhinitis with eosinophilia). The patient seems to have allergic rhinitis, and a nasal smear test reveals an elevated count of eosinophils, blood cells that are associated with allergy. Many allergists feel that NARES is an allergic reaction to an unknown allergen or allergens in the environment.

TREATMENT

The management of allergic rhinitis consists of avoidance, medication, and immunotherapy (allergy shots).

Chapter 4 describes in detail what measures to take if your rhinitis is caused by allergens in your home. But in treating seasonal rhinitis, you must focus more on allergens from the great outdoors. If you can keep pollen and mold spores out of your home and office, the chances are that your hay fever will not be too severe. (If you do not improve much even when avoiding pollen and outdoor mold spores, one possibility that an allergist would investigate is whether you also have an asymptomatic sensitivity to one of the indoor allergens that is exacerbating your seasonal allergy.)

Usually, the first step in controlling seasonal symptoms is to invest in an air conditioner, at least for the bedroom. If you have been, working out of doors, gardening, raking leaves, or the like, wash your hair and put your clothing in the laundry before going to bed. You do not want to carry pollen and mold spores into your bedroom or bed.

Check out the plant life around your home. For years, people with respiratory illnesses were sent to Arizona and New Mexico for their health. Soon, however, the fashion for growing Eastern lawns and gardens, in combination with the population's genetic inclination toward allergic sensitivities, produced a sort of chronic-allergy emergency. Droves of Sun Belt residents developed hay fever and/or asthma. Now, laws prohibit the sale of a variety of trees, including mulberry and olive trees, and fines may be assessed against homeowners who let bermuda grass grow tall enough to flower.

In addition to olive and mulberry trees, acacia, juniper, elm, box elder, walnut, sycamore, ash, oak, birch, and maple are also heavy pollinators. However, the tree-pollination season comes early in spring and usually is relatively brief.

Late spring to early summer is the time when grasses begin to pollinate, with the duration of the season depending on location. In late summer and fall, plants of the ragweed family pollinate. These are the most problematic plants for allergy sufferers.

If you live in the country or near a vacant lot and suffer from hay fever, be sure that you do not have a ragweed crop right on your doorstep. In the United States, the only almost-ragweed-free areas are the Pacific Coast, the southern tip of Florida, and northwest Maine.

Incidentally, alcoholic beverages sometimes cause increased allergic sensitivity; so when the pollen count is high, you may want to keep your alcohol consumption low. Ragweed pollen also may boost sensitivity to melons and other fruits and vice versa (see chapter 7).

Moving to a different part of the country in order to avoid exposure to the plants and molds to which you are sensitive is rarely worthwhile and often an expensive disappointment. You may well develop new allergies to the plants—even desert plants—in your new home region. However, if you have successfully visited in a region for several months and you always feel better there, this may be the exception to the rule. Typically, the seashore is the best bet.

As for medication or immunization, your doctor should be willing to take the time to explain the costs and benefits of a variety of approaches to reducing rhinitis symptoms. Unless the rhinitis is associated with some other more-serious condition, such as asthma or perhaps sinus disease, you can safely begin with a minimalist approach to treatment, working up to more expensive treatment or immunization only if necessary. Helpful medications include the nonsoporific antihistamines (which may be combined with a decongestant) and topical corticosteroid or antihistamine nasal sprays (see chapter 5). Remember, it is extremely important to use the sprays only as directed. Also, the antihistamines, as well as corticosteroid sprays, work best when started in advance of an outbreak of allergy symptoms; they (especially the sprays) are essentially preventives.

Immediate relief from nasal stuffiness can be obtained by use of normal saline solution (one-eighth teaspoon of salt in eight ounces of water). With a bulb syringe, irrigate the nasal passages to wash away mucus and allergens. Do one nostril at a time and allow the water to flow in gently. Don't force the water through the congested areas. Saline solution can also be used to wash out itchy, inflamed eyes. Various premixed saline solutions in the form of nasal sprays are available OTC as well.

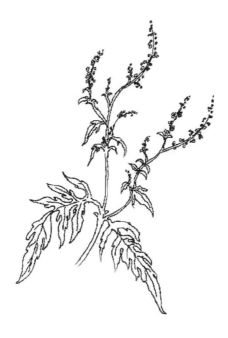

Ragweed

Most often, if you take steps to reduce exposure to the allergens that provoke your rhinitis, a moderate amount of medication can bring adequate relief. But if you have a number of allergies and year-round symptoms, then you might reasonably consider immunotherapy for a more thoroughgoing improvement. The decision whether or not to take this step may turn on exactly which allergens affect you (as revealed by skin and/or blood tests). Immunization is achieved more readily for some allergens than others, and your doctor should discuss this with you.

Also, for various reasons, some patients cannot tolerate the drugs normally used to treat rhinitis, so immunotherapy and very strict avoidance of allergens must be attempted.

POLLINATION SEASONS

The following summary of pollination seasons lists general pollination dates for significant varieties of plants in the United States. The seasonal dates will vary from region to region and will also change from year to year, depending on weather conditions. Finally, you may be allergic to plants in your region that are not listed here. So if you have hay fever, take the time to do a little botanical investigation of your neighborhood. Your local health officer, botanical gardens, or forestry service should be able to help you to identify troublesome plants.

In many places, the pollination period for trees overlaps with that of grass, and that of grass overlaps with that of ragweed. Therefore, the many people who are allergic to more than one type of plant are susceptible to a double whammy in summer and early fall. Molds (not listed here) also are prevalent in summer and fall, especially in damp weather.

If you are allergic to one grass, you are probably allergic to several. Related antigenically are timothy, orchard grass, redtop, sweet vernal grass, rye, fescue, and johnsongrass. Bermuda grass belongs to a different family. It is usually found in Southern states; and if kept trimmed, as in a lawn, it will not pollinate. But it also grows wild along roadways and in fields, where, of course, it does pollinate.

The pollination seasons listed below are generally for the southern part of each region; they will occur later in the more northerly sections.

NORTH ATLANTIC STATES

Connecticut, Maine, Massachusetts, New Hampshire, New Jersey, New York, Pennsylvania, Rhode Island, and Vermont

Trees. Trees in this region pollinate from March through June, with box elder and maple pollinating early (March through May) and oak being the latest (May and June). Other significant trees are ash, birch, cottonwood, elm, hickory, poplar, sycamore, and walnut.

Grasses. Grasses (many of which are grown as hay) pollinate from May through July. They include bromegrass, fescue, johnsongrass, June grass (Kentucky bluegrass), orchard grass, redtop, rye, timothy, velvet grass, and vernal grass.

Weeds. Early-pollinating weeds are plantain (not the banana plant but an herb of the genus *Plantago)* and dock (sorrel), May through July. Late pollinators are cocklebur, lamb's-quarters, pigweed, and ragweed (August through October).

MID-ATLANTIC STATES

Delaware, District of Columbia, Maryland, North Carolina, and Virginia

Trees. Trees pollinate from February through May, with box elder, maple, and elm being the earliest and hickory and pecan the latest. Others include ash, birch, cedar, cottonwood, juniper, oak, poplar, sycamore, and walnut.

Grasses. May through July is the grass-pollinating season. The following grasses are important: bermuda grass, johnsongrass, June grass (Kentucky bluegrass), orchard grass, redtop, rye, timothy, and vernal grass.

Weeds. Among weeds, dock (sorrel) is an early pollinator (May through July), along with plantain (May through August). Cocklebur, lamb's-quarters, pigweed, and ragweed pollinate from August through October.

SOUTH ATLANTIC STATES

Florida, Georgia, and South Carolina—the southern tip of Florida is one of the few places in the United States that does not have much ragweed. Plants characteristic of subtropical Florida to which people are allergic include palm trees, Brazilian pepper trees, bayberry, and melaleuca trees, which pollinate from December through April. Grasses pollinate year-round in subtropical Florida.

Trees. In this region generally, trees pollinate from January through May, with cedar and juniper being early pollinators and walnut pollinating in May. Privet pollinates all year. Other trees of interest to the allergy prone include ash, birch, box elder, cottonwood, elm, hickory, maple, oak, pecan, pine, poplar, and sycamore.

Grasses. Grasses pollinate from March through October. They include bermuda grass, canary grass, fescue, johnsongrass, June grass (Kentucky bluegrass), redtop, rye, timothy, and vernal grass. The subtropical grasses include Bahia grass and salt grass. As mentioned, at the tip of Florida grasses pollinate year-round.

Weeds. Weed pollination starts in May and continues through October. The significant weeds include dock (sorrel) and plantain (early pollinators), as well as cocklebur, lamb's-quarters, pigweed, ragweed, and sagebrush, which pollinate from July through October.

GREATER OHIO VALLEY

Indiana, Kentucky, Ohio, Tennessee, and West Virginia

Trees. In this region, the earliest-pollinating tree is elm (February through April). Hickory trees pollinate as late as June. Others, which pollinate in the spring, include ash, birch, box elder, cottonwood, elm, maple, oak, poplar, sycamore, and walnut.

Grasses. Pollination of grasses is from April through July, with grass plants including bermuda grass, fescue, johnsongrass, June grass (Kentucky bluegrass), redtop, rye, and timothy.

Weeds. The peak weed-pollination season is August through October, with plantain pollinating as early as May and the all-important ragweed pollinating from August through October. Others include amaranth, cocklebur, dock (sorrel), kochia, lamb's-quarters, pigweed, Russian thistle, sagebrush, and water hemp.

SOUTH CENTRAL STATES

Alabama, Arkansas, Louisiana, and Mississippi

Trees. Tree pollination starts in February and runs through May. The significant trees include ash, box elder, cedar, cottonwood, elm, hackberry, hickory, juniper, maple, oak, pecan, poplar, and sycamore.

Grasses. April through September is grass-pollination season, with the following important plants represented: bermuda grass, johnsongrass, June grass (Kentucky bluegrass), orchard grass, redtop, rye, and timothy.

Weeds. In May through July, plantain and dock (sorrel) pollinate, followed by kochia and Russian thistle in June through August. In August through October, the pollinators include careless weed, cocklebur, lamb's-quarters, marsh elder, pigweed, poverty weed, ragweed, and sagebrush.

MIDWESTERN STATES

Illinois, Iowa, Michigan, Minnesota, Missouri, and Wisconsin

Trees. The elm opens the season, beginning pollination in February. The main months of tree pollination are March through June, with the following represented: alder, ash, box elder, birch, cedar, cottonwood, hickory, maple, oak, poplar, sycamore, and walnut.

Grasses. Grass-pollination season is April through August. Keep in mind that dates are given for the southern part of the region; the pollination season runs about a month later in the north. The main grasses to which people are likely to be sensitive are bermuda grass, bromegrass, Canada bluegrass, canary grass, corn, fescue, johnsongrass, June grass (Kentucky bluegrass), orchard grass, redtop, rye, and timothy.

Weeds. In May through July, plantain and dock (sorrel) pollinate, followed by kochia and Russian thistle in June through August. In August through October, the pollinators include amaranth, chenopod, careless weed, cocklebur, lamb's-quarters, marsh elder, Mexican firebush, pigweed, poverty weed, and ragweed.

THE GREAT PLAINS

Kansas, Nebraska, North Dakota, and South Dakota

Trees. Pollination begins in March and goes into June, with the main trees being alder, ash, birch, box elder, cedar, cottonwood, elm, hickory, maple, oak, poplar, pussy willow, and walnut.

Grasses. Grass-pollination season is May through July. The most important grasses are brome grass, fescue, June grass (Kentucky bluegrass), quack grass, redtop, rye, timothy, western and crested wheatgrass.

Weeds. Plantain and dock (sorrel) pollinate in May through July. Ragweed and other important weeds pollinate July through October. They include amaranth, cocklebur, lamb's-quarters, marsh elder, Mexican firebush, pigweed, poverty weed, Russian thistle, sagebrush, and water hemp.

SOUTHWESTERN GRASSLANDS

Oklahoma and Texas

Trees. Tree-pollination season lasts from February through April. Important trees include ash, box elder, cedar, cottonwood, elm, hickory, juniper, mesquite, mulberry, oak, pecan, poplar, walnut, and willow.

Grasses. Grass-pollination season is April through August. The most important grasses are bermuda grass, fescue, johnsongrass, June grass (Kentucky bluegrass), orchard grass, quack grass, redtop, rye, and timothy.

Weeds. Pollination season is May through October. Ragweed pollinates August through October. Other weeds include careless weed, cocklebur, dock (sorrel), kochia, lamb's-quarters, marsh elder, pigweed, plantain, Russian thistle, and sagebrush.

ROCKY MOUNTAIN STATES

Arizona (mountainous), Colorado, Idaho (mountainous), Montana, New Mexico, Utah, and Wyoming

Trees. The pollination season begins as early as December in the southern part of this region (for the mountain cedar). It lasts through June. In addition to the mountain cedar, other significant trees are alder, ash, aspen, birch, box elder, cedar, cottonwood, elm, hickory, juniper, mesquite, mulberry, oak, olive, pine, poplar, and willow.

Grasses. Pollination of grasses is April through September (April through August in the south and May through September in the north). The following grasses are represented: bermuda grass, bromegrass, fescue, June grass (Kentucky bluegrass), orchard grass, quack grass, redtop, rye, and timothy.

Weeds. Pollination season is May through October. Ragweed pollinates July through September. Other weeds include amaranth, careless weed, cocklebur, lamb's-quarters, marsh elder, pigweed, plantain, Russian thistle, sagebrush, saltbush, and sugar beet.

SOUTHWESTERN DESERT

Arizona (desert) and Southern California

Trees. The pollination season begins in January and lasts through May. Important trees include ash, cedar, cottonwood, cypress, elm, juniper, mesquite, oak, poplar, and sycamore.

Grasses. Pollination of grasses is virtually year-round. The following grasses are represented: bermuda grass, bromegrass, canary grass, June grass (Kentucky bluegrass), and rye.

Weeds. Pollination season is May into November. Ragweed pollinates in March and April and in September and October. Other weeds include careless weed, lamb's-quarters, pigweed, Russian thistle, sagebrush, and saltbush.

INTERMOUNTAIN WESTERN STATES

Idaho (southern) and Nevada

Trees. The pollination season is February through May. Significant trees are alder, ash, birch, box elder, cedar, cottonwood, elm, juniper, mesquite, poplar, and willow.

Grasses. Pollination of grasses is May through July. The following grasses are represented: bermuda grass, brome grass, fescue, June grass (Kentucky bluegrass), orchard grass, quack grass, redtop, rye, salt grass, and timothy.

Weeds. Pollination season is primarily July through October, with dock (sorrel) and saltbush beginning pollination early (in May). Other weeds include cocklebur, kochia, lamb's-quarters, Mexican firebush, ragweed, Russian thistle, and sagebrush.

CALIFORNIA (NON-DESERT) AND THE PACIFIC NORTHWEST

California, Oregon, and Washington

Trees. Pollination begins in February and lasts through June. Major trees are acacia, alder, ash, birch, box elder, cottonwood, elm, hazelnut, poplar, sycamore, walnut, and willow. **Grasses.** Pollination of grasses occurs from February through November (primarily May through August in the north). The following grasses are represented: bermuda grass, bromegrass, canary grass, fescue, johnsongrass, June grass (Kentucky bluegrass), oats, orchard grass, redtop, rye, and timothy.

Weeds. Pollination season is May through October. There is very little ragweed here, although it does exist. Other weeds include careless weed, cocklebur, dock (sorrel), kochia, lamb's-quarters, pigweed, plantain, Russian thistle, sagebrush, saltbush, and sheep sorrel.

ALASKA

Airborne allergens are not a great problem here. There is a tree-pollination season from March through June, overlapping with a brief time of grass pollination in certain areas in June and July.

The most important trees are alder, birch, and willow. Others include aspen, cedar, hemlock, pine, poplar, and spruce. The grasses include June grass (Kentucky bluegrass), orchard grass, redtop, and timothy.

HAWAII

Pollen season is essentially all year.

Trees. A few trees contribute sufficient airborne pollen to be a problem. These include acacia and eucalyptus.

Grasses. Significant grasses relative to allergy include Bermuda grass, corn, finger grass, johnsongrass, June grass (Kentucky bluegrass), love grass, redtop, and sorghum.

Weeds. Pollen of English plantain, lamb's-quarters, and pigweed is a problem in some places.

Chapter 11

SINUSES, EARS, AND EYES

Allergies, especially allergic rhinitis, can be associated with chronic or acute infection or inflammation of the sinuses, ears, or eyes. When a patient has chronic sinus disease or earaches, often it is not initially clear whether allergies play a role or not.

Both allergists and ear, nose, and throat specialists treat disorders of the sinuses and ears, and sometimes eyes, as do doctors with a wider practice, such as pediatricians and internists. (The technical term for an ear, nose, and throat doctor is *otolaryngologist*. ENT is the popular shorthand designation.)

Ideally, there should be cooperation among different specialists. For example, if sinusitis keeps recurring after antibiotic treatment, tests for allergic sensitivities should be done to see whether allergic reactions may be causing blockage of the sinuses, thereby contributing to the development of infection. Similarly, an allergist who is treating sinus disease without much luck should consider referring the patient to a sinus specialist (ENT). In some cases, for instance, surgery is needed to help the sinuses to drain.

As a patient or as a parent of a patient, be aware that it is appropriate to seek a second opinion if a health problem continues. Often it is helpful to go to a doctor in a different specialty.

NASAL POLYPS

One condition for which it is important to see both an allergist and an ENT is the presence of nasal polyps. The symptoms are usually severe enough that the person realizes a visit to the doctor is needed. They are typically chronic nasal congestion, headaches, sinus aches, loss of the senses of smell and taste, and recurrent ear congestion or infection.

Luckily, polyps are relatively uncommon, for they are troubling and sometimes serious. They are usually associated with nasal disease or asthma, often asthma combined with aspirin sensitivity. If you have asthma and polyps, it is very likely that you are also allergic to aspirin and to other nonsteroidal anti-inflammatory drugs as well. Asthma attacks caused by aspirin allergy are often exceptionally severe when nasal polyps are present. Therefore, you must avoid all aspirin and NSAID-containing products.

Polyps afflict people with the atopic allergic diseases (allergic rhinitis, asthma, and eczema) more than they do the general population and are twice as common in men as in women. The great majority of polyps occur after age forty. In a child under age ten, the growth of polyps is highly suggestive of cystic fibrosis.

Polyps are growths, typically benign, off the side walls of the nasal passages or in the sinus cavities. Malignancy is relatively rare, although it is much more likely if the polyps appear only on one side of the nose or if they bleed easily. But in all cases, the possibility of a malignancy should be ruled out by an ENT; this is mandatory if the polyps are on one side only.

It is not clear exactly what causes polyps to grow, except that they often seem to do so when patients are allergic or when there is some recurrent infection or irritation of the nose and sinuses.

Formerly, surgical removal was the standard treatment; but since polyps tend to grow back, even after surgery, it is usually better to try less-intrusive medical treatment first. Today we have effective treatment that is not so aggressive. The most useful medical treatment is with topical nasal steroids. Antihistamines and decongestants do not help. Since polyps are so often linked with allergies, it is a good idea to see an allergist to determine whether or not you have allergic sensitivities. Sometimes, good environmental control of the allergens in your home is treatment enough to control the allergic factor in the condition. In other cases, immunotherapy (allergy shots) may be helpful. The latter two interventions will not reverse the polyps but can decrease the chances they will regrow following steroid treatment or surgery.

If steroid treatment does not work, surgery may be needed; but immediately after surgery, it is important to proceed with medical treatment to prevent the polyps from growing back. Allergy treatment should also begin if allergies have been detected.

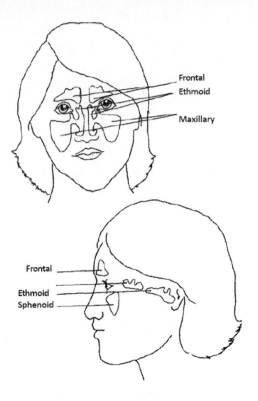

The Sinuses

SINUSITIS

Sinus disease is a much more common condition than most people realize. It is more common, for example, than arthritis.

Sometimes people fail to recognize sinus pain as an indication of a sinus infection for the simple reason that they are not sure where their sinuses are.

The sinuses are spaces in the skull bone surrounding the inner nose; each sinus has an opening that drains into the nose. These openings are called the ostia.

There are four pairs of sinuses. The frontal sinuses are above the eyebrows; the maxillary sinuses are in the cheekbones below the eyes; the ethmoidal sinuses are beneath the sides of the nose; and the sphenoidal sinuses lie deeper in the head, behind the ethmoidal sinuses.

Only the maxillary and sphenoidal sinuses are present at birth. The frontal sinuses develop at about age five, and in some individuals they do not develop at all. The sphenoids appear at about age nine.

The precise evolutionary function of the sinuses is not known. Perhaps their main purpose is to lighten the head so that it is easier to walk upright. (Apes, who have heavier skulls than humans do, do not have sinuses.) Possibly, sinuses play a role in smelling, in the production of mucus, and in phonation (forming sounds).

The cause of sinus disease is mucus congestion in the sinus cavities, setting the stage for infection. The sinuses are lined with a mucus-producing membrane and cilia, or tiny waving hairs, which move a thin layer of mucus over the lining of the sinuses. Bacteria and particles of dust, pollen, and so on are normally trapped in the mucus and propelled out of the sinuses into the nasal cavity.

Interference with this normal flow of mucus can cause sinusitis. The interference can be blockage of the ostia so that the sinuses cannot drain, or limitation on the movement of the cilia, or an overproduction of mucus.

Blockage of the ostia is the most common cause of sinusitis. It occurs most commonly after, an upper respiratory infection (a cold) or from an allergic reaction causing inflammation and swelling of the nasal tissues. Other causes of blockage are overuse of topical nasal decongestants, swollen adenoids, a deviated septum (a shifting of the cartilage that runs down the center of the nose), polyps, and tumors or foreign bodies. Smoking cigarettes interferes with action of the cilia and predisposes the smoker to sinus infection, and some types of immune system deficiency may predispose a person to develop sinusitis.

CHRONIC AND ACUTE RHINOSINUSITIS

Our understanding of the nose and sinuses has led us to consider these as sort of one airway in recent years. What we called sinusitis in previous editions is now referred to as rhinosinusitis, since studies have shown that there is usually simultaneous involvement of both the nasal cavity (rhino) and the sinuses in a viral infection. For simplicity we will still call it sinusitis. Sinusitis appears in four forms: acute, recurrent acute, chronic, and acute exacerbations of chronic. Typically, acute sinusitis arises after an upper respiratory tract infection. CAT scan studies have shown us that the majority of common colds or upper respiratory infections (URIs) result in sinusitis. However, it is estimated that only about one out of twenty-five cases of acute sinusitis require antibiotics, the rest being viral and resolving on their own with some requiring anti-inflammatory treatment with corticosteroids. The truth is that probably the overwhelming majority of antibiotics prescribed for URIs "complicated by sinusitis" are unnecessary.

Acute sinusitis usually sets in after you have had a cold for several days and your nasal discharge becomes yellow or dark green, thick, and perhaps foul smelling. The symptoms can last up to twelve weeks. Recurrent acute sinusitis is defined as episodes occurring more than four times per year and each lasting up to twelve weeks.

The patient is fine in between these bouts. The symptoms of acute sinusitis vary and can include any or all of the following scenario. You feel persistent pain high in your cheeks, around and behind the eyes, and in the forehead, over your eyes. If you lean forward, the pain is often worse. You may find spots that are tender to the touch. Sometimes the sinuses even puff out slightly. You may also have a fever. One recent set of guidelines to help physicians with this diagnostic dilemma is the following. Acute bacterial rhinosinusitis can be diagnosed if two major or one major and two minor symptoms of sinusitis persist beyond ten days or worsen after five to seven days (major symptoms include yellow/green nasal discharge, nasal obstruction/congestion, facial pain/pressure, hyposmia/anosmia [reduction of or loss of smell] or postnasal yellow/ green drainage; minor symptoms include ear fullness/pressure, fever, sore throat, fatigue, headache, and cough).

The American Academy of Otolaryngology has tried to outline the distinct symptoms of a cold, an allergic rhinitis, and sinusitis. But as you can see, there is overlap of symptoms between these conditions and the diagnosis can be difficult. Therefore, we often err on the side of precaution and prescribe antibiotics.

- Facial pressure and often pain is present invariably with sinusitis, only sometimes with a cold or allergy.
- The symptoms of sinusitis last at least ten to fourteen days. A cold clears up in less than ten days. The duration of allergies varies.
- The nasal discharge in sinusitis is thick and yellow green, compared to a thin, watery discharge due to allergies and a similar thin discharge or thicker whitish discharge due to a cold.
- Headache is characteristic of sinusitis and occurs only sometimes in allergies and colds.
- Pain in upper teeth and bad breath sometimes afflict sinusitis sufferers but are not characteristic of colds or allergies.
- A cough combined with nasal congestion is more likely with sinusitis or a cold than with allergy unless, of course, the patient has asthma.
- Sneezing indicates allergy or a cold but not sinusitis.

If you have a cold and your cold symptoms worsen after five days or persist for longer than ten days or if symptoms of sinusitis appear, you should see a doctor promptly. Occasionally, although very rarely, sinusitis can spread to the area around the eyes (in an orbital abscess) or into the bone, around the sinuses (osteomyelitis). Even more rarely, the infection may spread to the brain (as a brain abscess). These side effects were fairly common in the days before antibiotics.

Visible, palpable swelling of the sinuses occurs more often in children than adults and calls for an immediate visit to the doctor. The swelling will be around or near the eyes. But usually, the presentation of acute sinusitis is less dramatic in children than in adults. The youngster may have a purulent nasal discharge and bad breath, but the most important symptom may be a cough. A nasty, persistent cough, whether or not the other symptoms are present, may mean that a child has sinus disease. One seven-year-old boy recently treated turned out to have this problem. He had a nagging, dry cough, but a chest X-ray showed nothing. The parents were wondering whether to try a psychiatrist or an allergist. They decided on an allergist. CT scan of the sinuses revealed a bad infection.

In chronic sinusitis, which in adults is defined as sinusitis persisting longer than twelve weeks with persistent CT scan changes even after adequate medical treatment, the symptoms are generally undramatic. The pain is dull rather than sharp, and there is a feeling of fullness from congestion in the sinuses. Often the patient has a steady post-nasal drip, which can cause coughing and an irritated sore throat. The breath may be fetid. This unpleasant but generally not life-threatening disease affects some 15 percent (forty-five million) of people in the United States, according to the Department of Health and Human Services. Many patients do not even have symptoms and are unaware that they even have it, or have symptoms occasionally when they have an "acute exacerbation of chronic sinusitis, the fourth category of sinusitis."

Nevertheless, chronic sinusitis can occasionally become a serious health problem, especially for asthmatics. Sinus inflammation and congestion can make asthma much worse. Any asthmatic who is not doing well should have a CT scan done at some point to determine if sinus disease is involved.

There is no evidence that acute sinusitis leads to chronic sinusitis, and it follows that there is no evidence that treatment of acute sinusitis will prevent a person from getting chronic sinusitis. It is not even clear that chronic sinusitis is a result of a bacterial infection. In some patients, there are underlying abnormalities of the immune system (particularly antibody deficiencies) that allow bacteria to take hold and chronic sinusitis to develop. Recently, the role of fungal infections is being looked at to see if they play a role in some patients. Also, biofilms (layers of many bacteria) that line the sinuses in the majority of patients are being studied to see if we can come to understand why chronic sinusitis develops in some people.

TREATMENT

The treatment of an acute bacterial sinus infection includes pain medication, topical or oral corticosteroids and decongestants to help unblock the ostia and promote drainage, hot compresses for the front of the face over the sinuses to stimulate blood flow and drainage, increased fluid intake, and most important, antibiotics.

Normally there are no bacteria in the sinuses. When acute bacterial sinusitis is suspected because of the reasons outlined above, amoxicillin/clavulanate (Augmentin) and a cephalosporin (such as Ceftin) are reasonable antibiotics to try first. For both allergic and nonallergic patients, the fluoroquinolone drugs such as levofloxacin (Levaquin) and moxifloxacin (Avelox) may also be tried.

The treatment must continue longer than for many other sorts of infections. A course of three weeks or more may be needed to ensure eradication of the infection.

Chronic sinusitis infections typically respond less well to antibiotics and current medical thinking questions the use of antibiotics in chronic sinusitis unless you suspect an acute exacerbation. Sometimes intranasal steroids are helpful in reducing swelling that is blocking the ostia and in promoting sinus drainage.

If you have chronic sinusitis, you should see an allergist to determine if you have allergies that are causing rhinitis, which in turn is causing the sinus disease. Frequently, allergies do underlie sinus disease. You might also be checked for antibody deficiency as a possible contributing factor.

If you have been suffering from a sinus infection relating to allergies, medication is also likely to be needed, including nasal steroids, antihistamines, and decongestants. If your allergies cause severe or year-round symptoms, immunotherapy (allergy shots) may be required.

Although you can sometimes successfully self-medicate mild allergies, if you have sinus disease, you should see a doctor. Nasal corticosteroids, available by prescription only, can be helpful in both of these conditions.

Sometimes, surgery is needed for chronic sinusitis in which the infected sinuses simply do not drain adequately despite vigorous medical treatment. There are many surgical techniques, but the goal is to improve the opening from the sinuses into the nasal cavity. Nowadays, this is usually done using an endoscope for surgery; this is more precise and results in less tissue damage than the older, more-radical surgeries.

Surgery usually has to be followed up by aggressive medical treatment to prevent recurrence of the inflammation. If you are allergic, both immunotherapy and strict environmental control of your exposure to allergens should be considered.

EAR INFECTIONS

Earaches and ear blockage may be caused by numerous conditions, including allergic rhinitis. Serous otitis media (a persistent or recurring collection of fluid in the middle ear) is especially common in childhood, affecting 50 percent of all children at some point in their young lives.

With the advent of antibiotics, serous otitis and middle ear infections have not generally been regarded with much concern. But recent evidence suggests that ear ailments in infants and toddlers may cause a loss of hearing at critical stages of language development.

These early-childhood ear disorders can be related to allergy. Sometimes, though rarely, a food allergy such as milk allergy contributes to the problem. Whatever the cause, every parent should discuss with a pediatrician what signs indicate a possible hearing blockage. If language development or responsiveness is impaired, the reason may be a hearing problem related to chronic serous otitis media or recurring ear infections.

The reason that children, particularly under age seven, are more prone to ear blockage and infections than adults is that the smaller size of the child's skull sets the Eustachian tube at a different angle than in adults. The Eustachian tube runs from the middle ear to the nasal cavity, and in children it is set less vertically than in adults. It is more prone to obstruction, and fluid from the nose may leak into the ear more readily, especially when the child is lying on his or her back.

In adulthood, the likelihood that the ears will collect fluid or become infected varies from individual to individual, but it is generally less than in childhood. Chronic ear infections, especially on one side only, should be evaluated by an ENT specialist. The cause, rarely, may be a malignant tumor. These tumors tend to be more common among Asians.

The simple collection of fluid in the ears, without infection, is experienced mainly as a sense of fullness in the ears, sometimes with popping and a loss of hearing. (The Eustachian tube serves to equalize air pressure between the middle ear and the outside air. When the change in pressure is sudden, as when ascending in an elevator, popping occurs. Chewing gum helps to open the tube, which is why gum used to be handed out in airplanes during takeoffs and landings, when rapid pressure changes may happen.)

If the collected fluid helps an infection become established, pain and usually fever result and antibiotic treatment is needed. Sometimes even surgery is required. Adenoids may be obstructing the tubes, and they may have to be removed. Sometimes it is necessary to create a drainage passage surgically through the eardrum. Chronic allergic rhinitis may contribute to chronic serous otitis in children and adults. Although allergic rhinitis varies in seriousness and does not always require aggressive treatment, it should be taken seriously if it is associated with ear problems.

Finally, there have been some reports of foods producing symptoms resembling Ménière's disease. This disease involves poor function of the balance mechanism of the inner ear; the patient experiences vertigo (a sensation that the room is spinning), hearing loss, painful ringing in the ears, and sometimes nausea and vomiting. This disease affects some seven million Americans. But there is absolutely no evidence that food allergy plays any role in Ménière's disease.

EYES

Allergies often lead to symptoms involving the eye. Indeed, allergic rhinitis is sometimes apparent almost solely in eye symptoms, such as itching and swelling. But luckily, allergy-based eye problems are rarely so serious as to threaten eyesight.

Allergy symptoms may arise very noticeably in the eyes because the conjunctiva contains mast cells. The conjunctiva is the mucous membrane covering the front of the eye and the inner part of the eyelids. Mast cells carry histamine and other chemical mediators that cause the typical allergy reactions of swelling, inflammation, and itching.

When an allergen links up with an allergy antibody and a mast cell, then histamine and the other mediators are rapidly released. For example, if a pollen-allergic person is exposed to, say, a heavy dose of ragweed pollen, the eyes may begin to itch, burn, water, and sting. They also may become very light sensitive, and swelling may occur.

Treatment is essentially the same as for allergic rhinitis. Antihistamines (topical or oral) may be sufficient, or the full spectrum of medication and desensitization may be needed. There are many topical medications available for allergic conjunctivitis.

The use of vasoconstrictors, tetrahydrozoline (Visine), naphazoline (Naphcon, Vasocon) provides no antiallergy benefit but may serve to delay diagnosis and, upon discontinuation, may cause rebound redness.

Over-the-counter antihistamine-decongestant combinations naphazoline/ antazoline (Vasocon-A) naphazoline/pheniramine (Visine-A, Naphcon-A) are useful only in very-short-duration allergic episodes such as when junior rolls around in the grass at Grandma's house and gets itchy/red eyes.

The nonsteroidal anti-inflammatories (NSAIDs) block prostaglandin formation, which is one chemical in the eye responsible for itching. These include ketorolac (Acular) and diclofenac (Voltaren). These NSAIDs block prostaglandin in the late-phase reaction but don't impact histamine in the early phase, which also causes itching. Therefore, they are not consistent in benefit, working in some but not all patients.

The ocular antihistamine (emedastine (Emadine) is mainly effective for the symptom of itching. However, redness may occur with long-term use. This may be due to membrane toxicity or because they don't prevent mast cell release and subsequent formation of other mediators. For symptoms longer than two weeks, other drugs may be more useful.

Mast cell stabilizers, such as cromolyn (Opticrom, Crolom), lodoxamide (Alomide), nedocromil (Alocril), and pemirolast (Alamast), which prevent the release of allergy mediators from the mast cells, are available for optical use. It is best to begin using these medicines well before exposure—for example, before the onset of the season in which allergy symptoms usually develop. Results with these mast cell stabilizers have been less than stellar, mostly because they require frequent dosing three to five times daily and beginning treatment weeks before an allergy season begins.

Most recently, the mast cell-stabilizing antihistamine eyedrops have greatly improved our ability to control allergic-conjunctivitis symptoms. These include olopatadine (Patanol and once-daily Pataday), ketotifen (available without prescription: Zaditor, Claritin ocular, Zyrtec ocular), and azelastine (Optivar). These are very effective because they treat the acute histamine symptoms and also prevent further mast cell release.

All these topical eye medications should be used on advice of your physician.

Severe cases may require the use of topical steroids; but this should be decided by an ophthalmologist (eye specialist), as steroid use may be associated with the development of glaucoma, cataracts, or infections. Contrary to what you might hear, there is no such thing as an ocular steroid that is "safer"; they are all associated with side effects, especially with usage beyond one to two weeks.

Atopic dermatitis (eczema) also can involve the eyes, in which case the name of the disorder is atopic keratoconjunctivitis. Red lesions appear on the eyelids, followed by crusting and scaling. In severe cases, the eyes produce excess tears, and patients become so sensitive to light that they have difficulty opening their eyes in full daylight. Ultimately, the cornea may be damaged or cataracts may form.

The treatment is with steroids, under the direction of an ophthalmologist. Optic cromolyn may be of some help. If infections arise in the lesions, antibiotic treatment may be needed.

Obviously, if allergy is contributing to this condition, it should be dealt with promptly to avert the serious complications.

Children often develop a seasonal type of conjunctivitis, arising in spring and summer, with very intense itching of the eyes and sensitivity to light. In this disease, called vernal keratoconjunctivitis, there is a characteristic cobblestone appearance of the conjunctiva under the eyelids.

Sometimes the condition lasts year-round. Happily, it usually disappears at puberty, although adults too may be affected. Males are three times as likely as females to suffer from vernal keratoconjunctivitis. This is more common in drier countries like the Mediterranean and Africa and is not commonly seen in the United States.

The cause of the disease is not known for certain, but there are strong clues that it is related to allergy. First is the seasonal pattern. Second, eosinophils are present in the conjunctival fluid. (These are the blood cells whose number is characteristically elevated in allergy.) Also, most patients have other atopic illnesses, such as allergic rhinitis or asthma.

This condition can usually be managed with a mast cell stabilizer. Studies have shown nedocromil to be the most effective. Flares of the disease and complications such as ulcers require the use of ocular corticosteroids. Recent reports show a benefit from cyclosporine, an immune suppressor. Even though the patients may be very young, they must be followed by an ophthalmologist and checked for glaucoma. Use of steroids for the shortest possible duration and lowest dose is advisable, in order to reduce the chances of developing glaucoma and cataract.

Wearing contact lenses, especially soft lenses, is often associated with an itchy eye condition called giant papillary conjunctivitis. Often, the patient must give up use of the lenses. Sometimes a change of lens type or more frequent cleaning of the lenses prevents the condition from recurring.

Women in particular are prone to contact dermatitis of the eyelids as a result of an allergic reaction to cosmetics or other substances. The eyelid blisters and then thickens and turns red. The eyes itch. The conjunctiva may also be affected, with tearing and redness of the eyes.

The cause of contact dermatitis on the eyelids may be a sensitivity to (1) makeup or skin cleansers; (2) eye medications, including prescription drugs such as neomycin or antiviral agents; (3) solutions for wetting or cleaning contact lenses, especially if they contain thimerosal and some other anti-infective substances; (4) airborne agents, including hair spray, substances found in the workplace, pollen, and nail polish (when the person touches the lids with the polished nails); and (5) dust mites.

Diagnosis may require patch testing to determine what substance is causing the problem, but if you are a contact lens wearer, the most obvious first step is to use a different lens solution or to switch to thermal rather than chemical disinfection of the lenses.

Local corticosteroid creams applied to the lids will probably help, but again, *never use these steroid medications without the supervision of an eye doctor.*

Chapter 12

Skin Disorders

Hives and Angioedema

Hives are a nuisance, the acute variety affecting more than 20 percent of people at some point in their lives. The condition, technically called urticaria, is ordinarily harmless although uncomfortable. But you should always try to determine what has caused hives to appear, because sometimes they signal the development of a dangerous sensitivity to a food or drug that might lead in the future to an anaphylactic reaction. Sometimes they may be a sign of exposure to a toxic substance.

A hive is usually a relatively small, itchy red elevated spot that resembles a mosquito bite. The hive may be just one or two millimeters; however, they can grow to several centimeters in diameter and can appear anywhere on the body.

You may suffer from just one hive or many. Hives tend to come and go in a matter of one to several hours. If a single hive lasts for more than twenty-four hours, notify your doctor. Such persistent lesions may be a sign of vasculitis, which is a swelling of the blood vessels and requires medical attention. Some forms of thyroiditis—to be discussed later—as well as other autoimmune disease may also present as urticarial lesions that last more than twenty-four hours.

An attack of hives may last from several hours to several days or even weeks. Hives that persist for longer than six weeks are categorized as chronic.

Both chronic and acute urticaria may or may not be allergic in nature. Acute outbreaks of hives, however, are quite often traceable to specific allergies, such as an allergy to drugs or to foods. Chronic hives are less likely to be related to allergy.

Chronic hives generally last less than five years, but unfortunately, twenty percent of hives can last up to twenty years. As a general rule, the more severe the hives, the longer they tend to last.

Angioedema is similar to hives in that it involves swelling and may be caused by allergies. But in angioedema, the swelling is subcutaneous—that is, it occurs deeper under the skin and there is usually little or no itching.

Women develop angioedema more frequently than men do, and the condition often arises in adulthood. It may occur in conjunction with hives or alone. The swelling can last for a few hours to three days (in hereditary angioedema).

Angioedema without hives most often involves the face, tongue, extremities (hands and feet), or genitals. When hives are present, the angioedema may affect the tongue and pharynx. In anaphylactic reactions and in the hereditary form of angioedema, the respiratory tract may be affected.

Any kind of choking reaction or swelling of the throat should be brought to a doctor's attention, even if the episode passes safely. The next time, the reaction may be more severe. Your doctor may prescribe an EpiPen or a Twinject for you to carry; these are devices that contain a dose of injectable epinephrine (Adrenalin).

The physiological mechanisms underlying allergic hives and angioedema are essentially the same as in all other allergic reactions. But as you might expect in reactions involving the skin, the most-active mast cells (releasing histamine and other chemical-allergy mediators) are located primarily in the skin or in tissue just under the skin.

The redness of the skin is caused by swelling of the blood vessels and by blood leaking from the smallest vessels (the capillaries). Both effects are due to the vasodilatation caused by histamine and its chemical relatives.

In most cases, the release of histamine in outbreaks of hives and angioedema is not caused by the standard allergic linkage of allergen to IgE antibody to mast cell, although involvement of the immune system apart from IgE action has been demonstrated in some cases. In many instances, the mechanisms producing hives and angioedema are not fully known.

About 80 percent of cases of chronic urticaria are classified as idiopathic urticaria; *idiopathic* means that the cause of the hives is not known.

The "physical allergies" include attacks of hives brought on by cold, pressure, sunlight, and other factors. Frankly, there is still much to learn with respect to both the causes and mechanisms of urticaria. It is known, however, that alcohol, stress, and hormonal fluctuations during the menstrual cycle all can aggravate urticaria, no matter what the underlying cause. Other factors are outlined below.

CAUSES OF HIVES AND COMBINED HIVES AND ANGIOEDEMA

Drugs, foods, and food additives. In an acute outbreak of hives, a common culprit is a drug, especially penicillin, the related cephalosporin drugs, other antibiotics, aspirin, and the NSAIDs. In the *extremely sensitive* patients, even the minute amounts of antibiotics present in some meats and dairy products can cause hives. The reaction can appear within seconds of ingesting the drug or up to ten days later. The attack may last up to two months after the drug is stopped.

Amoxicillin can cause delayed hives, at times first appearing several weeks after the drug is taken and sometimes lasting a few months. Many other drugs are on the roster of usual suspects, including sulfonylurea drugs (used for treating diabetes), many diuretics, and certain local anesthetics.

Aspirin can cause hives or aggravate existing hives, but sensitivity to aspirin is not a true allergy; it is, instead, an intolerance that includes other NSAIDs (nonsteroidal anti-inflammatory drugs), such as meloxicam and ibuprofen. If you get hives from anti-inflammatory drugs, you very rarely may be sensitive to the food-coloring additive tartrazine (FD&C Yellow No. 5). Other additives that rarely may provoke hives are salicylates and benzoic acid (see chapter 7).

This cross-sensitivity to aspirin and additives can be the cause of both acute hives and some cases of chronic hives. The usual method of pinpointing the offending substances is to restrict food intake for a week to an additive-free canned, prescription nutritional supplement and see if the hives go away. Unfortunately, there is no skin or blood test for this sensitivity.

Because aspirin and other NSAIDs so often aggravate hives even if they are not the actual cause of the condition, it is probably just as well to avoid these drugs if you have chronic hives. If you need medication, consult with your physician. In place of these drugs, you may find that you can use choline trisalicylate (Trilisate) and related drugs.

Food allergies commonly cause acute outbreaks of hives and angioedema as well, but they can be blamed for chronic hives much less often.

When a food is the suspected cause, the suspicion can sometimes be confirmed by skin testing and/or RAST. With acute hives, food in the same family as the offending food may have to be eliminated. For instance, if you are allergic to one kind of bony fish, you may be allergic to all bony fish (see chapter 7).

With chronic urticaria, a single food—or even a combination of foods—is rarely the cause. Testing for allergy to a vast number of foods may merely yield false positives, which can be a considerable waste of time and money. Instead, you can try keeping a food diary listing all the foods you eat so that an allergenic food can be identified. In some cases, patients are asked to go on a restricted diet, starting with rice, lamb (or chicken), and water for three days. A more rigorous test would be no food, instead using an elemental, balanced food product made up of basic amino acids, simple carbohydrates, and digested fats, such as Pregestimil, Tolerex, or Vivonex. After a week, new foods would gradually be introduced to see if they cause the hives (see chapter 7). This is only used when all else has failed and a food-induced urticaria is suspected. However, before one uses this method of total food elimination, first the patient should have extensive food testing (either with skin tests or, in some cases, RAST testing) to guide in the choice of foods to eliminate. If this fails, then the total-elimination method might be tried.

Exercise. Exercise-induced hives can be a danger sign, indicating the onset of anaphylaxis. The mast cells are involved, but the cause is not really understood. In some patients, the risk exists only if they have eaten within a few hours of exercising; with others, the risk is dependent upon their having eaten certain specific foods, such as shrimp or celery. For these latter patients, neither eating the food alone nor exercising alone is risky; but doing both can be dangerous, especially eating and then exercising (see chapter 7).

In some people, the heating of the body during exercise produces very itchy small hives, sometimes associated with wheezing but not anaphylaxis. See the section on cholinergic urticaria below.

Underlying illness. Hives sometimes signal an underlying infection. The possible underlying conditions range from mild viral infections to, in rare circumstances, cancer. However, with the exception of the previously discussed autoimmune syndromes, thyroiditis and vasculitis, other underlying illness are very uncommon.

In rare cases, hepatitis B may present as hives. If a patient develops hives and undefined illness, the diagnosis of hepatitis should come to mind.

Since we published this book ten years ago, an association with thyroid autoimmunity (thyroiditis or Hashimoto's thyroiditis) and chronic urticaria has become evident. This type of urticaria is usually the more severe and persistent type. Most physicians today will order thyroid-antibody titers as part of a chronic urticaria workup. The exact relationship is unknown, and usually, treating the thyroiditis—which often requires no treatment—is of no benefit in treating the hives. However, in patients who have thyroiditis, once that is known, it is usually pointless to pursue other causes.

As mentioned above, vasculitis (inflammation of the blood vessels) may be a cause of hives, especially when individual hives tend to persist in one location. A variety of other underlying bacterial, viral, and fungal infections may cause hives, as may infestation with parasitic worms.

An adverse reaction to a blood transfusion, serum sickness from drugs, as well as disorders of the mast cells all can lead to hives.

Physical allergies. These are allergic-type reactions to a physical stimulus, such as heat or cold, that produce hives. An important diagnostic point is that the individual hives rarely last more than a few hours.

Cold sensitivity. Some people suffer hives and angioedema when their skin is exposed to cold. Often the symptoms get worse when the area is warmed again. Frequently, the reaction is limited to contact with cold air, but some people develop swelling of the lips or throat when they eat or drink cold foods.

Of particular concern is the fact that a cold-sensitive person may react dramatically to swimming in cold water, with a drop in blood pressure, loss of consciousness, and even drowning. There are many reasons a person should never swim alone, and this is one more.

Sensitivity to cold syndromes can start at any time of life, but it is rare and easy to self-diagnose. Hold an ice cube on your forearm for a minute or two, no longer than that, and observe the area after removing the cube. If a hive or swelling appears a few minutes after removing the ice cube, you have developed this physical allergy.

The condition *must* be evaluated by a doctor to rule out underlying complications, which may include infections and blood disorders. Antihistamines, usually in high doses, are often effective treatment. Sometimes the condition disappears on its own.

Currently, we recommend treating all urticaria, including cold urticaria with the second-generation H_1-antihistamines. The reason for this is it is much more comfortable for the patient as very often, the high doses of antihistamines that may be needed can induce extreme somnolence in the patient, unless a second-generation antihistamine is used.

Cholinergic urticaria. These are hives that occur when the skin is heated, whether by direct exposure to heat or hot water or through exercise or anxiety. The hives are different from most varieties, being very small and round (one to four millimeters in diameter) and surrounded by redness, but they certainly itch like other hives do. They can appear anywhere in the body except the palms and soles and rarely in the axillae. It is more common from ages ten through thirty and more so in women.

Asthmalike symptoms may appear after exercise in patients with cholinergic urticaria, and as a result, it is often confused with exercise-induced asthma. Cholinergic urticaria can be quite serious. Patients with this problem can have significant systemic symptoms such as fainting, abdominal cramping, diarrhea, increased salivation, and headaches. Because a hot shower can bring it on, patients sometimes speculate that they are allergic to soap or shampoo. It can be confused with aquagenic urticaria (discussed below). The actual inducing factor is sweating. Of interest is the higher incidence of this condition in patients with atopic dermatitis. The treatment of choice are all the second-generation nonsoporific antihistamines such as loratadine (Claritin or Alavert), cetirizine (Zyrtec), desloratadine (Clarinex), levocetirizine (Xyzal), and fexofenadine (Allegra), all of which are usually prescribed in fairly high doses.

If this is not sufficient, then other treatments are beta-blockers such as ones used for blood pressure control, Danazol, a modified androgen, which is also used for cold urticaria and ultraviolet light (we are reluctant to suggest this because of skin cancer and other risks). Finally, avoid hot foods, beverages, highly spiced foods, as well as alcohol.

Sensitivity to pressure on the skin. Some people have skin that is unusually sensitive to pressure. One form of this sensitivity is called dermographism, a condition in which one can write or draw on the skin. Mild pressure or scraping may quickly cause redness, swelling, and itching. If your skin is this sensitive to pressure, you are likely to develop hives in any area where clothing is tight—for example, under elastic in undergarments or around the beltline.

Some patients with pressure urticaria will react to pressure with swelling in a few minutes. In delayed-pressure urticaria, the hives or swelling appears usually six to eight hours after the pressure has been applied. Often these patients have chronic idiopathic hives (the cause of the hives is unknown) as well.

The condition should be evaluated by a doctor. It occurs more commonly in men in their twenties and thirties and, fortunately, is rare. It is difficult to treat, although antihistamines may help, but often not completely, because histamine is not the only mediator involved in causing this syndrome. Prednisone is often effective, but the long-term side effects are a serious issue, and it is only used if the lesions are incapacitating. As always with steroids, you want to use the lowest-possible dose, preferably on alternate days. Singulair may be of benefit as well. NSAIDs, only under the supervision of a physician, may be helpful on occasion and are worth trying. Loose clothing is certainly the dress style of choice.

Some patients have a rather-serious pressure sensitivity that can cause delayed swelling and lesions in such places as the bottoms of the feet, under a bra strap, even under a wallet carried in a back pocket.

This is a chronic disease that can impair lifestyle and last for five to ten years, sometimes longer.

Solar urticaria. This is a rare disease in which exposure to certain forms of light, in some cases sunlight, causes hives to appear within several minutes. In most cases, avoidance is the only effective treatment. One must not expose the skin to the kind of light to which one is sensitive. When sunlight is the cause of the problem, windowpanes or similar glass usually filters the light adequately for protection. Out of doors, unclothed areas of skin must be protected with sunblock.

The mechanism for this syndrome is unknown, but it is possibly caused by an antigen-antibody reaction that occurs only in the presence of the appropriate UV band of light. It is imperative that a workup for associated and fortunately uncommon illnesses be done. Porphyria as well as autoimmune disease is associated with this phenomenon.

The disease is characterized by itchy small wheals that occur severe minutes after sunlight exposure. It can also manifest as the rapid onset of very itchy flat areas. The lesions will recede several minutes after the exposure to sunlight occurs, and this characteristic distinguishes it from the contact solar dermatitis syndromes. The lesions can appear on any area of the skin exposed to light, including areas with thin clothing. Paradoxically, the face and the dorsum of the hands do not react, perhaps because of a natural desensitization, as these areas are the most exposed to sunlight.

This condition can be differentiated from all other light-induced conditions by the fact that there is a rapid onset after exposure to sunlight and equally fast remission after the exposure is eliminated. Solar urticaria is differentiated from contact photosensitivity, which follows the pattern of lesions occurring wherever the offending substances (such as aftershave lotion) were placed, and the rash lasts for several days after exposure.

The treatment is avoidance, which usually is impossible. So there must be as much avoidance as possible and the use of very effective sunblockers—although paradoxically and rarely, the sunblocker may be the cause of a contact photosensitivity. Also, clothing that has UV protection built into it can be helpful. There are companies that make this type of clothing. In addition, this condition is at least partially histamine mediated and can be helped by antihistamines. We suggest using a non-sleep-inducing

H_1-receptor-site blocker in high doses. Loratadine, cetirizine, as well as fexofenadine are effective. If they do not do the job completely, then an H_2 blocker such as ranitidine (Zantac) can be added.

Another helpful modality is the antimalarial drug Plaquenil; however, this can have significant side effects.

Aquagenic urticaria. In this very-rare disorder, the patient develops hives when soaked in water, regardless of the water's temperature. You must be exposed to the water for a considerable time; just washing your hands will not usually trigger the hives.

If you have this problem, do not plan to become an Olympic swimmer. Avoidance of immersion in water is the best treatment.

Hereditary vibratory urticaria. Your chance of developing this is about one in a billion, but it does illustrate the complexity of heredity and the immune system. The disease has been described in one family and in a few other sporadic cases. The hives are caused by vibration of the skin; they are not dermographic and are not induced by pressure. Avoidance of vibration is the treatment.

Contact with allergens. Occasionally, contact with inhalant allergens such as pollen can cause urticaria. The sensitivity, called contact urticaria, can at times be confirmed by skin tests or RAST.

In one case, a woman developed chronic hives; and after a futile search for the cause, a house visit revealed that she had an old-fashioned horsehair mattress. Further questioning revealed that the hives were their worst in the morning and tended to fade during the day.

Sure enough, the patient was allergic to horse dander and horsehair. When she got rid of the mattress, the hives disappeared.

Hives can uncommonly result from skin contact with a chemical substance to which you are allergic, such as a dry-cleaning chemical or fabric softener. Also, contact with toxic substances or simply strong chemicals can cause skin reactions, including hives.

DIAGNOSIS

Because urticaria can at times indicate an infection somewhere in the body, your doctor may recommend quite a few tests if you go in with a complaint of frequent or chronic hives and a cause cannot be quickly determined. A complete physical should be done. A urinalysis and blood analysis may be recommended. The blood work may include a test for blood complement if angioedema is present or vasculitis is suspected. X-rays of the sinuses, teeth, or chest may be ordered.

There is disagreement in the medical community as to how much testing is appropriate; and you, the consumer, should be aware of the issue. Some doctors will not advocate a comprehensive workup if your history and physical exam indicate normal health. Others take the view that some infections, such as certain sinus infections, are almost without symptoms and might be missed without X-rays.

Always feel free to question the necessity for tests and to give some weight to your own common sense. Factors that certainly can be taken into consideration are how troublesome the symptom is to you and whether you generally feel well or not. The workup should be tailored to your individual situation.

For either persistent or recurrent angioedema only involving the face, a CT scan of the sinuses and chest should be done. Sinus infections and some tumors of the chest can simulate angioedema of the face.

In one patient with recurrent angioedema only involving the face, a CT demonstrated an asymptomatic tumor of the lungs. Fortunately, it was discovered in time and removed. Had it continued to grow undetected at some point when it did become symptomatic, it could have been inoperable.

DRUG TREATMENT

In general, the best treatment for hives is avoidance of whatever triggers them. But if that is not possible, relief may be obtained in some cases from drug treatment.

In cases of acute hives, an injection of epinephrine (Adrenalin, in extremely bad hives) and certainly antihistamines, followed by a large oral dose of prednisone once again in severe circumstances and for a short period of time, can help to stop the ongoing reaction.

In rare instances, prednisone may be used to control severe outbreaks of chronic hives. But because of the serious side effects, steroids should be administered in the lowest dose possible, preferably every other day.

In most cases, H_1-antihistamines are the better choice for treatment of acute or chronic hives, although antihistamines do not work in all cases. The newer nonsedating antihistamines are tolerated best by most people. Often, the addition of an H_2 antihistamine (typically used for stomach problems related to acid) to the standard H_1-antihistamine will improve the effectiveness of drug treatment (see chapter 5).

CAUSES OF ANGIOEDEMA

Angioedema, or swelling, frequently accompanies allergy reactions of all sorts. It is prominent in severe, acute reactions to food and drugs. It is sometimes associated with milder allergies, such as allergic rhinitis. There is even a form of angioedema that corresponds to the rare urticaria caused by vibration. Occasionally, vibration causes swelling without hives.

Angioedema should always be seen by a doctor for diagnosis. One of the goals of the evaluation of the swelling is to be certain that it is indeed allergy related. Certain heart and kidney disorders can also cause swelling of a different sort.

Cellulitis is another condition producing swelling that may be confused with allergic angioedema. Cellulitis is an infection of the skin that requires antibiotic treatment.

If you are on blood pressure medication in the category of an ACE inhibitor (medications such as lisinopril, enalapril, ramipril) and you have angioedema, you must consult your doctor immediately and have her switch you to another class of medications. One of the side effects of these medications is angioedema. The other side effect to be discussed in chapter 8 is cough.

HEREDITARY ANGIOEDEMA (HAE)

In the past, people suffering from this rare but severe disease were likely to die suddenly of asphyxiation. Hereditary angioedema (HAE), which typically does not appear until adolescence or later, is of dominant autosomal inheritance, which means that it will affect men and women approximately equally and will affect many members of a family. Happily, we are now able to control the disease, so it is worthwhile to get a prompt diagnosis. There is considerable risk in delaying treatment.

Basically, hereditary angioedema involves a lack of a normal blood protein, C1 esterase inhibitor. In some cases, the protein levels are too low or the protein is present but does not function. This is an evanescent substance that can only be administered intravenously.

One of the signs of hereditary angioedema is that the angioedema is fairly long lasting, up to several days. It can be cyclic, occurring every ten days to two weeks, or it can be quite erratic.

As a first symptom, an extensive, burning red rash may erupt. In approximately 25 percent of patients, erythema may precede the occurrence of edema. An estimated thirty to fifty percent of patients with HAE reportedly have erythema marginatum (the presence of pink rings that are barely raised and are nonpuritic) preceding or accompanying the attacks. The swelling, which is not especially itchy, can take place anywhere in the body; but there is an unusual predilection for the throat and respiratory tract and the gastrointestinal tract. The condition thus causes hoarseness and choking; sometimes, intense stomach pain, nausea, and vomiting occur. Frequently, people with this disorder are given emergency abdominal surgery, which produces no findings.

Angioedema attacks may be triggered by soft-tissue trauma, such as dental work, oral surgery, or a tonsillectomy. Patients who have had attacks of this disease should never have surgery or dental work without first ensuring that appropriate precautions are being taken (see below).

In the past, the only way to treat hereditary angioedema was with the drugs stanozolol and danazol. These are androgens (male hormones) related to testosterone and so must be used under a doctor's supervision to avoid unwanted side effects.

Recently, new hope for the successful management of this serious disease has been generated by the development of three new treatments. The FDA recently approved Cinryze and Berinert, C1-inhibitor concentrate products, used both for attack prevention and treatment of attacks. This has been safely used in Europe for thirty years but took some time to be approved here since it is a blood product, and there is a theoretical small risk of infection with unforeseen new agents such as slow virus infections; however, the filtration process used in preparing this product and screening of donors removes all *known* infectious particles such as viruses. Some patients with HAE only have occasional attacks and do not require regular treatment. However, for those with more-frequent attacks (and the cutoff is usually one attack per month), Cinryze offers an alternative to androgen therapy, which can have a lot of side effects. It will likely be effective in preoperative management as well, but studies in this situation are not complete. Still in development is Rhucin, which, when approved, will likely become the treatment of choice. Rhucin is a recombinant (produced in a test tube) form of the protein, which is missing in this disease. Therefore, the protein can be replaced without the risk of transmitting infection. This is comparable to how we treat diabetes with insulin or thyroid deficiency with thyroid hormone.

The third is Kalbitor (ecallantide), an inhibitor of the kallikrein-kinin pathways). This drug works in a more peripheral manner than the other two agents do. However, it can be administered subcutaneously, which is convenient. The problem with Kalbitor—and a potential limit to its use—is that anaphylaxis occurs in almost 4 percent of the patients given this drug. Although all these drugs are new, we feel that Rhucin and Kalbitor will prove to be more useful. Anaphylaxis is a dangerous side effect, and it actually has very similar symptoms to HAE. When anaphylaxis occurs from Kalbitor, it could be very confusing to the medical personnel administering the drugs.

Epinephrine and antihistamine are not effective against this disease.

In preparation for surgery or dental work that can cause an attack, the patient can be treated with high doses of androgens before and after the procedure or a transfusion of fresh frozen plasma before, which will supply the missing C1 esterase inhibitor. It is likely that Cinryze, once studies are complete, will be useful in this situation and will become the treatment of choice. Another approach, used in patients who are being treated regularly with androgens for the disease, is to raise the dose of the androgens used for a period of time before surgery.

ACQUIRED ANGIOEDEMA

When angioedema caused by C1 esterase inhibitor deficiency appears in a person who does not seem to have a family history of the disease, it is called acquired angioneurotic edema. This condition may be a feature of certain malignancies and autoimmune diseases. The treatment is to control the underlying disease, if possible. Extensive laboratory studies including a chest X-ray are necessary in evaluating this syndrome.

PRURITUS

Sometimes, an itch will appear in your skin and there is no rash. The three most common causes of this symptom are atopic dermatitis (although the rash will appear at some point); urticaria, which comes and goes; and just plain-dry skin. In dry skin, the itch will respond to various emollients much as is described in the section of this chapter concerning the treatment of eczema.

Neurological problems can be associated with itching. Often, nerve-root compression in the spinal canal can produce itching along the nerve root. Herpes zoster (shingles), after it goes away, can often leave the patient with itching, pain, or both where the lesions were.

If pruritus responds well to the treatments discussed below, then there is usually nothing to worry about. However, if it does not and if you are on medication on a regular basis or you have fever, loss of appetite, or unexplained weight loss, then a consultation with your doctor is a very good idea. Pruritus can be caused by many medical illnesses, reactions to medications, as well as psychological causes.

Below we list the known diseases and issues associated with pruritus. Pruritus associated with a rash or a known disease state can often be easily dealt with. When the cause is not known, then diagnosis and treatment may be extremely difficult. To make matters worse, pruritus that does not respond easily to treatment can be associated with serious illness or drug reaction in 10 to 50 percent of cases.

The following disease states can cause pruritus. Liver diseases that cause a backup of the bile ducts will cause severe itching often associated with jaundice. Kidney failure can also cause pruritus. Usually, these illnesses present with other symptoms; but occasionally, itching is one of the first signs.

Carcinoid tumors (tumors of the neuroglandular system) can also appear first with generalized itching. Other symptoms are flushing, wheezing, diarrhea, abdominal cramping, and swelling of the extremities.

Both non-Hodgkin's and Hodgkin's lymphoma can either present with or be associated with itching.

Many endocrine problems can either present or be associated with itching. Both hypothyroid and hyperthyroid disease as well as parathyroid disease either present with or can be associated with itching.

Waves of intermittent itching with neurological symptoms can be caused by multiple sclerosis. Parasites can be picked up while vacationing in exotic locations, and some parasites can produce generalized itching.

So as you can see, itching that doesn't go away requires a doctor visit. The doctor should ask a lot of questions about your general health and what medications you are taking. This should be followed by an extensive physical exam. The doctor may order tests based on both the analysis of the information you give him and the physical examination.

The recommended tests for everyone with itching are complete blood count and chemistries, sedimentation rate, and thyroid studies.

Depending on your symptoms, age, and sex, a chest X-ray, a stool examination, HIV (AIDS), and parathyroid hormone tests may be done. Other blood tests (too numerous to mention) might also be done. Abdominal ultrasound and CT scans of the abdomen and chest may also be needed.

Treatment of pruritus can be frustrating for both the physician and patient. Moisturizing the skin can be crucial. This is discussed in the next section on atopic dermatitis.

Cooling counterirritants such as menthol, phenol, and camphor can be helpful. Topical anesthetics such as lidocaine or pramoxine have their place as well. Topical diphenhydramine (Benadryl) can be helpful, but there is a high risk of sensitization and should be avoided. Topical steroids are also helpful. Moderate-potency steroids can be used on the trunk and extremities. One percent hydrocortisone should be used on the face, groin, and axillae as the skin is thinner here. Although there may be issues with long-term use, topical calcineurin inhibitors (tacrolimus [Protopic] and pimecrolimus [Elidel]) may be helpful.

ATOPIC DERMATITIS AND CONTACT DERMATITIS

The second most common allergic skin disease—after urticaria, or hives—is eczema (AKA atopic dermatitis).

The term *eczema* is from ancient Greek and means "to boil over" or "to erupt." This refers to the inflammation and weeping (leaking) of the eczema rash. Actually, any inflamed, crusty, itchy rash may be called eczema; but several different conditions can produce such a rash, including atopic dermatitis, which tends to be inherited and is often associated with an allergy to some substance ingested or inhaled, and contact dermatitis, which is caused by contact with some substance to which you are sensitive or allergic, such as the resin of poison ivy. Most often, however, eczema refers to atopic dermatitis.

Atopic means "not having a place," which is an excellent description for this allergic rash because it may appear almost anywhere on the body. It was an American pioneer in allergy, Arthur Coca, who in the early 1900s discovered that atopic dermatitis is associated with allergic rhinitis and asthma. A tendency toward developing these atopic diseases runs in families, and if you develop one, you are likely to develop another (although it is rare to have all three forms).

The itching, especially in childhood forms of the disease, is intense; and the skin lesions and related complications seem to arise primarily from scratching the affected area. The itching is often made worse by stress, sweating, irritants, and other factors, and may flare up at bedtime.

Dr. Coca and others felt that patients suffering from this disease had easily irritated nerve endings in the skin. Sometimes, therefore, the disease was called neurodermatitis. From this the public got the idea that people with atopic dermatitis are neurotic. This is not so, even though stress may aggravate the symptoms.

INCIDENCE

Reliable figures on the incidence of atopic dermatitis are not available, but approximately 4 percent of infants and children are afflicted. The disease tends to get better in about half to two-thirds of affected infants as they get older, although adults may go on to develop irritant dermatitis—a tendency to develop rashes from exposure to dishwashing detergents, certain chemicals, and the like.

Only about 1 percent or less of adults are afflicted with atopic dermatitis, but many mild cases probably are not reported. A tendency to dry skin may be the only lingering sign of the disease. When skin is more than normally dry—say, as a result of low humidity or frequent washing with soap and hot water—the skin may become uncomfortable or a rash may flare up. A mild tendency to rashes may be aggravated by working in wet conditions or occupations in which one must wash one's hands frequently; water tends to dry the skin by removing natural oils.

Almost all cases of the disease begin before age five, two-thirds arising under age one. In infants, the face is typically affected first, along with the lower abdomen. A few months later, a rash is likely to appear on the legs and forearms. In older children and adults, the insides of the elbows and backs of the knees are the most common sites. The backs of the hands and feet are also frequently affected. One sees more boys than girls with atopic dermatitis in early childhood. This reverses as children get older.

The rash is typically in the form of red patches, followed by thickening and scaling of the skin, with the affected areas becoming a darker red. In infants and in children aged up to three or four, the rash is likely to weep (leak fluid). Thereafter, weeping may stop, but the disease may cause a thickening of the skin (lichenification).

PHYSIOLOGICAL MECHANISMS

Medical researchers are still working to discover the exact mechanisms underlying flare-ups of atopic dermatitis. Numerous studies indicate that the immune system in these patients is abnormal in several subtle ways. There may be abnormal lymphocytes and mast cells that infiltrate the skin of such patients.

Also, the blood flow to the skin is abnormal, leading to a condition called white dermographism. Dermographism is the tendency for the skin to develop red streaks under even slight pressure. (These streaks may swell and develop as hives.) In atopic dermatitis, when you rub the skin, red streaks appear; but then they quickly turn whitish, and this white dermographism persists for several minutes.

About 80 percent of the people with atopic dermatitis have very high levels of the allergy antibody IgE in their blood. Many atopic dermatitis patients show an unusual number of positive results when given skin tests for allergies. Frequently, these results have no clinical significance—they are unrelated to the disease. In some patients, however, allergic sensitivity is linked to flare-ups of the rash.

Food allergy has long been recognized as a cause of some cases of atopic dermatitis. In addition, research by Drs. Alan Adinoff and Richard Clark at the National Jewish Medical and Research Center in Denver, Colorado, suggests that an allergic sensitivity to environmental allergens, such as pollen, dust mites, and dander, also may cause a rash to flare up.

The immune mechanism underlying this kind of dermatitis is not well understood, but it is known that the mechanism is not the same as the standard mast cell-mediated reaction that governs most allergies.

Finally, atopic dermatitis patients have impaired cellular immunity, with a susceptibility to developing viral and bacterial skin infections. If you are prone to this kind of dermatitis, you should be aware of the risk and get to a doctor promptly if a rash is more severe or more persistent than usual.

If the rash is weeping, crusted, or has small pustules (white bumps), it should be checked by a doctor. Also, a doctor should look at any rash that lasts more than a week. Staphylococcus bacteria are common infectious agents. The next most-likely villain is the streptococcus type of bacteria. Antibiotic treatment is required to clear up these infections.

Viral infections can be more complicated to treat. For instance, infection by herpes simplex (eczema herpeticum) was once very difficult to treat; there were potentially fatal complications. Oral acyclovir now is used to control the herpes. But a doctor should supervise the care of the rash.

Other complications of atopic dermatitis that require expert medical care are nipple lesions and involvement of the eyes. Patients are also prone to develop cataracts (even early in life), abrasions and infections (especially by a type of herpes virus) of the cornea, retinal detachment, and harmful rashes on the eyelids.

Eating citrus fruit may cause lesions around the mouth and occasionally even furrows on the lips.

DIAGNOSIS OF ATOPIC DERMATITIS

There is no single test or sign by which to identify atopic dermatitis. A doctor will look for the following characteristics. Three are considered adequate to make the diagnosis.

- The rash is itchy.
- The rash begins as red patches; these thicken and darken, and the skin scales. In infants, particularly, the rash may weep (leak fluid).
- The rash follows a typical distribution for the age of the patient.
- The rash tends to be chronic. It repeatedly flares up or follows a seasonal pattern, worsening in winter, when the air is dry.
- The patient or the patient's family has a history of atopic diseases (allergic rhinitis, asthma, and atopic dermatitis).

The presence of three or more of the following features will tend to confirm the diagnosis:

- Positive results in skin testing for sensitivity to allergens such as pollen and dander.

- Elevated levels of the allergy antibody IgE.
- A tendency to develop skin infections.
- Lesions of the nipple.
- In the eye, a distortion of the cornea (keratoconus) and a certain type of cataract.
- Itchiness when sweating.
- Intolerance of wool on the skin.
- Intolerance of certain foods.
- White dermographism.
- Exacerbation by stress or other emotional factors or by environmental factors, such as chemical fumes in the workplace.

An eczema-like rash that is sometimes misdiagnosed as atopic dermatitis is caused by scabies. This disease, produced by a skin infestation of tiny scabies mites, is extremely itchy and can seriously undermine the patient's health. A clue to the diagnosis may be given in the location of the rash, as scabies prefers certain tender areas of the skin: wrists and armpits, between the fingers, the groin, and toes. In infants, they often go for the scalp, face, palms, and soles of the feet. Confirmation of the diagnosis is by microscopic examination of a small skin sample.

Psoriasis, a nonallergic disease involving excess production of skin cells, causes a much-scalier rash and sometimes joint pain and swelling. It tends to affect the arms, scalp, ears, and groin.

ALLERGY TESTS

Food allergies in about 10 percent of patients are associated with flare-ups of atopic dermatitis. Therefore, avoidance of problem foods can be helpful, even though food is rarely the sole cause of atopic dermatitis.

The foods associated with the rash can usually be identified through the history that you give your doctor, but sometimes an elimination diet or challenge testing is needed to detect the food or foods to which you are sensitive (see chapter 7). The most common problem foods are eggs, cow's milk, soy, wheat, peanuts, and fish.

If avoidance of a given food helps to clear up the rashes, part of your problem is probably solved! But no one, especially a child, should be kept for long on a restricted diet without double-checking that the apparent allergy really is present. If you have never shown any violent reaction to the suspect food, you may simply try some from time to time to see if it still causes flare-ups of dermatitis, but discuss this with your doctor.

If your food sensitivity has ever caused a severe reaction, with swelling or other systemic symptoms, then of course you should not experiment on your own. But an allergist, using care, can run a challenge test with small amounts of the suspect food to verify the diagnosis.

Testing is complicated with atopic dermatitis patients because their skin is often highly reactive to any stimulus. This makes reliable skin tests, both for food and for inhalant allergens, more difficult to accomplish. In these patients, skin testing may yield more false positives than is normally the case. However, skin testing can be performed if the doctor finds the negative control is not any more reactive than normal skin is and the doctor can find areas of normal skin to work with.

In vitro testing of a blood sample (RAST) may be recommended for patients with significant skin disease, but these tests also yield false positive results.

Both in vivo and in vitro tests are more reliable in children, and the positive tests have much greater validity. But *negative* RAST or skin tests in both children and adults are helpful in that they rule out an allergy to that food. What kind of tests to run and in what sequence and combination are questions about which capable, well-trained allergists still frequently disagree. As always, not too much reliance should be put on any one test.

TREATMENT

Our skin is made up of a lot of water, held in place by various proteins and carbohydrates. Because of the underlying immunologic defects in eczema, the skin does not hold on to this moisture and it becomes dry, causing rashes and making it prone to infection. In some patients, there may be triggers such as food and inhalant allergens as well as skin irritants that make things worse.

The treatment of atopic dermatitis associated with inhalant allergens (dust mites, dander, pollen, or the like) is by avoidance of the allergens, in combination with treatment of the rash itself. A daily skin-care program is of the utmost necessity in managing eczema. This skin-care program is often necessary year-round to control chronic rash and to prevent flare-ups. **We cannot emphasize enough the importance of a regular skin care program.** There are more comprehensive skin-care instructions at the National Eczema Association's website (www.nationaleczema.org) and its associated skin-care site (www.easeeczema.org). We caution against the use of various remedies available in health-food stores as they have not been properly studied and their efficacy is unknown.

Unless the patient also has other allergic conditions, such as rhinitis or asthma, it is not a good idea to treat atopic dermatitis patients with allergy shots because they are not effective. Generally, treatment of atopic dermatitis, when it is chronic, requires a variety of approaches. An allergist will often work with a dermatologist on treatment.

People with atopic dermatitis have extremely dry skin because water does not bind properly in the skin and is rapidly lost. Thus, replacing water is the key to therapy in any stage of the illness. There is a pervasive myth that daily bathing is contraindicated for children with eczema because it dries the skin. In fact, daily bathing in plain lukewarm water, followed by patting the skin until it is damp and applying a moisturizer, is recommended to help maintain an intact skin barrier because water hydrates and cleanses the skin. The patient should take a soaking bath or shower for fifteen minutes at least once if not twice a day. Pat the skin dry (do not rub) and then apply any prescription medications that have been prescribed followed by an emollient (moisturizer) to all the skin (Alpha Keri, Aveeno, CeraVe, Keri, Lubriderm, Vanicream, etc.) to prevent water from evaporating from the skin.

Topical steroids may be prescribed, and the time to apply them is within several minutes of bathing (because they penetrate better when the skin is moist). Apply the steroids first and then the moisturizer over the entire body. In severe cases, wet wraps may be used after bathing.

Hot water should be avoided. Bath oils do not help the dermatitis, and they also make the tub slippery, increasing the possibility of an accident. The addition of oatmeal (Aveeno) to the bath, however, can be soothing. The best choice of soap may require a little experimenting, although studies have suggested that Dove for sensitive skin (unscented) may be the best soap for cleansing in eczema.

For wet, weepy lesions, your doctor may suggest compresses with Burow's 1:40 solution or one packet of Domeboro powder per quart of water. Such a compress works as an astringent and antibacterial agent. But these compresses should not be used for more than two or three days because they can be drying.

Infection, of course, is a constant concern and may require antibiotic therapy. This should be under the supervision of a physician. Only oral antibiotics can be used. Neither over-the-counter nor prescription antibiotic creams or ointments are helpful. Bleach or vinegar baths can also be of benefit to reduce the levels of bacteria in the skin, but again, physician supervision is required if there is infection.

Topical steroids, which are the mainstay of pharmaceutical treatment, must be used with caution because of their side effects. The guiding principle is to use the weakest concentration that will work.

The most-potent topical steroids cause thinning of the skin and cannot be used daily over long periods of time. The potency of the steroid is related to the degree of fluorination (which makes the steroid molecules stronger) and to the amount of the steroid in the cream or ointment.

Except under the direction of a dermatologist, do not use anything stronger than 1 percent hydrocortisone cream or ointment on the face, neck, or any body-fold area, such as the groin or armpit. These areas have the thinnest layer of skin and are very vulnerable to atrophy.

Incidentally, the choice of whether to use a cream or ointment is best made by your doctor. Ointments decrease water loss but may increase itchiness. Creams spread more easily but may cause drying.

A medium-strength steroid preparation is ordinarily the drug of choice. Very potent steroids have to be used with great caution. One sound approach is use of the strongest steroids in the early, severe stages of the rash, switching to weaker concentrations as the condition improves. For a guide to relative strengths of steroid preparations see the list in Chapter 5.

Over-the-counter cortisone preparations typically come in 0.5 and 1 percent strengths. You may be able to use these to treat very-mild rashes yourself, but if the problem persists for more than a week or two, you should see a doctor. Another type of topical treatment rarely used today is the application of tar-based ointments, such as Estar Gel. These help some patients. Others find them irritating and the odor unpleasant. Sometimes it is helpful to use them at bedtime and then wash them off in the morning bath or shower so that you do not carry the odor all day.

Some people report partial relief from antihistamines, but that may be because the sedating effect reduces the intense itching. Curiously, high doses of aspirin may also calm the itching in some patients, but aspirin must be administered under the guidance of a doctor because of the side effects of large doses.

Sunlight helps to clear some cases of atopic dermatitis; but the patient must avoid sunburn, high humidity, and getting too warm, which can worsen the rash. Sunlamp treatment helps in some cases, but it should be done only under the guidance of a physician.

Immunomodulators. A class of medications called calcineurin inhibitors, which are of the broader group of immunomodulators and includes tacrolimus (Protopic) and pimecrolimus (Elidel), suppresses a component of the immune system and may help maintain normal skin texture and reduce flares of atopic dermatitis. These prescription-only medications are approved for children over the age of two and for adults. Due to possible concerns about the effect of medications that suppress the immune system when used for prolonged periods of time, the Food and Drug Administration has issued the following warning: Continuous long-term use of topical calcineurin inhibitors, including Protopic and Elidel, in any age group should be avoided and application limited to areas of involvement with atopic dermatitis. They are also quite useful used on the face and on the eyelids as well as near the eyes. Great care should be taken as with all topical preparations not to get them into the eyes as tacrolimus (Protopic) and pimecrolimus (Elidel) can be *transiently* irritating to the eyes.

Another "old new type" of treatment that recent research suggests is helpful is bathing a child in a dilute bleach or vinegar solution for five days in a row, along with applying a nasal antibiotic ointment mupirocin (Bactroban) for the same five days in a row each month. These five-day bathing and nasal treatments are preceded by a two-week course of cephalexin (Keflex). This sequence of treatments significantly reduces the colonization of the eczematous skin by staphylococcal bacteria. There are excellent skin-care instructions at the National Eczema Association's website (www.nationaleczema.org) and its associated skin-care site (www.easeeczema.org) The results looked very promising at the time of publication of this book. Do not attempt this yourself—discuss it with your physician!

Most people with atopic dermatitis find that they have to avoid certain substances and activities that irritate the skin. Soap and detergents, cleaning solvents, wool and nylon clothing, plastic covers on bedding can all cause flare-ups of the rash. All clothing, sheets, and fabric that are in direct contact with the skin should be 100 percent cotton.

Frequent washing with hot water is apt to cause a reaction, as will sweating, in patients with severe dermatitis. Exposure to hot, dusty environments; to animals; and to many chemicals may exacerbate the disease.

Some doctors recommend not washing in water and using antiseptic lotions instead. But as a rule, it seems more effective to bathe and clean the skin well, using a hypoallergenic or lubricating soap and a hypoallergenic moisturizer to prevent drying. A good, economical moisturizer, sold in some drugstores and at the manufacturer's website (www.psico.com) is Vanicream. CeraVe (www.cerave.com) is a newly developed moisturizer that helps to restore the skin barrier. Old standards include Aquaphor, Cetaphil, and Eucerin. Be careful of little-known products without good track records, often sold in health-food stores and on the Internet. The soap you use does not have to be expensive as research by dermatologists suggests that Dove unscented sensitive-skin bar soap may be the best soap for eczema.

CONTACT DERMATITIS

Rashes caused by contact with irritants or with substances to which you are allergic are called contact dermatitis. Technically, allergists are concerned only with allergic contact dermatitis (ACD), not irritant contact dermatitis. But since the exact cause and nature of the dermatitis often cannot be quickly determined—and since the patients want relief whatever the cause—allergists and dermatologists typically treat both sorts of rashes.

Actually, a number of substances, such as cement and industrial chemicals, can act as both allergic agents and irritants; and irritant dermatitis is often a complication of some other skin disease, such as atopic dermatitis or psoriasis. Patients with atopic dermatitis are at increased risk for contact dermatitis and should avoid topical antihistamines, antibiotics, and anesthetics, which frequently cause contact dermatitis.

ACD does not arise on first exposure to a substance but only after you have already become sensitized to it. But exposure to one substance to which you build up a sensitivity may also give rise to an allergy to a related substance.

The physiology of this type of allergy response depends on the sensitization of certain white blood cells—T cell lymphocytes—to particular substances that are then recognized as antigens when they enter the body. When a T cell meets a molecule of an antigen, it produces substances called lymphokines. Among the functions of the lymphokines is attracting hungry big macrophages to the region; these are white blood cells that specialize in gobbling up and destroying foreign substances in your body, whether they be bacteria or otherwise-harmless molecules of poison ivy antigen.

Incidentally, one of the lymphokines is interferon, a substance that is being used widely to fight a number of diseases.

The response that underlies ACD does not involve the allergy antibody, IgE, but it is an immune system response. It is also called a cell-mediated response or delayed hypersensitivity, the latter because it takes about two days to develop.

LATEX ALLERGY

Allergic reactions to latex have become a major health problem in the last decade or so. Health-care professionals, police, and even teachers are now trained to don rubber gloves whenever there is chance of infection from contact with someone who may be infected with HIV or hepatitis. Sexual partners use condoms much more frequently than in the past.

Latex gloves and condoms may sensitize the wearer, as well as the person touched, to allergens in latex.

Latex is also present in catheters, enema tips, household rubber gloves, balloons, and vehicle tires. Tires shred with use, and rubber particles fill the air. However, tires are not usually a problem (fortunately). One needs to understand how latex is processed to understand this difference.

Natural rubber can be processed in one of two ways: *dipped* or *dry* rubber. Gloves, condoms, and balloons are made by the dipped method whereby rubber tree sap is processed into liquid latex and the products are made by dipping a mold into the liquid latex. The allergenic proteins are readily available in these dipped products to react with the body's immune system and cause allergic reactions. Products made with dry rubber are thick, less stretchy, and include tires, belts, sports equipment, hoses. Dry rubber is tree sap that is cured at high temperatures to remove the water, and the heat also changes the latex proteins so they are not allergenic. Recent testing shows that latex-allergic individuals exposed to dry rubber products do not have allergic reactions. Further studies have shown it is unlikely that particulate matter from tires in road dust is unlikely to sensitize people to latex. An interesting study was published recently by Dr. R. G. Hamilton at Johns Hopkins about the risk of sensitizing children exposed to rubber-surfaced playgrounds. These researchers found that the playground material contained one allergy unit per gram (AU/g) of sample. This was compared to a latex glove that had almost two million allergy units per gram!

Cornstarch or other powder used in the gloves absorbs the latex and becomes airborne when one pulls the gloves on and off, which means that in many hospitals and laboratories, latex-sensitive people are breathing in latex allergens.

The increase in demand for latex may be indirectly related to the allergenic potency of the substance. Latex is derived from the sap of trees and is produced in only a handful of countries, many in Southeast Asia.

The latex is collected in buckets, much as New Englanders collect sap from sugar maples. The buckets contain chemicals to prevent bacterial contamination of the latex. These chemicals may also make the latex less allergenic. But with skyrocketing demand for the product, the latex is being transferred out of the buckets with increasing rapidity. Thus, rushing the process probably yields a more allergenic type of latex.

Speculation aside, there is no doubt that people allergic to latex may develop contact dermatitis, often in a severe form; they may develop latex-induced asthma, again often very severe; they may develop hives and swelling; and worst of all, they may suffer anaphylactic shock.

The reaction to latex may be more powerful if the person has already been exposed to a related protein in food, especially in what are considered the high-risk foods: bananas, kiwis, avocados, and chestnuts. Moderate-risk foods are apple, carrot, celery, papaya, potato, tomato, and mangoes. There are many others that are low risk. These foods would be of concern to a highly latex-sensitive individual. We refer you to the American Latex Allergy Association website for these foods (www. latexallergyresources.org).

About 7 percent of the general population is allergic to latex. The people most at risk are health workers; 10 to 20 percent of them have some form of latex allergy, and some have died or had to take up another line of work. Children with spinal bifida or urogenital disease are highly likely to develop an anaphylactic latex allergy, which makes their already difficult lives even more frightening. Also at risk are medical and dental patients of any age who undergo multiple procedures in which latex comes into contact with mucosal tissue.

One of our patients went into anaphylactic shock during a barium enema. Fortunately, the radiologist was sharp and quickly initiated effective treatment. The culprit, we discovered later, was the rubber tip of the enema apparatus.

Symptoms. Contact dermatitis caused by latex allergy usually appears within a day or so of contact and takes the form of an itchy, eczema-type rash with small red blisters.

However, an irritant reaction to latex can also occur. **Irritant contact dermatitis.** This common reaction to protective gloves isn't an actual allergy. It's most likely due to sweating or rubbing under the gloves or from detergents left on your hands before wearing them. This rash occurs most often in people who wear protective gloves, such as dental and health-care workers. Irritant contact dermatitis usually makes your skin appear red, dry, and cracked.

Asthmatic reactions appear most often (but not exclusively) in connection with exposure to airborne latex allergen.

Immediate-type reactions include asthma and nasal symptoms (rhinitis) but also include hives, swelling, and anaphylaxis. For example, you pull on latex gloves and get hives at once. Or you blow up a balloon and your lips swell.

If you have any type of immediate reaction to latex, report this to your doctor. The next exposure might bring on anaphylactic shock.

Diagnosis. Confirming latex allergy is a tricky business because the patient may be so sensitive that a skin test is potentially fatal. Skin testing, with extra safety precautions, can be done with patients who have experienced only contact dermatitis. But at the time of publication, no FDA-approved skin-test material was available in the United States. If there is any chance that the patient may have an immediate or anaphylactic-type reaction, only in vitro testing (usually RAST or some variant of RAST) should be performed. Currently, some physicians will place a small amount of latex on your forearm and then prick your skin with a needle. A small amount will be injected, and if you are allergic, you will react as with other skin tests. The authors rely on RAST to evaluate their latex-sensitive patients.

Treatment. The treatment is avoidance, which is difficult but usually possible to some degree. A good general rule for everyone is stay away from latex if you can.

There is a growing recognition that latex gloves should be unpowdered or lightly powdered. Some hospitals, such as the Mayo Clinic in Rochester, Minnesota, have taken dramatic steps to reduce exposure to the latex allergen in gloves and powder and all other forms. Some brands of gloves seem to be less allergenic than others. Substitute materials, such as vinyl, may be acceptable in some cases, although they do not provide as good protection against infections as latex does.

Researchers hope to use genetic engineering to produce nonallergenic rubber. However, until they do, a complete list of latex-free products is available from the American Latex Allergy Association (www.latexallergyresources.org). However, at the time of publication of this book, the following breaking news occurred and is too soon for us to evaluate. The U.S. Food and Drug Administration has cleared for marketing the first device made from a new form of natural rubber latex, guayule latex. The product, the Yulex patient-examination glove, is derived from the guayule bush, a desert plant native to the southwestern United States.

Traditional latex gloves are made from the milky sap of a rubber tree, *Hevea braziliensis*, which triggers the allergic reaction. Available data on the new guayule latex show that even people who are highly allergic to traditional latex do not react on first exposure to guayule latex proteins. This is very good news for health-care workers as well as all latex-allergy patients as it is likely that this product will become widely available if this product is as good as it sounds. The Yulex glove is made by the Yulex Corporation of Maricopa, Arizona. And is the first major change in the allergenic nature of latex gloves since they began to be used by health-care workers in 1890. We had mentioned the research on the above-mentioned product in our previous book.

POISON IVY

Poison ivy is a good example of an itchy ACD rash. Also, if you have become sensitized to any member of this plant family (poison ivy, poison oak, and poison sumac), you are likely to be sensitive to all members.

When they have been pulled up, these plants should be buried or else discarded in the wild. Burning them creates dangerous fumes.

If you live in poison ivy country, it is best to police your property fairly regularly so that the vines do not proliferate. They are quite difficult to kill off once they are well established, and for some people, even slight contact will provoke a rash.

TREATING POISON IVY

If you are sensitive to poison ivy, poison oak, or poison sumac, there is a nonprescription topical cream containing TEA stearate and stearate MEA, called Ivy Shield, that you can apply before exposure to reduce the severity of a reaction by up to 50 percent. Of course, avoiding these plants is best; but if you want to hike or camp out, complete avoidance may be difficult.

Researchers are currently studying whether organoclay may provide an even more effective shield. This substance is used as a filler in deodorant, but do not try to use deodorant as a shield. The filler is not present in large-enough quantities to help against poison ivy.

The sensitizing substance in poison ivy and its cousins is an oil, uroshiol, that sticks to all surfaces. Isopropyl alcohol, which tends to deactivate it, can be applied to skin, clothing, and work tools as needed. Washing down with alcohol or plain water after exposure may help, but soap may spread the oil on your skin. The oil may also be spread if you take a hot bath.

Pets can carry the poison-ivy oil, and children who hug and kiss dogs, baby goats, and other lovable animals may develop whopping cases of poison ivy. A child or anyone with a dramatic case of poison ivy should be seen by a doctor, especially if there is swelling, of the hands or lips or large areas of skin, are involved.

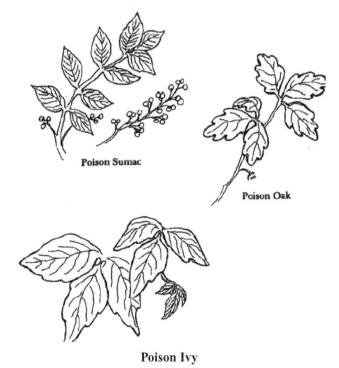

Poison Sumac

Poison Oak

Poison Ivy

For mild outbreaks of poison ivy, over-the-counter cortisone ointments are probably the best treatment.

There is a possibility of desensitization through shots and oral immunization, but this treatment approach has not been fully studied yet and is not recommended. Avoidance is still best.

OTHER CAUSES OF ACD (ALLERGIC CONTACT DERMATITIS)

ACD is a fairly common industrial complaint, and in some industrial factories, as much as 10 percent of the workforce has this disease. If your work environment seems to cause rashes or hives in a significant number of those who are on site, you should probably try to find out whether the situation also may pose more-serious health risks.

ACD affects older people more frequently than it affects the young. To take an example of one of the most-common sensitivities, 14 percent of women over age fifty are allergic to nickel, but only 2.2 percent of girls under age ten react to nickel. This is evidently because in most, though not all, cases of ACD, it takes months or years of exposure to develop the sensitivity. But we should add that the fad for body piercing apparently has changed the traditional picture somewhat. There are reports of extreme sensitivity to nickel following piercing.

Because of the danger of infection and the risk of allergic reactions, we urge persons wishing to undergo body piercing of any sort to use extreme caution, seek care in a very reputable place, and use only jewelry containing no nickel although that is typically more expensive. The European Union has taken further steps by limiting the amount of nickel allowed in products that come into contact with skin.

In some cases, sunlight breaks down a substance that ordinarily causes no problem into components that may produce a reaction. This is photo contact dermatitis. For instance, you may wear a perfume on your body with no problem until one day, you splash a little on your neck and temples before going out to watch a tennis tournament. Later, a rash appears on your face.

SYMPTOMS

The ACD rash often begins as redness of the skin, with bumps and blistering following. It usually appears within a few days after contact with the offending substance. Typically, the edge of the rash is sharp, or clearly defined, which is a clue to the diagnosis. The rash itches, and if it is situated near the eyes, swelling resembling angioedema may occur. In chronic forms of the disease, there is less blistering and more crusting and scaling.

The rash is most likely to appear on the neck, eyelids, and groin. Perspiration and rubbing will make the skin more susceptible to the rash.

DIAGNOSIS OF ACD

The basic evidence for the diagnosis is the history of the circumstances in which the rash erupts and the clinical appearance of the rash: Is it well demarcated? Are there small blisters? In addition, patch testing can be done to confirm a diagnosis.

In patch testing, an adhesive patch with a suspect substance is applied to the skin. The patch is left in place for forty-eight hours then removed, and the skin is examined for a reaction. The area should be checked again in a day or two and then again a week later, to see if there is a late reaction.

If you start to itch intensely before the forty-eight hours is up, call your doctor. The patch should probably be taken off early.

Often several patches are applied at once, but one drawback to patch testing is that your skin may become "excited" and react to a number of substances whether you are allergic to them or not. Therefore, if there are multiple positive tests, it is often advisable to retest a suspect substance alone at a later date to be sure that the test result was accurate.

Accuracy of the patch tests is improved by avoiding vigorous physical activity and baths during the time the patch is in place.

Rare side effects of patch testing include anaphylactic reactions. These occur within minutes after contact. Also, again rarely, the test procedure may sensitize the patient to the substance being tested.

There are countless substances that may cause ACD, so random testing may be useless as well as quite expensive. But there is a screening set of tests for twenty substances most often implicated in ACD. These are chemicals and drugs commonly encountered in cosmetics, in cleaning fluids, as local anesthetics, in hobby shops, and so on. They are benzocaine, 2-mercaptobenzothiazole, colophony, p-phenylenediamine, imidazolidinyl urea, cinnamic aldehyde, lanolin alcohol, Carba rubber mix, neomycin, formaldehyde, thiuram rubber mix, ethylenediamine, epoxy resin, mercapto rubber mix, black rubber mix, butylphenol formaldehyde resin, potassium dichromate, quaternium-15, balsam of Peru, and nickel sulfate.

The place on the body that the rash appears often gives clues as to the possible cause. A general body rash is likely to be caused by resins, dyes, formaldehyde in synthetic fabrics, or rubber in garments. The following table gives the most-likely causes of rashes that are confined to various sites.

Area of the Body Affected	Most-Likely Causes
Feet	shoes, foot-care products, shower sandals, medication for athlete's foot
Genitals (male)	jock-itch medication, condoms, vaginal or contraceptive medication used by sexual partner
Genitals (female)	contraceptive medication, rubber diaphragm, scented sanitary pads, deodorants, douches, condoms
Anal region	hemorrhoid medication
Hands	hand-care medicines and lotions, latex or other rubber gloves, metal jewelry, plants
Underarm region	deodorants, fabric or rubber in garments, perfume
Forehead, neck, and shoulders	hair dyes, hair-care products, cosmetics, sunscreens, topical medicines, perfumes, nickel in jewelry, garments, hatbands
Ears	nickel in earrings, perfumes, earplugs, earphones, cell phones, and the like.
Eyelids	cosmetics, eyedrops, nail polish, hair spray and other hair products, chemical fumes such as those from epoxy resins
Lips	lipstick, lip protectors, toothpaste, mouthwash, fruits or other food, rubber erasers
Face in general	cosmetics, topical medications, plants, shaving aids, fumes such as those from epoxy resins, sunscreens, nickel in jewelry, and cell phones

The history that you give the doctor should cover occupation, hobbies, and habits. Sometimes a normally benign item, such as a nibbled-upon pencil eraser, turns out to be the culprit.

A savvy physician, however, will hope to find the cause quickly by focusing on the following questions:

- Do you wear jewelry containing nickel?
- Do you work with cement or in the tanning, dyeing, or printing industries? The common ingredient that causes trouble in all these occupations is chromium salt. Other elements and chemical compounds used in these industries may also cause skin reactions.
- Do you work with or frequently handle plants?
- What cosmetics and hair products do you use?
- What perfumes and deodorants do you use? (There are so many substances present in cosmetics, hair products, perfumes, body lotions, and so on that you may have to write the company that makes the product for a complete list of ingredients.)
- Do you have pets? (They can carry resin from poison ivy on their coats.)
- Are you using any topical medications, such as an antibiotic cream, local anesthetic or anti-inflammatory ointment, eyedrops, antibacterial agents? Be aware that it may not be the main ingredient but a preservative—for example, parabens—that is the problem.
- Are you frequently in contact with soaps, detergents, bleaches, furniture oils, paint and paint thinner, and other common cleaning and painting products? Do you rinse clothes thoroughly to remove cleaning agents?
- Are you exposed to formaldehyde in your work, clothing, or environment? Health-care and lab workers formerly were widely exposed to formaldehyde used as a preservative. Since it is now recognized as a carcinogen, it is used less. But it is also present in some common products, including certain kinds of wallboard and newly purchased permanent-press clothing. With wallboard, the formaldehyde is supposed to be subject to treatment that fixes it in the board. Reportedly, defective wallboard is sometimes installed.

TREATMENT

In acute contact dermatitis, with an extensive rash, cold wet dressings with dilute Burow's solution may be recommended.

In later stages of the rash, topical steroids are very effective, but be sure to follow the safety precautions outlined above in the discussion of atopic dermatitis. You must follow the prescription directions and never use a strong topical steroid cream or ointment on your face or other parts of the body where the skin is thin.

Oral steroids may be needed for a short period. Antihistamines may relieve the itching. If an infection superimposed on the rash threatens, your doctor may prescribe oral antibiotics.

If you have sensitive skin—if, for example, you already suffer from atopic dermatitis—you should avoid coming in contact with substances that tend to produce irritations. Some topical drugs very frequently cause sensitization and should be avoided. These include topical antihistamines, antibiotics, and benzocaine and other local anesthetics.

One patient being treated for nasal allergies and atopic dermatitis (primarily by allergy shots) responded well for several years but then developed an eczema-like rash on her hands, eyelids, and to a small extent on her face. One approach would be to stop using all cosmetics, perfumes, face creams, and so on; but who wants to live that way? Finally, after a lot of work, her doctor isolated the problem. She had an unusual contact allergy to sorbic acid, which was in a perfume that she used.

Armed with a list of things that contain sorbic acid, she avoided trouble. But one day she had an EKG, and eight hours later, there was dermatitis on every spot where the electrodes had been placed. She had told the technician of her allergies, including the sensitivity to sorbic acid, but he had not thoroughly checked the label on the EKG jelly. This illustrates an important point: if you have allergies, it is always risky to take anyone else's word for the ingredients in anything. Luckily, no real harm was done.

Chapter 13

ANAPHYLAXIS

Food allergy and anaphylaxis are so interrelated that it will be helpful to read this chapter in conjunction with the food-allergy chapter. It is extremely important to be alert to the possibility that an allergic reaction may take the form of anaphylaxis, that is, a rapidly developing systemic allergic reaction that can lead to shock and even death. The silver lining is that the total number of deaths from anaphylaxis is relatively low, approximately 1 for every 2.5 million people per year. It is estimated that between one out of two thousand to one out of fifty persons experience anaphylaxis in their lifetime (prevalence). It is also felt that the actual incidence is underreported since there usually is no specific evidence of anaphylaxis when an autopsy is performed. The incidence of anaphylaxis is highest in younger persons, with a rate of seventy per one hundred thousand person years in the age-zero-to-nineteen group. More importantly, the incidence has doubled in this age group in the past twenty years.

Among the most-common causes of anaphylaxis discussed so far are allergies to foods (peanuts in children and shellfish in adults); drugs, most commonly penicillin and other antibiotics, NSAIDs or nonsteroidal anti-inflammatory drugs (including aspirin); and latex. Even when treated, anaphylaxis has a mortality rate of up to 10 percent, so the recommended approach when anaphylaxis is suspected to be occurring is to administer epinephrine and, when it is suspected to have occurred in the past, to provide the patient with an epinephrine autoinjector (EpiPen, Adrenaclick, Twinject).

The incidence of the various causes is not easily obtained, but some of the numbers that have appeared in our literature recently are reported here so the reader will have an idea as to how common these are. Nonfatal penicillin-induced anaphylaxis affects between two million and twenty-seven million Americans. The incidence of latex allergy had been rising in the past twenty years but is now felt to have stabilized because of efforts to reduce exposure to latex, for example, by using nonpowdered latex gloves and gloves made of other materials. The incidence of latex allergy is between three million and sixteen million Americans.

Severe reactions to dye used in X-ray procedures (ionic-contrast media) occurs in one to two per one thousand procedures using the older dye (hyperosmolar media) and three per ten thousand procedures using the newer, nonionic, low osmolar agents. The latter is more expensive, and insurers are reluctant to pay for them. However, if you have a history of a reaction in the past or have asthma, allergies, or eczema, you are more at risk to have a reaction to these dyes; and you should insist on their use. *An allergy to shellfish has nothing to do with reactions to X-ray dyes.*

Anaphylaxis can be induced not only by certain food and drug allergies but also by hypersensitivity to insect stings, accounting for some forty deaths annually in the United States. It is estimated that six out of one thousand children and three out of one hundred adults are at risk for serious reactions to insect stings.

Under some circumstances, anaphylaxis can be brought on by a reaction to vigorous exercise. There is also a form of anaphylaxis called idiopathic, which means that we don't know what causes it. In adults, idiopathic anaphylaxis is probably the most commonly encountered type. Idiopathic anaphylaxis in children is rare.

Anaphylaxis has been recognized as a syndrome since ancient times, but it is only in the past one hundred years that we have developed an understanding of the physiology of the reaction. In 1900, Charles Richet and Paul Portier undertook research that ultimately clarified the cause of many mysterious deaths.

Occasionally a patient will have a severe allergic reaction to a muscle relaxant or other drugs used in general anesthesia. This is scary because the patient is already asleep and the reaction is somewhat difficult to spot, unless it shows up clearly in the skin—with hives, for example. But an alert anesthesiologist will note a change in the patient's blood pressure or breathing status, indications that the patient is in trouble, and quick action can be taken. Anaphylaxis occurs in one of fifteen thousand instances of anesthesia, but only 5 percent of anaphylactic reactions during surgery result in death. Perioperative anaphylaxis accounts for 10 to 20 percent of complications of anesthesia. Of these anaphylactic episodes, muscle relaxants account for two-thirds and latex about one-sixth. Other medications account for the other one-sixth.

The possibility of an allergic reaction is one of the many reasons to be very conservative in using general anesthesia—but most people would heartily agree that it is not a reason to forgo necessary treatment that requires a general anesthetic.

There is also the rare danger of an allergy-immunization treatment causing anaphylaxis. Many impatient patients feel that their doctors are being overcautious when they insist on the half-hour waiting period in the office after an allergy shot.

CHARACTERISTICS OF ANAPHYLAXIS

True anaphylactic reactions result from the action of IgE on the mast cells in connective tissue and the basophils in blood, which release chemical mediators that cause allergy symptoms.

It is important to reserve the term *anaphylaxis* only for reactions that fit the definition. This is true for any illness, that it has to fit accepted criteria for diagnosis. This may be especially true for anaphylaxis, which is not so easy to diagnose in some patients. Exactly how to define what anaphylaxis is has been evolving in recent years. Our current definition revolves around whether or not exposure to a known or suspected allergen has happened before the symptoms develop.

If there is *no known allergen exposure*, then we define anaphylaxis as the acute onset of an illness (minutes to several hours) with involvement of the skin, mucosal tissues, or both (e.g., generalized hives; itching or flushing; swollen lips, tongue, uvula) and at least one of the following: (1) respiratory symptoms (e.g., shortness of breath; wheezing; stridor, which is a gaspinglike sound associated with closing of the upper airway; reduced pulmonary tests; or low oxygen measured in the blood) and (2) reduced blood pressure or associated symptoms of end-organ dysfunction (e.g., loss of muscle tone [collapse], fainting, incontinence).

If there is a *likely allergen exposure*, then we define anaphylaxis as two or more of the following symptoms occurring rapidly (minutes to hours) after exposure: (1) skin/mucosal, 2) respiratory, (3) reduced blood pressure, (4) gastrointestinal (crampy abdominal pain, vomiting).

In the situation where there is a *known allergen exposure*, such as when a peanut-allergic person accidentally eats a peanut, then the criteria for diagnosis become different still and we accept just a 30 percent reduction in blood pressure as enough to make a diagnosis. Of course, there could be additional symptoms.

The point of the above definitions is that we don't want to overdiagnose or underdiagnose anaphylaxis. For example, let's say that a ten-year-old boy has a severe peanut allergy but is not allergic to tree nuts. One day he eats a few walnuts and complains that he feels a little dizzy and that his mouth is maybe a little itchy. The mother is a nurse and checked the blood pressure, and it was normal. Is this anaphylaxis? This is the situation of a *likely allergen* as peanut-allergic children are often allergic to tree nuts. This child does not have two of the above criteria. While dizziness can be a symptom of lowering of blood pressure, in this situation, it is not, as the blood pressure was normal. While this child should be reevaluated for tree-nut allergy, this situation does not represent anaphylaxis. A similar process not involving IgE used to be called anaphylactoid, meaning "like anaphylaxis." However, in conjunction with the evolving criteria for diagnosis described above, we now refer to these reactions as *nonallergic anaphylaxis* and no longer use the term *anaphylactoid*. Allergic anaphylaxis refers to reactions that involve the immune system (IgE, IgG, or immune complexes). One of the most common causes of nonallergic anaphylaxis is the use of radiographic contrast media ("dye") in taking X-rays. Some people are sensitive to these dyes; and no sooner is the contrast medium injected than when the patient reacts with symptoms of anaphylaxis, such as hives, angioedema (swelling), and in very serious cases, swelling of the trachea and/or shock. Since this ordinarily happens in a hospital setting, the patient usually can be brought around quickly with injections of epinephrine, antihistamines, and steroids. Otherwise, the mortality rate might be high indeed.

Another cause of nonallergic anaphylaxis is sensitivity to aspirin and other nonsteroidal anti-inflammatory drugs.

The distinction between allergic anaphylactic and nonallergic anaphylaxis reactions is of no great importance to the patient; but in theory, the former requires some prior exposure to the reaction-causing substance, whereas a nonallergic anaphylactic reaction can occur—and often does occur—on the first exposure.

There have been isolated reports of allergic anaphylaxis seeming to occur upon first exposure, but most likely, the patient was exposed to the substance or a related substance earlier without realizing it. This can occur from trace amounts of penicillin in milk or, in a child, prior exposure to the substance in breast milk.

The symptoms of anaphylaxis are unforgettable to anyone who has been through them. They typically begin to appear within seconds to about fifteen minutes after exposure. In response to the histamine and other chemical mediators that are flooding into the body, capillaries open, the bronchial tubes constrict, and there is excess mucus production and swelling (edema), sometimes accompanied by hives and itching. Swelling of the throat and larynx, which causes hoarseness, choking, and difficulty swallowing, is particularly dangerous. It may first be felt as a lump in the throat or, if the reaction is to food, as a numbness or tingling in the mouth. The skin flushes. Blood pressure drops. The patient feels lightheaded, faint, breathless, and sometimes nauseated and sick all over. Cramps and diarrhea may ensue. The patient may have increasing difficulty breathing, the skin may take on a cyanotic (bluish) tinge—indicating oxygen deprivation—and the heartbeat may become irregular. The patient may feel anxious and sense impending doom.

Occasionally, an anaphylactic reaction may be delayed for an hour or several hours.

Most deaths occur among adults, and it seems that risk of anaphylaxis increases somewhat with both age and the presence of comorbid disease, especially asthma, COPD, and heart disease.

People with atopic illnesses (i.e., rhinitis, eczema, or asthma) are considered more likely to develop anaphylaxis from foods, exercise, idiopathic, radiocontrast media, and latex but are probably not at increased risk from insulin, penicillin, or stinging insects. Among asthmatics, especially if they are not well controlled, the reaction may be more severe. For example, people with asthma may suffer slightly worse anaphylaxis from a reaction to penicillin and certain other drugs, even though their risk of reacting is the same as that of the population in general.

Occupation and location may also put you at greater risk for anaphylaxis. For example, beekeepers lead dangerous lives. If you come from the South and have fire ants in your backyard, you are more at risk than a native of Alaska is. Intermittent exposure to a given substance is more likely to trigger an anaphylactic attack than if something is given continuously. As a matter of fact, when someone is desensitized to something that has caused anaphylaxis, such as aspirin, they must be maintained on daily doses to keep the allergy from reoccurring. People having their blood flow through artificial membranes, such as in heart surgery and in kidney-dialysis treatments, sometimes have nonallergic anaphylactic reactions as protein components of the blood react with the membranes. The list of substances that might trigger anaphylaxis is infinite. In addition to stinging insect venom, discussed below, the following is a list of some more common substances that have caused anaphylactic reactions:

Antibiotics. Penicillin, cephalosporins, tetracycline, nitrofurantoin, streptomycin (see chapter 8 on drug allergies).

Local anesthetics. We include this because historically this was thought to be a frequent cause. There are more than one hundred kinds, but reactions to these are extremely rare, although there are common complaints of reactions that prove to be unrelated to the local anesthetic. We have seen thousands of cases of suspected reactions to local anesthetics but have never seen a case of anaphylaxis secondary to local anesthetic reactivity.

Nonsteroidal anti-inflammatory drugs (NSAIDs). Aspirin, ibuprofen, indomethacin, fenoprofen, naproxen, tolmetin.

Enzymes. Chymopapain (once used to treat herniated spinal disks), chymotrypsin (used to treat digestive problems), streptokinase (used to dissolve clotted blood and thus a treatment for heart attacks).

Psyllium. Present in laxatives and added to cereals.

Hormones and serums. Insulin, ACTH (adrenocorticotropic hormone), parathyroid, cortisone, horse antibody (horse serum).

Diagnostic agents. Iodinated contrast media and dyes, such as Bromsulphalein (BSP), which is used in liver testing.

Food. Peanuts and other legumes, eggs, fish and shellfish, milk, tree nuts, and sesame seeds. Less commonly, grains, other seeds, and fruits (see chapter 7).

Latex. In rubber gloves, condoms, and so on (see chapter 12).

Wheat contaminated with mites has also been reported to cause anaphylaxis. The contamination is most likely to occur in warm climates. In temperate climates, mite-infested food is uncommon, even though it is virtually impossible to keep food completely insect-free.

Recently, there have been reports of delayed anaphylaxis occurring in persons after eating red meat (beef, pork, lamb). The reaction occurs four to six hours after ingestion, so it can be easily overlooked. Perhaps some patients who have been told that they have idiopathic anaphylaxis have to be reevaluated now since perhaps consumption of red meat caused their reactions. This delayed anaphylactic reaction to red meat occurs more frequently in persons who have large skin reactions to tick bites. Some of the patients had immediate reactions to tick bites, ranging from hives to anaphylaxis. The details of this new phenomenon are being worked out.

Health-food stores carry "bee pollen" (mostly dandelion pollen), as well as sunflower seeds and chamomile tea, all of which can occasionally cause a systemic reaction in hypersensitive persons who are often also sensitive to ragweed pollen. Sulfites used to preserve food and drinks may also cause anaphylaxis.

Anaphylaxis can occur during the transfusion of blood or blood products. This can be the result of antigens, such as in egg protein, in the donor's blood to which the patient is sensitive. The reaction is more apt to occur among people who lack one of the immunoglobulins, IgA.

Protamine, a protein which used to be derived from sharks, is now artificially made by recombinant DNA technology. It is added to certain insulin (NPH) to stabilize absorption and also to reverse the actions of blood thinners (heparin) particularly during open-heart surgery. Patients exposed to it in one version can have reactions when exposed to it for another reason.

Seminal fluid can cause an anaphylactic reaction in a woman. The culprit is a protein in prostatic fluid. The only protection is for the man to use a condom. Desensitization is available experimentally for couples who want to have children.

EXERCISE-INDUCED AND IDIOPATHIC ANAPHYLAXIS

As noted previously, *idiopathic* means "of unknown cause." It is appropriate to link idiopathic anaphylaxis with exercise-induced anaphylaxis since the latter is quite mysterious too.

Anaphylaxis after vigorous exercise is rare but well documented. It is sometimes associated with eating prior to exercise or with eating certain foods before exercise. Several foods have been implicated, including wheat, shellfish, fruit, milk, celery, and fish. If you have ever had an anaphylactic attack associated with exercise and eating, you should consult a physician knowledgeable in this entity, and they will likely advise you not to eat anything for two to four hours before exercise; and some doctors would advise leaving a longer period. (See chapter 7.)

Many patients who have experienced exercise-induced anaphylaxis also have one of the atopic allergic diseases (asthma, rhinitis, eczema), and even more have relatives with these diseases.

It is more common in females and those in their late teens to early thirties.

If you develop hives or itching or other allergy symptoms while exercising, stop at once. If you have had an anaphylactic reaction while exercising, carry emergency medication—autoinjectable epinephrine (EpiPen, Adrenaclick, Twinject)—and never exercise alone.

If you have had one or more anaphylactic reactions for no known reason, you too should carry autoinjectable epinephrine (EpiPen, Adrenaclick, Twinject).

A typical case of idiopathic anaphylaxis is that of a healthy woman, aged thirty-five, in New York City, who on a normal afternoon was speaking on the phone with her stepson, who lived about twenty blocks away. He began to realize that she seemed to be ill and fading, and then she hung up. He called 911, found a taxi, and arrived to find her unconscious with the paramedics working on her.

The diagnosis at the hospital was anaphylaxis, but since no cause was found, the diagnosis was idiopathic anaphylaxis. In the following three years, the incident did not recur; but following the advice of her doctor, the woman carries epinephrine (Adrenalin) and, in her wallet, a card identifying her problem.

In patients with frequent episodes of idiopathic anaphylaxis, daily medication may be used to prevent or reduce the frequency of these scary attacks.

Prior to making a diagnosis of idiopathic anaphylaxis, a very careful search for a cause must be made. The obvious, such as insect or peanut allergy, will have already leaped out at both patient and physician when they are the cause. However, more obscure causes, such as the delayed response to red meat and, even more important, food preservatives or sulfites in wine, should be excluded. Even when nothing is found, as long as the attacks continue, an ongoing search for a cause must be done.

However, as far as prevention and preparation are concerned, the patient with idiopathic anaphylaxis should at a minimum carry one of the epinephrine autoinjectors (EpiPen, Twinject) that should be equipped to deliver two doses if needed—and most importantly, they or someone they are with should know how to use it. They should wear a MedicAlert bracelet in case they lose consciousness. They certainly should try to stay out of obscure regions of the globe where they are hours away from the nearest medical facility, if they are lucky enough to find two fast llamas to transport them. This is discussed in much-greater detail below in the section on anaphylaxis from insects.

They should certainly consult an expert in allergy familiar with anaphylaxis, whose advice should supersede ours. They should be given a medication regimen, which often starts with daily second-generation antihistamines. However, if the attacks continue since they are so dangerous, daily or alternate day steroids may have to be used. This is your physician's call as each case is different.

Insect Stings

Insects, which are far more numerous than *Homo sapiens* and probably better adapted for survival, add injury to insult by stinging and biting us whenever possible (or so it sometimes seems). The stings can cause anaphylactic and toxic reactions, with about 1 to 3 percent of the population believed to be susceptible to anaphylaxis following a sting.

If you get stung, you should get a tetanus booster if it has been more than five years since your last one. If you cannot get the booster within twenty-four hours, then discuss with a physician what precautions you might take. The risk of tetanus from a sting is low, but the death rate following a tetanus infection is high.

There are three major families of stinging insects in the Hymenoptera order: apids (bees), vespids (wasps), and formicids (ants). The apid family includes honeybees and bumblebees, both of which are mild-mannered and tend not to sting without a lot of provocation; however, they sting when stepped on with bare feet. The vespid family includes hornets and yellow jackets, as well as wasps. The members of the formicid family that concern us most are fire ants, which are found predominantly in the South. For those of you planning trips to the South, it is estimated that 50 percent of the population in some areas of the South are stung each year! Fire ants have been found as far north as Maryland. Harvester ants, a mere quarter inch in size, also sting (they can paralyze and kill small animals) and can cause anaphylaxis. They live primarily in desert areas of the western and southwestern United States, Canada, and Mexico.

Rarely but occasionally, other bugs cause systemic reactions as well. Those lesser-bad guys include kissing bugs (found in southwestern states and California), mosquitoes, horse flies, and deer flies (the latter two usually cause painful bites). Given how common a mosquito bite is, it is surprising that anaphylaxis from a bite is extremely rare. The more common reaction is swelling (Skeeter syndrome) and responds well (if treatment is begun early enough) to either steroid cream or antihistamines.

The venom that stinging insects inject into their victims is composed of enzymes, amines, and proteins. The exact mix varies from species to species, but related insects may carry types of venom similar enough to cause cross-sensitivity. Thus, if you are allergic to one member of the vespid family, you may be allergic to others. This is particularly true of yellow jackets and hornets.

Various components of insect venom are allergenic, but the most important allergens are the enzymes phospholipase and hyaluronidase.

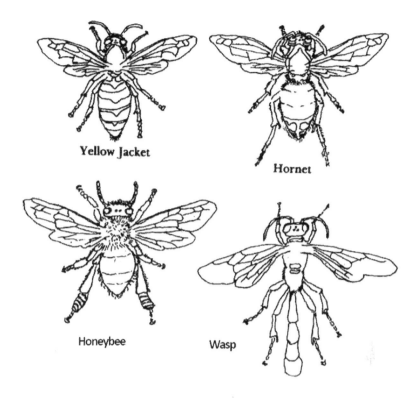

Yellow Jacket

Hornet

Honeybee

Wasp

COMMON STINGING INSECTS

Insect venom can be sufficiently strong (especially with multiple stings) to cause serious toxic reactions even in people who are not allergic. Sometimes the typical local reaction of swelling and redness can become alarmingly more extensive. For example, a hornet sting on the hand will ordinarily result in swelling and soreness in the hand. But if the arm swells up also, that can be a matter of concern. Multiple stings can put a person in mortal danger, with or without an allergy reaction. About forty persons die in the United States each year from allergic reactions to stings, but it is possible that many go unreported or unrecognized. Most deaths occur in people above age forty-five. One-half of fatal reactions occur with no history of a previous allergic reaction to a sting.

Honeybees leave their stingers and venom sacs in the skin of their victim; only rarely do vespids do this. In the past, we recommended that you flick away the stinger with a fingernail or knife. The idea was to avoid squeezing the venom sac, thus inadvertently forcing more venom into the skin.

The most important first step is to get the stinger out as fast as possible, which usually requires taking hold of it with a tweezers and pulling. In the case of multiple stings, try to get all the stingers out quickly. Speed is the key.

The reason it is so important to remove the stinger is that typically attached to the stinger are enough muscle and nerve tissue to keep pumping venom and driving the barbed end of the stinger deeper.

The next step is to be sure that you can get medical help if needed. Get to a doctor's office or hospital or other type of urgent-care clinic. If in doubt, call 911 and report what has happened. Do not pause to apply meat tenderizer, mud, ice, or other traditional remedies that are worthless.

> **If you know that you are allergic and you have Adrenalin (epinephrine), use it immediately after being stung by an insect. Then call 911 or an ambulance service, as advised above.**

To illustrate how quickly one must sometimes take action, consider the case of a pharmacist from Los Angeles who was traveling to a convention in the South some years ago. He was alone in his car when a yellow jacket made a direct hit on his face. He winced, but there was no awful pain, so he kept driving. About five minutes later, he became aware of tightness in his chest, he felt hot, and his face had puffed to about twice its normal size.

He considered pulling over to the side of the road but realized that he had to try to get to the nearest hospital, which he estimated to be about five minutes away. He kept driving fast and held his hand hard on the horn. Luckily, a state trooper saw him and pulled him over; and even more luckily, the officer recognized the emergency and in about two minutes delivered him to the hospital, where he received epinephrine and other lifesaving treatments.

After a serious sting and anaphylactic reaction, your body is depleted of IgE and probably you will not have another major allergic reaction for several weeks, even if stung again. Don't bet your life on this—individuals do vary, but you should be aware of the possibility of IgE depletion because if you are tested for venom sensitivity in this period, the results may be falsely negative. The tests should not be run until a month or more after the episode. In the meantime, do see an allergist and get instruction on how to use epinephrine autoinjector (EpiPen, Adrenaclick, Twinject).

Unfortunately, delayed reactions to stings can lead to such serious problems as kidney disease, vascular disease, fever and serum sickness, neuritis, and arthritis-like symptoms.

Identifying the type of insect that stung you is not reliable and is usually unnecessary as there is cross-reactivity between the types, and if you need immunotherapy, you will be treated with all the types to which you test positive.

It is helpful to know a little bit about these insects in order to help you avoid stings, however.

Big fat bumblebees are easy to identify. Honeybees are small, usually yellow or brownish, and chunky, with a round thorax (the part of the body near the head).

Vespids are recognizable by their narrow waists between thorax and abdomen. Yellow jackets have rather handsome bands of yellow and black and are relatively svelte in build. They are the insects most often seen buzzing around garbage bins in picnic areas. They love sweets.

Hornets usually have white or yellow stripes and a white face. Their large conical gray or tan nests are typically located at a considerable height, in a tree or under eaves, for example.

Yellow jackets ordinarily nest in or near the ground, although in unusually rainy seasons they may nest higher up, on a porch, for example. If you see them in your neighborhood, try to spot their nesting place. Disturbing a nest can cause the yellow jackets to attack in a swarm. Such accidents are common during gardening, mowing lawns or fields, and while horseback riding through fields.

Brown and black wasps, often found around and in houses, are less inclined to sting. Accidents will happen, however, especially in the spring or fall, if the creatures are a little drowsy from the cold. It is then easy to step on one. They are also apt to lie concealed in clothing or in shoes. Shake out clothing and shoes before putting them on. Finally, keep in mind that wasps are also likely to sting if disturbed: when you are painting a house, putting in storm windows, cleaning gutters, and so on. As often as not, it is your hands or head that gets the sting. To avoid this, scout the region where you will be working the day before and destroy the nests at night. (Follow the directions on the pesticide carefully.)

Fire ant bites can usually be identified because the ant grabs on to the skin with its jaws and then, nastily, pivots in a circle, stinging as it goes. In about twenty-four hours, characteristic little blisters appear at the site.

Fire ants live in Texas, Louisiana, Arkansas, Mississippi, Alabama, Georgia, the Carolinas, and Florida. Up to 60 percent of the human population in these areas is stung yearly, with a 1 percent anaphylaxis rate!

Venom Immunotherapy (Shots)

People sensitive to insect stings can be desensitized with shots, and this usually affords good protection. The desensitization procedure for wasps and bees is now more effective than it was thirty years ago. In the past, doctors used whole-body extracts, which did not reliably build the desired venom immunity; but now the venom itself is used, and these shots are 95 to 100 percent effective eliminating or at the very least reducing the reaction to a future sting.

Fire ant allergy is still treated with whole-body extract of the ants, but a standardized extract is in the testing stage.

In patients who have significant reactions to a stinging insect, testing is indicated so that desensitization shots can be given. Since there is such a crossover in sensitivity among vespids (yellow jackets, hornets, wasps), your doctor will test for all five of the relevant stinging insects and, if you test positive, will recommend immunotherapy based on these tests. If skin tests are entirely negative, then RAST (blood) tests should be done. If these RASTs are also negative, the skin tests should be repeated in three to six months.

A seemingly obvious allergic sensitivity, based on a severe reaction following a sting, should still be confirmed by skin tests. Sometimes an apparent anaphylactic reaction is really a severe toxic reaction. In such a case, you should carry epinephrine but need not be immunized.

A strong but strictly local reaction, such as a finger or arm that is very swollen and sore after a sting, is not an indication of susceptibility to anaphylaxis from future stings.

Adults who develop hives in reaction to an insect sting should count that as a significant reaction and consider getting immunized. However, children who develop hives but no other anaphylactic symptoms after a sting are not considered to need immunization. But this issue is still under study.

Venom immunotherapy shots are administered in basically the same manner as other allergy shots are. Gradually increasing doses of venom are injected once or twice a week until a maintenance dose is reached. This takes from two to six months. Thereafter, the injections are given every four to eight weeks. Research centers may attempt a more rapid desensitization.

There is disagreement in the medical community as to whether the shots should be continued indefinitely (i.e., for life) or whether they can be stopped after about five years or after skin tests or RAST show no further sensitivity. More studies are needed to settle the question. Probably someone who is at a special risk of death from anaphylaxis—for example, someone with heart disease—should keep up the shots indefinitely. Someone who had a particularly severe reaction initially to a sting should continue the shots longer. Also, honeybee allergy may require longer therapy. After stopping shots, there is a 10 to 20 percent risk of reactions to another sting, but they are usually considerably milder.

What is presently certain is that if you have a history of insect anaphylaxis, you should always be prepared to cope with an emergency reaction. You should carry an epinephrine autoinjector (EpiPen, Adrenaclick, Twinject) and you should not hike, canoe, or mountain-climb alone.

Avoidance

Beekeeping is one of the most profitable, easily managed forms of farming for the small entrepreneur, but it is not the career of choice for the insect-allergic person. Important research on bee allergy has been done using the blood of beekeepers.

In addition to not working with bees, allergic persons should be sure there are no bee or wasp nests in or near their homes. It is always best if a nonallergic person gets rid of the nests, but with the products on the market now (powerful, long-distance spray insecticides), the process is pretty safe. Just be sure to follow directions and wait until well after dark before spraying the nests.

Try to get rid of the nests as early in the spring as possible. The residual pesticide tends to discourage further building, reducing the amount of spray needed later.

Because it can be very difficult to spot ground bees (yellow jackets), be careful about going barefoot, gardening, hiking, mowing, field riding and trail riding on horses, and other outdoor activities.

If you have wasps flying around your house, try to locate the nest and get rid of it, rather than just spraying the individuals.

Do not go out in summer wearing scented cosmetics or hygienic products. Do not picnic or snack outdoors. Bees and wasps love soda, sweet iced tea or tea with orange, corn on the cob, watermelon, and other sweet foods.

Do not drink out of doors from soda cans, straws, or dark bottles. A bee or wasp may have flown into the container. Stings to the throat or tongue can be serious even in nonallergic individuals.

Be careful around compost heaps and while handling garbage.

If you have an article of clothing that seems to attract bees (and any strong or bright color or pattern—even black—may do so), do not wear it in daylight during the summer. Neutral shades, such as tan, may be safer. Insect repellants provide little or no benefit.

It is best not to have honeysuckle or other very sweet plants near your home.

Be careful when painting a house, cleaning gutters, and so on.

Inspect your car for bees before driving. If a bee flies in while you are on the road, pull over, get out, open the windows, and let the creature fly out. ***Do not try to deal with it while driving.***

TREATMENT OF ANAPHYLAXIS

For almost all varieties of anaphylaxis, there are basically three treatments: avoidance of triggers, avoidance of medications that complicate anaphylaxis, and emergency treatment measures. The main exception is insect stings, for which immunization therapy can be used, as we just described above. Currently there are efforts being made to orally desensitize persons allergic to various foods. A drug with similar characteristics to Xolair may be used in the near future to control peanut and tree-nut allergies, so these potential treatments should be included as well. Idiopathic anaphylaxis often can be suppressed with medication as described above. Occasionally, an effort is made to desensitize a drug-allergic person so that the drug can be used in treatment. This must be done under constant medical supervision in a hospital.

Persons who are at risk for anaphylaxis should, if possible, avoid taking certain medications. These include (1) beta-blockers (used mostly for high blood pressure, migraine, and glaucoma therapy), which decrease the effectiveness of epinephrine, making an episode more severe; (2) ACE inhibitors and ARB (angiotensin receptor blockers) drugs (used mostly for high blood pressure therapy). These drugs block the body's response to a fall in blood pressure and can make an episode of anaphylaxis more severe; (3) monoamine oxidase (MAO) inhibitors, which can cause severe life-threatening reactions to epinephrine; (4) some tricyclic antidepressants, which also can have negative interactions with epinephrine and thus complicate an episode of anaphylaxis.

The key in emergency treatment is injection of epinephrine (Adrenalin) as soon as possible after the reaction begins.

> You should *never* wait to see if the reaction is going to be severe to take the epinephrine, nor should you take an antihistamine first to see if that will control it. Delaying administration of epinephrine is a major cause of mortality in anaphylaxis and may increase the likelihood of a biphasic response (where the reaction resolves only to begin again one to seventy-two hours later).

Injection of epinephrine (Adrenalin) stops the release of the chemical mediators of the allergic reaction, and it buys time to get to the hospital or to call medical personnel to the scene. The patient should be in an emergency room or under the care of trained emergency medical technicians within five to fifteen minutes of the onset of the attack if possible and should use the autoinjectable epinephrine on the way there. This is because about one third of reactions start up again immediately after the epinephrine (Adrenalin) wears off. The epinephrine autoinjectors (EpiPen, Adrenaclick, Twinject) now take this fact into account and come with two doses.

Epinephrine (Adrenalin) injections can be repeated every fifteen minutes. Antihistamines and bronchodilators (beta$_2$-agonist) may be added. Intravenous medications and fluid replacement are often indicated. Oxygen therapy and the insertion of a tube into the trachea to keep it open are frequently necessary. Corticosteroids are used to prevent a late-phase reaction later.

Anyone who has had an anaphylactic attack, indeed perhaps anyone in an isolated household, should have at hand emergency epinephrine (Adrenalin) in autoinjectable form. This applies even to patients on venom immunotherapy. We usually speak of having an EpiPen because that is the device most patients use most easily. There is also an EpiPen Jr for children. A newer autoinjector is Twinject, which has one syringe that contains one autoinjectable dose and then the syringe needs to be partially disassembled to administer the second dose.

You must follow the instructions given with the kit and given by your doctor. Your doctor should show you how to use the epinephrine autoinjector (EpiPen, Adrenaclick,

Twinject). In particular, be sure to replace the drug when it expires or as stipulated in the instructions.

You should also wear a MedicAlert bracelet or carry a card stating that you are allergic and that you have had anaphylaxis, as well as stating the cause of the anaphylaxis.

Chapter 14

OCCUPATIONAL ALLERGIES AND "SICK BUILDINGS"

Noxious substances in the workplace are a common problem. We will concentrate on allergic or other immune system reactions to substances that can indicate a potentially critical health problem in the working environment, such as a contaminated air-conditioning system. Sometimes even allergic reactions, if not recognized and treated, can cause life-threatening damage, usually to the lungs.

FRESH AIR

Benjamin Franklin wrote, "No common air from without is so unwholesome as the air within a closed room that has been often breathed and not changed." Indeed, good air exchange is essential to avoiding pollution of interior air.

Since the 1950s, the trend in architecture has been toward sealed buildings in which natural airflow is replaced by climate-control systems. These systems don't always function as well as they should because of poor design, poor maintenance, poor operation, or all three. The number of allergens, toxins, bacteria, and viruses floating around in the air in some buildings is truly amazing.

In a 1988 article on building-related illnesses in *Clinical Reviews in Allergy and Immunology* by E. J. Bardana Jr., Anthony Montanaro, and M. T. O'Hollaren, the authors note that indoor air pollution in the United States became even worse after the energy crisis (oil shortage) of the 1970s. Professional engineering standards for indoor ventilation were reduced from ten cubic feet replaced per minute per person to five cubic feet per minute. Moreover, the ten-cubic-foot standard was itself a reduction from thirty cubic feet per minute, the standard earlier in the century. The American

Society of Heating, Refrigerating, and Air-Conditioning Engineers now recommend replacing twenty cubic feet of air per minute per person.

Among the infectious diseases transmitted through ventilation, heating, and cooling systems is Legionnaires' disease, which killed twenty-nine people staying at the same hotel in Philadelphia in 1976 during an American Legion convention. A similar disease is Pontiac fever. Q fever, usually contracted from animals, also can be transmitted in a building's climate-control system.

Two of the most-serious allergic or immunologic diseases caused by substances circulating in closed environments are occupational asthma and hypersensitivity pneumonitis.

OCCUPATIONAL ASTHMA

Occupational asthma is fairly common, but only a minority of cases are allergic in nature. Nonallergic occupational asthma typically involves the release of chemical mediators that provoke an allergy-like response. But the allergy antibody, IgE, does not play a role.

The distinction may seem academic from the patient's point of view, but making the correct diagnosis of the type of asthma can be important in designing the treatment. Avoidance is usually the treatment of choice, but if the asthma has an allergy component, allergy immunotherapy may be helpful.

The mechanism of nonallergic occupational asthma is not completely known. The harmful substance may irritate nerves in the lungs. Or it may act by opening up the space between cells in the lungs' lining, exposing, and stimulating underlying mast cells and the release of chemical mediators. Either way, the result is asthmatic bronchoconstriction and inflammation.

Workers who already have one of the other atopic allergic diseases (allergic rhinitis or atopic dermatitis) are at a greater-than-normal risk of contracting allergic occupational asthma. This is also true of people with a family history of atopic diseases.

If the asthma is allergic, then the diagnosis can be made by skin tests or RAST. If not, one must narrow the field through a careful case history and other means. Naturally a pattern of illness associated with the workplace is an indicator of the likely diagnosis. The patient may complain of coughing or wheezing at work, sometimes with rhinitis symptoms (sneezing, stuffy nose, burning eyes), then report that at night; or on the weekends, the symptoms fade. The association is not always so clear, however, because late-phase reactions sometimes take place away from work.

A doctor should ask whether your work exposes you to any of the well-known culprits in occupational asthma. The offending substances that cause allergic asthma very often come from animals. For example, one-fifth of laboratory workers who handle animals have symptoms of allergic rhinitis or allergic asthma related to their work.

Plant proteins also can cause allergic asthma. For example, proteolytic enzymes used in the manufacture of detergents cause adverse reactions in many workers. (Exposure to detergents at home as well as work makes the onset of asthma more likely.) Mold spores in very large quantities from grains, grasses, and wood can also cause asthma.

Rhinitis usually precedes the asthma, so if you are getting symptoms resembling hay fever or a cold at work, try to determine as early as possible whether the problem is exposure to an allergen. You do not want to progress from rhinitis to asthma, so pay attention if your eyes are burning and you are sneezing and sniffling. If the symptoms continue for more than two weeks, see a doctor.

If the problem is exposure to allergens circulated through a humidifier or other climate-control mechanism at work, the diagnosis and treatment can be quite difficult, as they may require the cooperation of management. You may have to change jobs. Ideally, air sampling of the workplace should be done. For many allergens and toxins, the National Institute for Occupational Safety and Health has established guidelines for permissible levels in the air.

Hypersensitivity Pneumonitis

In its acute form, this disease is an explosive reaction to inhaling some type of organic dust or vapor. The disease is just as likely to hit someone who is not allergic as someone who is. Even if you have no allergies and come from an allergy-free family, you may still be affected.

Among the hundreds of inhalants that may cause pneumonitis are numerous plant and animal proteins (as in urine, feces, and dander) as well as mold spores and microorganisms from food, hair, hay, sawdust, and so on.

Pneumonitis is the result of an intense sensitization that can take months or years to develop. But once you have become hypersensitized to a particular substance, you are liable to experience a severe immunologic inflammatory reaction in the lungs if you inhale that substance. This reaction typically occurs within four to six hours after exposure. The symptoms are cough, difficulty breathing, fever (sometimes as high as 104 degrees Fahrenheit), with chills and aches. The symptoms may persist up to eighteen hours. If the cause of the disease is a sensitivity to bird droppings, there may be a two-phase reaction, with asthmalike symptoms preceding the more typical flulike reaction.

Thermoactinomyces bacteria, found in damp hay, straw, and other vegetation, can also infest certain air-conditioning and humidifying systems (including room humidifiers in which stagnant water and debris collect). When this substance vaporizes and is circulated, it can cause hypersensitivity pneumonitis, called in this case ventilation pneumonitis.

Recovery from a pneumonitis attack is spontaneous, but the symptoms will reappear at the next exposure. Repeated attacks may lead to loss of appetite, weight loss, and severe breathlessness.

DIAGNOSIS

A doctor listening to your chest during an acute attack will probably hear distinctive sounds called rales. Blood studies are likely to show an increase in immunoglobulins and white blood cells, as if you had a severe infection. Pulmonary function may be markedly changed from your normal performance.

Unpleasant as all this may be, at least the severity of the symptoms tends to drive people to seek medical help. Unfortunately, there is a chronic form of hypersensitivity pneumonitis, in which the patient suffers similar but very mild symptoms. Often the main sign of trouble is nothing more than a nagging cough, which seems like some kind of stubborn bronchitis. The signs of chronic pneumonitis are shortness of breath and weight loss over time. In the meantime, the lungs are becoming fibrotic (scarred). They can become so damaged, in fact, that the patient may die.

Obviously it is important not to ignore persistent health problems. There is always a reason for a cough and breathlessness. It may be minor or it may be critical, but it should be found.

In order to establish the diagnosis, it may be necessary to run special challenge tests using the suspect substance, such as debris from a humidifier or, if the patient is a farmer, dust from moldy hay. Such tests are usually done in a hospital. After inhaling the suspect substance, the patient is monitored for twenty-four hours on a variety of factors, including pulmonary function. A lung biopsy may be helpful in checking for lung-tissue damage. Challenge is difficult and is only done in a few centers. There is danger to this procedure as well. Research continues to find less-invasive ways to definitively diagnose these illnesses.

TREATMENT

Treatment of hypersensitivity pneumonitis is first of all avoidance of the offending substance. Sometimes, improved ventilation, air filtration, a cleaning of the climate-control system, or wearing a breathing mask can provide adequate protection. But a change of occupation, job, or residence may be necessary.

Pharmaceutical-treatment centers on the administration of oral corticosteroids (cortisone), but steroid treatment should never be substituted for avoidance since it does not halt the progress of the disease when there is chronic exposure.

WORKERS AT RISK

The following are some of the occupations in which one may be exposed to substances causing hypersensitivity pneumonitis or asthmatic reactions.

ANIMAL WORKERS

People who work with animals in laboratories, veterinary offices, farms, or elsewhere or who simply have pets may develop allergic asthma or hypersensitivity pneumonitis from exposure to the dander, urine, or feces of the animals. People working with birds, for instance, may develop what is called pigeon breeder's (or bird breeder's) disease, or hen worker's disease. The dried feces of pigeons, parakeets, chickens, and other birds can enter the air and be inhaled, causing hypersensitivity pneumonitis. Similarly, jockeys are more likely than those in the general population to come down with asthma.

BAKERS

Baker's asthma, which affects as many as 10 percent of bakers, may be caused by allergenic proteins in flour and grains. Fungi of the *Aspergillus* and *Alternaria* genuses and other organisms such as storage mites have also been linked to baker's asthma. The disease, which may take years to develop, is usually preceded by allergic rhinitis; and there seems to be a genetic aspect—that is, those from atopic families are more likely to get it.

COSMETICIANS AND HAIRDRESSERS

The beauty business is not all glamour. Hairdressers have been reported to develop rhinitis and asthma as a result of allergy to human hair or dander. Persulfates in bleach can cause asthma, and many other chemicals used in treating hair and in cosmetics cause both respiratory and skin reactions.

DETERGENT WORKERS

A sensitivity to subtilisin (an animal enzyme in detergents) can cause respiratory distress among people involved in manufacturing detergents. Exposure at home can also be an inciting factor in the development or continuation of the illness.

DOCKWORKERS AND GRANARY WORKERS

Grains of all sorts contain allergens that may affect the sensitive person, leading to asthma and eventually, if untreated, to serious lung disease. Grain fever is essentially the same as baker's asthma.

FARMERS

Farmers frequently breathe in bacteria and fungi in hay, straw, and grains. The *Aspergillus* fungus and *Thermoactinomyces* bacterium are common farm menaces, causing pneumonitis, often called farmer's lung. Working with wet baled hay or in a closed barn in winter may cause intense exposure.

Farmers who handle animals are susceptible to the afflictions of animal workers described above.

FOOD PROCESSORS AND COOKS

People preparing many kinds of food develop allergic rhinitis and asthma.

Allergies to plant proteins and plant enzymes also afflict food processors. Mushroom worker's disease is a type of hypersensitivity pneumonitis and is secondary to exposure to *Thermoactinomyces* bacteria.

Dust from coffee beans and cocoa beans can also be a fairly potent allergen, as can moldy malt, in which the allergen *Aspergillus* mold may be present. The result is malt worker's disease.

Cheese worker's lung is caused by an allergy to cheese mold. Sensitivity to eggs can cause allergy symptoms among food processors, bakers, and cooks. Simply inhaling vapors of a food to which one is allergic can set off a reaction.

Meatpackers occasionally develop asthma from inhaling the vapors of the polyvinyl plastic wrap used to package meat in supermarkets. The fumes, which come from heating the plastic to seal the wrap, can be avoided by using a wrap that can be sealed without heating.

FURRIERS AND TAXIDERMISTS

People working with fur and pelts are prone to a number of infections and adverse reactions caused by the pathogens in fur or by chemicals used to prepare the furs. These problems are difficult to avoid, even when strict cleanliness is practiced.

METALWORKERS AND WELDERS

Sensitivity to fumes from heated galvanized steel may cause metal fume fever among welders. The symptoms are respiratory distress and fever. Allergic asthma is an occupational hazard among those involved with processing and plating chromium, nickel, or platinum.

PAINT AND INK MANUFACTURERS AND PAINTERS

Asthma caused by castor bean dust is a hazard in the manufacture of substances such as certain paints, varnishes, inks, and cosmetics, which use the castor bean. Painters and woodworkers also may develop lung disease due to sensitivity to these substances.

PHARMACEUTICAL WORKERS

The same allergic sensitivity that causes some people to have adverse reactions to penicillin and other antibiotics affects workers in the pharmaceutical industry who inhale dust or vapors from these drugs.

PLASTICS, GLUE, AND CHEMICAL WORKERS

Diisocynates (such as toluene 2,4-diisocyanate, or TDI) used in the manufacture of various chemicals, foam, plastics, and adhesives can cause allergic asthma and, less commonly, hypersensitivity pneumonitis. Workers exposed to these chemicals include not only those in factories but also spray painters, people who work with plastic food wrappings, and many others. Reactions to epoxy resins afflict both plastics workers and woodworkers. Exposure to fish-based glue, which is common among bookbinders and postal workers, can cause reactions in people allergic to fish.

POTTERS AND OTHER ARTISTS

Potter's lung, a reaction to clay dust, is only one of many dozens of ailments that affect artists. Clay, glazes, paints, solvents, fixatives, metal fumes, inks, and so on all are likely to produce adverse toxic or immunological reactions, some permanent or fatal. When buying art materials for children, be sure that they are nontoxic.

An organization that provides information on safety in art materials is Arts, Crafts, and Theater Safety (ACTS, www.artscraftstheatersafety.org); we assume the pun is intended.

PRINTERS

Printing involves exposure to a variety of chemical fumes and vegetable gums that may cause allergic respiratory or skin disorders.

REFRIGERATION AND AIR-CONDITIONING WORKERS

Exposure to chemical fumes and to microorganisms, especially the bacteria *Micropolyspora* and *Thermoactinomyces,* can lead to humidifier lung, or air-conditioner lung.

SUGARCANE WORKERS

Bagasse is, collectively, fibers and residues remaining after sugarcanes are crushed for syrup. Sensitivity to *Micropolyspora* and *Thermoactinomyces* in the bagasse causes sugarcane worker's fever, or bagassosis. This can lead to hypersensitivity pneumonitis.

TEXTILE-MILL WORKERS

Byssinosis, sometimes called mill fever, is a lung disease common among workers exposed to cotton fibers, flax, or hemp. The symptoms are breathlessness, wheezing, cough, and often, fever. If not treated for the disease, even an initially healthy person may eventually become very ill with respiratory blockage and emphysema. The condition can be fatal.

It is believed that the cause may be at least in part a sensitivity to toxins produced by bacteria in the plant fibers.

WOODWORKERS AND BUILDERS

Sawmill workers, carpenters, and furniture makers are exposed to wood dust and to a variety of strong chemicals used to treat and finish wood. The dust of Western red cedar, probably the most-studied wood dust, is a well-documented cause of asthma. The substance in the wood causing the harm is believed to be plicatic acid. Unfortunately, years may pass before the asthma recedes, even after no further exposure to the dust. Wood molds can also cause respiratory damage. Sequoiasis, a type of pneumonitis, is caused by moldy redwood. To the best of our knowledge, this is the only word in the English language that has a Greek and Cherokee root.

WATER TECHNICIAN

People responsible for treating drinking water may be exposed to hydrazine, which causes symptoms that initially mimic a cold or allergy: sore throat, sniffles, and eye irritation. In October 1995, the *Mount Sinai Journal of Medicine* reported the case of a hospital water technician who was treated with antibiotics for these symptoms. Unfortunately, this worker suffered far worse damage (memory loss, autoimmune damage, and impotence) before the cause of his illness was discovered.

SICK-BUILDING SYNDROME

There are some modern buildings, both residential and commercial, where the tight, energy-efficient but low-ventilation system results in polluted, contaminated air. In such buildings, infectious organisms in the climate-control system and even in water pipes and shower heads can cause serious respiratory disease.

Fumes from construction materials, carpeting, and potent cleaning substances can cause headaches, fatigue, upper respiratory irritation, asthma, and a variety of other disorders. Poor ventilation may be associated with these fumes as well as with high levels of carbon dioxide and even carbon monoxide, which, of course, are dangerous toxins. Fiberglass particles in the air irritate the skin and eyes and are unhealthy to breathe. Mites and molds thrive in damp indoor environments, possibly contributing to allergies and asthma. Pesticides and fungicides used to eliminate the mites and molds can linger in an airless space, sickening those who must work or live there.

Fumes associated with dry cleaning work are particularly stubborn, sometimes causing problems even after the cleaner has shut down. For example, in New York City in 1997, a new elementary school in Harlem had to be closed temporarily because of fumes. The building had formerly housed a dry cleaning business. The toxic agent was perchloroethylene, a cleaning solvent.

A family house may be a sick building; but the term is most often used for an office building, school, apartment house, factory, or other structures in which those who must spend time there have little control over their environment. Typically, sick buildings are the focus of longstanding complaints from workers or others inside while management maintains that the workers' symptoms are trivial or the result of mass suggestion or malingering.

In recent years, the federal Occupational Safety and Health Administration (OSHA), corresponding state agencies, and insurance companies have become more sophisticated in identifying factors that may be the cause of a building's being sick. And building managers are somewhat more aware of the need for ventilation following the installation of carpet or a visit from the exterminator. Nevertheless, individuals and even workers collectively may face an uphill fight in trying to arrange adequate tests for a suspected sick building. For example, years of complaints preceded the discovery of high levels of carbon monoxide at the Sloan-Kettering Cancer Center in New York City in 1997. Seven hundred workers were moved to new quarters.

On the other hand, while sick buildings clearly do exist, complaints regarding sick buildings sometimes are difficult to verify, both with respect to the building and the symptoms of those affected. Claims that buildings have caused "multiple chemical sensitivity," rendering the person allergic to almost all synthetic materials, understandably have created anxiety among building managers and their insurers concerning their liability for questionable disorders (see chapters 14 and 19). In the twenty-first century, many of the claims about multiple chemical sensitivity have been debunked. There have been several position papers by the American College of Physicians and the American College of Occupational and Environmental Medicine as well as the Council on Scientific Affairs of the American Medical Association, which take the position that most of the claims concerning multiple chemical sensitivity are nebulous at best.

HUMIDIFIER FEVER

Humidifier fever is sometimes categorized as a type of hypersensitivity pneumonitis, approximately identical to ventilation fever. But the term can also be used generally to refer to flulike reactions to molds, bacteria, and other contaminants spread by humidifying systems. The disease may have an asthma component. Typically, when a workplace humidifier is involved, the symptoms—which can include fever, chills, headaches, chest tightness, and shortness of breath—flare up early in the week and subside when one has time off.

FORMALDEHYDE AND OTHER CONSTRUCTION MATERIALS

Use of formaldehyde has declined in recent years since it has been identified by the Environmental Protection Agency as a probable carcinogen. No longer are high school biology labs filled with an unforgettable odor from barrels of formaldehyde and dead frogs awaiting dissection. Nevertheless, formaldehyde is still used in no-press textiles, plywood, and a number of other construction and furnishing materials, including materials for drapes and carpets. It is believed to be the cause of numerous adverse reactions (evidently not IgE mediated), including bronchitis, hives and rashes, and headaches.

There is a certain amount of skepticism in the medical community concerning reports of formaldehyde sensitivity. Nevertheless, chemicals entering the air from construction materials or textiles must be on the list of suspects when one encounters the sick-building syndrome.

In an embarrassing incident in 1988, workers at the Environmental Protection Agency building in Washington, DC, fell ill with flulike symptoms, sore throats, and burning lips. Apparently, the new carpet being installed was irritating the workers. The chemical most likely to have caused the problem was identified as 4-PCH, a by-product of the latex used in carpet backing and glue. This chemical is now being used less in carpet backings, and manufacturers are said to be airing out their products more thoroughly before installation. Nevertheless, during carpet installation, it is advisable to keep a good flow of air through the area being carpeted.

It is not possible to avoid all the hazards that might arise from exposure to chemicals in construction materials and office furnishings. But if you or your coworkers have a problem with a particular product, the U.S. Consumer Product Safety Commission (CPSC) may be able to provide relevant information (www.cpsc.gov).

RADS (REACTIVE AIRWAY DYSFUNCTION) AND IIA (IRRITANT-INDUCED ASTHMA)

RADS and IIA are both types of irritant-induced nonallergic asthma. Both are caused by the inhalation of irritating substance, such as smoke, dust, fumes, gases, and vapors. The most common substances causing RADS are chlorine, TDI, and oxides of nitrogen. RADS occurs in a person within twenty-four hours of exposure, whereas IIA occurs after more than twenty-four hours of exposure but usually after at least several weeks of exposure with low-grade symptoms developing. Both syndromes last several months to years. If they go away within a few days, the involved person is lucky, but then their reaction is probably not RADS or IIA.

We will discuss both syndromes below. However, if you are exposed to a toxic substance in a confined space and developed asthma symptoms of wheezing cough and shortness of breath within twenty-four hours of exposure, see your doctor or go to the emergency room immediately. The list of possible substances is extensive but includes chlorine, ammonia, acetic acid, and sulfur dioxide. The list of potential causes continues to grow. Other common causes are bleaching and cleaning agents as well as fire and smoke. Spray and heated paints, floor sealants, and metal removers are also potential troublemakers. Finally, formalin has been reported to cause respiratory illness. The others are rare, and if you are having the symptoms described below, you should already be at your physician's office.

The criteria for these illnesses are the following:

1. A documented absence of preceding respiratory symptoms for at least the past two years. However, even if you currently have asthma and the exposure occurs and your symptoms increase, then consult your physician immediately.
2. The onset of symptoms occurred after a single specific exposure or accident. However, to complicate matters, multiple low-grade exposures can cause this syndrome. So if you think you are getting low-grade noxious exposures (in that your symptoms are mild and tolerable), then you should also consult with your physician if the exposure was to a gas, smoke, fume, or vapor that was present in very high concentrations and had irritant qualities to its nature. The onset of symptoms occurred within twenty-four hours after the exposure and persisted for at least three months.
3. Symptoms simulated asthma with cough, wheezing, and dyspnea predominating.
4. Pulmonary function tests may show airflow obstruction.
5. Positive methacholine challenge, which is a diagnostic test in which a patient inhales methacholine in increasing concentrations and performs repeated pulmonary tests before, during, and after. Normal persons tolerate higher doses of methacholine before they get bronchoconstriction.
6. Other pulmonary diseases are ruled out.

Both diseases were defined in 1985 but were undoubtedly present for many years before that. The World Trade Center tragedy in 2001 induced both illnesses depending on degree of exposure in many first responders and others who were involved with the early cleanup as well as people who lived or worked in the immediate vicinity after the attack and before it became apparent how dangerous this was.

Treatment is symptomatic and is the same for asthma.

However, prevention should really be the goal. So do not work with noxious substances in enclosed spaces with poor air exchange and never without proper protection. If workers come into your office or home and are working with a noxious agent, especially if they are dressed in space-age garb, then you need to either get out of the area (preferably) while the work is being done or at least suit up with the appropriate mask and protective gear.

Chapter 15

PSYCHOLOGICAL ASPECTS OF ALLERGY

With any chronic disease, especially when the symptoms are relatively mild, the person affected is probably going to have to put up with an occasional suspicion on the part of family or friends that the ailment is "psychological." This is true of lower-back pain (which always seems to flare up at the worst moments), arthritis, ulcers, and of course, asthma and allergies.

Actually, there very likely is a psychological component to all or most diseases. If you have suffered a loss or shock, such as death of a spouse or unexpected unemployment, you are at greater risk of developing any number of diseases, including cancer.

There also seems to be a conditioning mechanism at work in some types of allergy. With hay fever, for example, research has shown that if you have been exposed to a potent allergen in a particular locale, you may undergo an allergic reaction upon returning to that place, even if the allergen is no longer present. This is a conditioned response.

In an experiment with asthmatics allergic to cats, a significant number showed changes in pulmonary function when inhaling a solution in a nebulizer that they were told contained cat dander but that did not.

In perhaps the most-surprising experimental result in this field, laboratory rats were given intradermal skin tests for various allergens and then certain musical sounds were played for forty-eight hours as the tests developed in the skin. Subsequently, animals that tested positive were subjected to the same test—but using only a water solution—and the same musical sounds. The animals tested positive to the water.

The interaction between the mind and the immune system is stronger than generally realized. But this does not mean that the immune system's reaction in a conditioned response is "psychological" rather than physical. In these conditioned allergic responses, your sensory and neural systems convey the message "allergen danger"; and your immune system responds with protective mechanisms, such as mucus production, bronchial constriction, mast cell activation in the skin, and so on.

This is not a neurotic response. It is as normal a physical reaction as any other. It does not mean that the disease is "just in your head" or that you can cure it if you "really want to." It means that our thoughts and emotions and the functioning of our bodies is inextricably intertwined.

The role of the psyche in disease is one of the world's most-debated questions. Luckily, one need not resolve it in order to use medical information constructively. For example, the symptoms of an asthma attack and the symptoms of an anxiety reaction are very similar. All too many people get in serious trouble with asthma because they try to "just calm down" when they should be calling a taxi or ambulance and heading for the hospital. If you have asthma, don't analyze the cause of the attack; treat the symptoms. After you are better, you can explore the cause.

PAROXYSMAL SNEEZING

Frequent sneezing, a typical symptom of allergic rhinitis, is a normal physiological response to an irritant in the nasal mucosa. The sneezing reflex is initiated by irritation of the trigeminal facial nerve.

Paroxysmal sneezing, which is sudden, violent sneezing of unusual frequency and duration, evidently is sometimes psychogenic in nature. Adolescent girls are particularly susceptible to this disorder. There may be a history of sexual abuse, and patients tend to be compulsive.

The symptom is not quite a full sneeze, and patients keep their eyes open while sneezing and may be able to carry on normal activities without apparent distress.

A full workup, including an MRI, should be done in these cases because there is a variety of possible physical causes, including (rarely) encephalitis and tumors, also epilepsy, allergies, and nasal septal deviation. The sneezing may be associated with pregnancy, sexual excitement, or exposure to light.

If the sneezing is mainly psychogenic in nature, the recommended treatment is likely to be some form of psychiatric medication, perhaps in conjunction with hypnosis or some form of psychotherapy.

SIGHING DYSPNEA

This disorder involves a breathing difficulty that is occasionally mistaken for asthma and is sometimes associated with it. Sighing dyspnea may also be associated with cardiovascular or thyroid disease and with sinusitis. However, it is usually psychogenic in nature.

Dyspnea means difficulty breathing or shortness of breath, and the patient's main complaint is usually inability to get a full breath. The disorder ordinarily affects girls and women in the second to fourth decades of life. The patient sighs deeply and repeatedly in an attack that can last up to several hours. The experience is uncomfortable and frightening, for the feeling is that one cannot get air. The chief cause, if there is one, appears to be stress. It can also be a symptom of anxiety, which is associated with many psychiatric disorders. Again, the recommended treatment is primarily psychotherapeutic.

Asthma Mimic (Vocal Cord Dysfunction)

There is a disorder that mimics an asthma attack and is due primarily to anxiety. This disorder involves a panic dysfunction of the vocal cords, in which the cords move in the wrong direction on exhalation, temporarily blocking air. The patient, who appears to be in danger of choking to death, would benefit at that moment from professional reassurance and distraction designed to give the vocal cords an opportunity to relax and assume a normal position. Instead, patients are often subject to extreme emergency treatment, including intubation (for a respirator) or tracheotomy.

There are several ways of differentiating between vocal cord (glottal) dysfunction and an asthma attack. With vocal cord dysfunction, patients can speak and hold their breath. If asked to cough, the patient can do so; and this response may actually set the vocal cords right, relieving the attack. In asthma attacks, patients cannot speak well and get worse if asked to hold their breath or cough. Another diagnostic test is that people with glottal dysfunction are not adversely affected by breathing mecholyl in a challenge test, whereas asthmatics begin to wheeze.

The most-effective treatment for glottal dysfunction is psychological counseling to help the patient overcome the anxiety or tension that causes the vocal cords to malfunction. Breathing training and voice training may also help. Most asthmatics, however, will not benefit from this approach, although learning breathing and relaxation techniques may be generally useful in helping the patient cope with the disease.

Habit Cough

Habit cough is a diagnosis of exclusion, meaning you have to rule out other possible causes of cough first. Since there is nothing physically wrong with the patient and because it responds to behavioral therapies, it is mentioned here. A more complete discussion about this condition is in chapter 16, as it most commonly occurs in persons less than age eighteen and is the second most common cause of cough in that age group.

Stress

The major villain among psychological causes of physical disease is stress. The stress can be physical as well as psychological in origin. For example, a maltreated child who is physically abused is also emotionally stressed. The overworked single parent may be both sleep deprived and chronically anxious over how to make financial ends meet.

People vary enormously in how much stress they can tolerate. Some are bored without constant pressure and challenges. Some need to work quietly, with lots of time to relax. Most at risk of suffering serious adverse effects from stress are those who physiologically do not handle stress very well—their blood pressure rises, for example—even though they may not consciously sense this reaction at all. They appear calm and they feel calm, but they are heading for a medical crisis.

Pioneer studies of the physical effects of stress were carried out in the 1930s by Hans Selye. He reported that rats that were severely stressed showed changes in their adrenal glands and in their immune systems and developed gastrointestinal ulcers.

The initial changes that take place in reaction to stress (a surge of adrenaline, increased heart rate, and so on) are designed to help you to overcome or escape a dangerous or painful situation, whether it is social (such as a sadistic boss at work) or physical (a bad automobile accident). But if the pain cannot be overcome or avoided and the stress is severe and long lasting, most people will eventually suffer exhaustion and dysfunction in one or more body systems.

Fear and anger act on the autonomic nervous system, which controls the functioning of internal organs and blood and lymph vessels, but it is not known why some people under stress are affected in one organ system rather than another—why, for example, some develop stomach symptoms while others develop respiratory illnesses. Possibly an original imbalance in the biochemistry of an organ makes it prone to dysfunction under stress.

The allergy diseases that seem to be influenced most frequently by one's psychological state are eczema, hives, and allergic asthma. There is no scientific estimate of what percentage of patients having these diseases might experience an improvement through reducing stress or increasing happiness, but a guess based on years of experience is that about one-third may be in that category. This third would include children. We often forget how stressful children's lives can be. Some children are severely depressed, and a recent study has indicated that depression in asthmatic children significantly increases their risk of dying of the disease.

With respect to asthma, stress lowers the level of the neurotransmitter CAMP, a substance that asthmatics need; for it counteracts bronchoconstriction and the release of histamine and other chemical mediators by the mast cells. Through its effect on the mast cells, the reduction in CAMP may also play a role in outbreaks of eczema, hives, and rhinitis (see chapter 12).

There is a type of perennial rhinitis, vasomotor rhinitis, which is similar to perennial allergic rhinitis, except that no allergic factor can be found. Psychological factors may play a role in this disorder.

Stress may play a role in the causation of chronic hives, although it is not the only cause. There is less evidence that stress influences acute hives.

MEDICINES AND MOOD CHANGES

Being sick undermines one's psychological well-being. People who have never suffered an asthma attack have difficulty appreciating how frightening and at the same time infuriating these episodes can be. No one is at their best when trying to cope with repeated episodes of what may be a life-threatening illness. To add to the patient's psychological burden, the medicines prescribed may cause mood changes as well.

Antihistamines, of course, are widely used in the treatment of allergies; and the H_1-antihistamines are famous for producing lethargy. Paradoxically, in some patients, especially children, antihistamines may stimulate the central nervous system, causing anxiety, difficulty sleeping, arid restlessness. The H_2 antihistamines, especially cimetidine (Tagamet), have been associated with confusion in elderly patients. Alcohol and other recreational drugs are likely to exaggerate these side effects.

Many of the problems traditionally associated with H_1-antihistamines can be avoided by using the new nonsoporific or nonsedating antihistamines, loratadine (Claritin), desloratadine (Clarinex), and fexofenadine (Allegra). See chapter 5.

Several of the drugs used to treat asthma and occasionally other severe allergic conditions may cause restlessness, anxiety, shakiness, and difficulty concentrating. The most tricky to handle are the oral corticosteroids, which may have to be taken over long periods. They can cause insomnia, mood swings from agitation to depression, and may even (although rarely) produce psychotic symptoms. Withdrawal, after long-term use, can lead to depression; and for both physical and psychological reasons, it should always be gradual.

Montelukast (Singulair), which is used for treating asthma and allergies, was in the news recently and generated a lot of concern. Several adolescents recently started on the drug had committed suicide. Keep this in perspective that millions of people have used this drug. The FDA issued a warning about a possible association between this drug and depression and suicide attempts. Further studies have been conducted, and although there is no absolute cause-and-effect relationship between montelukast (Singulair) and depression and suicide, the warning remains in effect. The warning also applies to the other two drugs in this class: zafirlukast (Accolate) and zileuton (Zyflo). The neuropsychiatric events that are included in this warning are agitation, aggression, anxiousness, dream abnormalities and hallucinations, depression, insomnia, irritability, restlessness, suicidal thinking and behavior (including suicide), and tremor. These drugs have been used safely in millions of patients. The significance of these reports and this FDA warning is still not known. In general, we do not prescribe these drugs to patients with a history of these psychiatric symptoms.

Theophylline, which is occasionally prescribed for both children and adults with asthma, is related to caffeine. The effects are variable, but jumpiness and difficulty concentrating are common. Needless to say, this may affect a child's schoolwork.

Beta$_2$-agonists and epinephrine may cause tremors and anxiety. Ephedrine too is a stimulant and may increase alertness, but it also may cause insomnia and irritability.

Some allergy patients, typically older patients, are also regularly taking medications other than those prescribed for the allergy. Your doctors and your pharmacist should be aware of every medicine you may be taking, including nonprescription ones.

Ask what precautions you should observe, what side effects to watch out for, and what is the best way to take each medication: with food? at night? Write down the information and keep it with your medicines. Do not feel embarrassed to ask these questions again frequently. New information on the effects of drugs is constantly being discovered.

TREATMENT

In the twelfth century, Maimonides wrote of the asthma patient, "In mental anguish, fear, mourning or distress, his agitation affects his respiratory organs, and he cannot exercise them at will . . . . The cure lies not in foods, in drugs alone, nor in regular medical advice; psychological methods are a greater help."

In our time, however, at the height of the enthusiasm for Freudian theory, the insight that emotions influence health was sometimes given too much weight. In the 1950s, for example, all too many people with treatable organic disorders were spending time and money on psychoanalysis that was not helping. Patients who deserved sympathy and effective medical treatment were at risk of being told how neurotic they were. Certain personality types were said to have a tendency to develop certain illnesses.

The medical community is now trying to strike a balance in its approach to treatment. Instead of tending to think that certain personality types are to "blame" for certain illnesses, there is attention to research that suggests that often it is the illness itself that alters the personality, producing the suspect characteristics. Today, rather than assuming that psychological disturbance underlies every allergic illness, the focus is more on the particular patient. Your doctor should consider and discuss with you whether stress or lifestyle may play a role in your allergy flare-ups.

To alleviate the anxiety that naturally comes with being sick, ask your doctor for information about the mood swings that ordinarily accompany illness or use of certain medicines. This holds for a children as well as adults. Both parent and child should have an understanding of how the disease and the treatment may affect their feelings and ability to concentrate and work. If you feel that your moods are becoming difficult to handle or that your personality is changing, as the result either of medication or of the disease itself, you have a right to expect a sympathetic and helpful response from your doctor.

Keep in mind, however, that in order to provide effective help, the doctor may have to ask about work conditions, family life, drinking or smoking habits, and other issues that ordinarily are private. It may be that an unhappy child should change schools or that an adult should join Alcoholics Anonymous.

If an intractable problem is identified, your doctor should be able to recommend for your consideration family counseling, a smoking clinic, psychiatric therapy, a 12-step program, or whatever is indicated.

To protect your interests, you should ask a therapist what results should emerge from the treatment and how long the process will take. If the treatment is goal oriented, you will be better able to assess whether it is working or not.

You might think that since some allergy responses apparently can be conditioned, therefore, behavior-oriented conditioning treatment would be especially promising. But the value of such conditioning has not been established. It is far easier to transfer a response to different situations than to eliminate it.

For example, in the classic conditioning experiment, Pavlov's dogs "learned" to salivate upon hearing a bell because many times in the past, that bell had sounded as food was given. One can retrain such dogs so that they do not salivate when a bell rings, but training them not to salivate at feeding time would be another story.

If most of your allergy symptoms are unconditioned—that is, if they are direct responses to allergens in the environment (just as salivating is a direct response to food)—then behavior or conditioning therapy may not be much help.

Turning to other modes of treatment, there is not much scientific evidence to show that psychoanalysis or the various forms of psychotherapy have much effect on the progress of asthma or other allergic conditions. Nevertheless, as we have mentioned, for some people the emotional support of a psychotherapist through this stressful illness can be helpful. Therapists who have a good record in curing panic attacks and phobias may be able to provide some help in reducing anxiety reactions associated with allergic asthma and other allergic diseases.

Physical exercise and some of the relaxation and breathing exercises done in yoga and other similar types of discipline are beneficial to many patients. Of course, if you are under a doctor's care, you should discuss any exercise or sports program with her or him before getting started. Vigorous exercise has both physical and psychological rewards for asthmatics, although it must be carefully managed (see chapter 9). Fresh air, adequate sleep, and a good, healthful diet are also important in coping with almost any illness.

Chapter 16

ALLERGIES IN CHILDREN

Asthma and the associated conditions of allergic rhinitis and eczema are the most-common chronic illnesses in childhood. In the twelve years since the previous edition of this book, there have been major advances, which we detail below.

Allergies in infants and toddlers are almost always handled by the baby's pediatrician, which is appropriate. A well-trained pediatrician is qualified to diagnose and treat most allergies in infants and young children. Allergists are rarely called in for children under age two, unless the case is unusually troublesome—for example, if the child has multiple allergies or allergic asthma.

Later in childhood, however, allergists often take an active role in treatment. One of the main types of allergy treatment, immunotherapy (allergy shots), is more likely to be successful in the five-to-sixty age group than in any other and is almost always undertaken by an allergist.

There are a couple of reasons for waiting until a child is about five to do immunotherapy. There is some concern that the immune system of younger children may not be adequately mature for such treatment and that complications, including anaphylaxis, might arise. Also, it is often not possible to be certain at so young an age that the symptoms will persist.

Nevertheless, in some cases in which an allergy is clearly established, immunotherapy, or allergy shots, may be recommended for a child under age five and may work very well. In particular, children aged two to six who are allergic to mites have been shown to benefit dramatically from allergy shots. The immunotherapy may reverse their illness.

CHILDREN'S ALLERGIES TO FOOD AND DRUGS

Food allergy is increasing in Western nations, and up to 6 percent of children experience allergies to food in the first three years of life. Allergy to cow's milk is common among young children; up to 2.5 percent of children up to age three have it.

That is a reason to breast-feed. Caring for a baby with cow's milk allergy is no fun. Common symptoms are diarrhea, stomach pain, and rashes. Moreover, in the first few weeks of life, breast milk also provides protection against respiratory, gastrointestinal, and meningeal (meningitis) infections.

Soy formula is the standard substitute for cow's milk and has vitamins and minerals added to make it nutritionally equivalent to milk-based formulas. It works 50 percent of the time, but when it doesn't or if the baby develops an allergy to soy as well, then it's time to try a hypoallergenic formula.

There are two types of hypoallergenic formulas: *extensively hydrolyzed* formulas and *elemental* formulas. In the extensively hydrolyzed formulas, the protein has been broken down so that they are more easily digested and less likely to cause a reaction. The following brands are extensively hydrolyzed: Nutramigen Lipil, Pregestimil, and Alimentum. Substitution with an extensively hydrolyzed formula should be the next step as partially hydrolyzed formulas are not acceptable. If this fails, then it's on to the elemental formulas, which are as follows: Neocate, Elecare, and Nutramigen AA Lipil.

If there is a family history of allergies or if your baby has already shown signs of allergy, discuss with your pediatrician the advisability of delaying or limiting the addition of solid food to the baby's diet.

CAN ALLERGY IN INFANCY BE PREVENTED BY ALTERING THE DIET OF THE MOTHER IN PREGNANCY?

Allergists have been intrigued by the idea that altering the diet of a mother during pregnancy could alter the development of allergic disease in a child with a potential to develop allergies. There is presently no sound scientific evidence that alteration of the diet during any stage of pregnancy will affect the allergic state of the developing fetus. However, this matter is still under investigation; therefore, if you are pregnant or about to become pregnant and there are allergies in your family or the father's, be sure to discuss this problem with your allergist and obstetrician. For a more precise definition of which children are at risk of becoming allergic, see below.

ALTERATION OF THE ALLERGIC STATE AFTER BIRTH

The term *atopic march* refers to the natural history of atopic manifestations, characterized by a typical sequence of IgE antibody responses and clinical symptoms that appear during certain age periods, persist over years and decades, and often show a tendency for spontaneous remission with time. Extensive studies have been done concerning the alteration of the atopic march (the development of allergic symptoms in an atopic individual from birth on) by avoidance of food and environmental factors. The results are still not conclusive. (See chapter 4 for a discussion of the environmental controversy.) There is some discussion in chapter 7 of the progression of food allergy in children. In our previous book, we made many suggestions concerning how to feed an allergic infant, and they are detailed below. We still practice those principals pending the resolutions of the various controversies. We suggest that you work very closely with your child's pediatrician as to how to handle feeding and environmental issues. One concept is clear: that smoking during pregnancy and exposing any child (and even worse, an allergic child) to passive smoke will increase the incidence of allergies and asthma (as well as other conditions) in the child.

We agree with Dr. Robert S. Ziegler, at the University of California at San Diego and an acknowledged expert on this subject, that the infants who most likely can be helped by dietary adjustments are those with (1) both parents allergic or (2) one parent allergic and at least one other sibling also allergic.

Such a child can benefit from breast-feeding for four to six months. During the time the child is breast-feeding, the mother should consult with a pediatrician on dietary matters. In general, she should avoid allergenic foods (eggs, milk, peanuts) and should supplement her diet with 1,500 milligrams of elemental calcium to make up for the lack of calcium in the milk that she can't drink (this should be discussed with her obstetrician or her internist).

Soy formula can be just as allergenic as milk. Therefore, if the baby needs a supplement, use a protein hydrolysate formula, such as Nutramigen. Do not introduce any of the allergenic solid foods until after the first year of age. Then the following allergenic foods should be added cautiously, if tolerated, at the rate of one every other week: milk, wheat, soy, corn, citrus, eggs, peanuts, fish. Delay eggs, peanuts, and fish even longer if the child has already shown signs of food allergy.

Foods other than milk are best added to a baby's diet one by one, starting with the least-allergenic foods (rice cereal and scraped banana). If a food allergy develops, the problem food should be withdrawn, although in a year or two, the child may grow out of the sensitivity. Eggs, fruit, chocolate, wheat, orange juice and other acid fruit, and shellfish are common causes of allergic reactions in infants and young children.

Be cautious about concluding on informal evidence that a child is allergic to sweets, "nonorganic" foods, or any other type of food. If you observe that your child does not do well on certain foods, try to keep them out of the child's diet. But before determining that a food should be eliminated altogether, get medical advice. The effects of overly restricting a child's food choices, particularly if based on unproven theories, can create their own problems.

From this point on, the material discussed is not controversial. Anaphylactic reactions to food are rare in childhood. But if one occurs, the child must be taught never again to eat the food that caused the reaction. Set an example by reading food labels with the child and asking questions in restaurants. If the child eats meals at school, be sure that the nutritionist knows of the youngster's allergy and supervises food preparation and consumption accordingly. Notify the school nurse as well.

A child who has had an anaphylactic reaction should carry an epinephrine autoinjector (EpiPen, Adrenaclick, Twinject) and wear or carry a MedicAlert bracelet or similar identification so that people will recognize a medical emergency if it occurs. These devices come in two sizes or dosages. The EpiPen Jr (0.15 milligrams) is for children thirty-three to sixty-six pounds, and the adult size (0.3 milligrams) is suitable for all children above sixty-six pounds. For the Adrenaclick and Twinject, the 0.15 milligram or 0.3 milligram strength must be specified on the prescription. Be sure that you—or in the case of an older child, they—know how to use the device.

Allergies to eggs and milk tend to disappear after age three; but other allergies, such as to peanuts (see chapter 7: more recent studies show that 20 percent of peanut allergies will disappear by age five), tree nuts, and shellfish, tend to last a lifetime. After a number of years have passed, an allergist may recommend a challenge test in a hospital or similarly safe setting to determine if the allergy is still present. The chapters on food and drug allergies contain more information on these subjects.

From a psychological perspective, it is important as far as possible not to make an allergic child feel or appear different from other children. Food allergies should be treated matter-of-factly.

You can help teach a child who absolutely must avoid one or more foods the social skills that will help him or her get through difficult times. A young person who talks incessantly about his or her allergies will soon have many social problems. Kids with smooth manners learn to sound regretful about having to pass on an offered food. Other children's parents are often not sympathetic enough to the needs of a small visitor with allergies.

As for over-the-counter medicines, it is best not to use any one medicine frequently without checking with your pediatrician or family doctor. Some should not be used on children at all. Aspirin is a wonderful drug but is rarely recommended now for people under age eighteen; if given in association with certain viral infections, it may cause Reye's syndrome (a disease affecting the brain and other internal organs). Aspirin sensitivity, associated with asthma and allergy reactions, such as hives, is also common.

If your child is treated with penicillin or another antibiotic, be aware of the possibility that an allergy may develop. In very rare cases an allergy reaction may appear on first exposure. In most or all such cases, there probably has been covert prior exposure in food or by some other means.

If a child is given a shot of any kind, it is best to keep the child in the doctor's office, or at least within reach of medical help, for a half hour in case an anaphylactic reaction occurs. Sometimes a child who is allergic to a drug or serum will complain of a sore throat or will vomit and the parent mistakenly assumes these symptoms are due to the sickness for which the youngster is being treated or are a normal reaction to the shot.

In the hour or so following your child's injection, pay close attention to any complaints involving a sore or swollen mouth or throat, itching or swelling anywhere on the body, hives, or difficulty speaking. If these symptoms start to appear following

**a shot, immediately bring the child back to the doctor's office or
to an emergency room.**

Rashes and Hives

Certain reactions affecting the skin are particularly common among young
children.

As just noted, children are prone to food sensitivities, many of which pass as time
goes on. A common symptom is an outbreak of hives, and acute hives occur more
often among children than in adults.

Not surprisingly, diaper dermatitis, or diaper rash, affects the younger set almost
exclusively. It results from leaving the baby too long in soiled diapers or from using
diapers in which there is a residue of soap or antiseptic. The condition's distinguishing
characteristic is that it affects the skin under the diaper and the adjacent areas of the
stomach and thighs.

The first step in treatment is to keep the child as clean and dry as possible. Change
the diaper frequently and wash the baby with mild soap and water—rinse well. If you
are using cloth diapers, give them an extra rinse to be sure that they are clean. Use only
a mild soap. If you are using a diaper service and you believe that soap or detergent is
the problem, notify them.

According to the Mayo Clinic, there is no compelling evidence that cloth diapers
are better for a baby with diaper rash or eczema. The best advice is to use whatever
agrees with your baby the most and works best for you. It is helpful to leave the baby
without a diaper whenever possible as that will give the irritated skin a chance to dry
and heal.

Zinc oxide ointment as well as petroleum jelly is the most-time-proven method
of providing a barrier to protect a baby's sensitive skin. A 1 percent hydrocortisone
cream is often effective in healing the rash, although use of this or stronger topical
steroids *absolutely must be approved by a doctor*. The stronger preparations should
not be used for more than a week unless the condition is severe, which is not usually
the case with simple diaper rash. If the symptoms persist for several days, the baby
should be seen by a doctor. There is always a possibility of bacterial or fungal
infection, and other more-serious skin diseases are occasionally mistaken for diaper
dermatitis.

Atopic Dermatitis

Atopic dermatitis (eczema) can flare in infancy and throughout early childhood.
In the past, many children endured long, miserable periods of eczema, during which
they were swathed in compresses and told not to scratch or were restrained to prevent
scratching.

Modern corticosteroids, although they must be used with great care, have taken much of the agony out of severe eczema. It is very important to remember, however, how potent these drugs are. Your doctor should not be casual about supervising treatment; and it is essential to pay close attention to medical directions from your doctor, from the pharmacist, and on the label.

Atopic dermatitis usually does not appear before the child is two months old. In the youngest children, it is apt to appear first on the face, especially on the cheeks. Later it may spread to the area of the hairline and behind the ears (see chapter 12).

The disease may clear up in infancy, but sometimes it progresses or reappears after a time of remission. Among toddlers and older children, the rash (dry lesions) characteristically appears in front of the elbows, where the arms bend, and behind the knees. The face is often spared, but the feet may not be, and the rash may be misdiagnosed as athlete's foot. In adolescence, the rash often becomes milder. Unfortunately, it occasionally becomes much worse and widespread, affecting large areas of the head, neck, chest, arms, and feet.

Statistically, more than half of children with atopic dermatitis at age three will still have the condition as adults. And as you probably know at this point in the book, the atopic diseases (allergic rhinitis, atopic dermatitis, and asthma) run in families; and if you have one, you may develop another. Up to three-quarters of youngsters with atopic dermatitis develop allergic rhinitis or asthma, but it is rare to have all three.

Children who have developed atopic dermatitis and are therefore at risk of developing asthma may get some protection through control of their exposure to allergens. *Reducing exposure to dust mites, animal dander, and cockroaches as well, may prevent the development of asthma in these children.* Similar precautions may be helpful for all children whose parents are allergic.

The treatment of atopic dermatitis is the same for children as for adults (see chapter 12).

CONTACT DERMATITIS

Children's skin is very delicate. Most of us can remember the awful discomfort of itchy woolen sweaters or trousers. If a child says that a piece of clothing makes him or her itch, believe it.

Wool is an irritant in and of itself, but chemicals used in the processing of fabrics and the manufacture of clothing can also cause contact dermatitis, especially in places where the garment fits tightly. Sometimes, washing or cleaning new clothes before wearing them solves the problem.

Poison ivy resin can imbue a fabric or be carried on an animal's coat for several days, with the potential of causing poison ivy dermatitis if the resin touches the skin. Teach your children to recognize and avoid this plant and to put clothing in the wash if they have been walking through poison ivy. If a pet has been running through poison ivy, the animal should not be hugged and kissed until it has had a bath.

Other plants, including chrysanthemums, can cause contact dermatitis. The disease also can be caused by substances containing plant products, such as turpentine and Vicks VapoRub.

Some children react to leather or rubber used in shoes or to nickel in the toes of certain shoes by developing contact dermatitis. To make diagnosis more difficult, atopic dermatitis caused by something as remote as a food allergy may also cause a rash on the feet.

If it is contact dermatitis, patch tests can identify the offending substance. Sometimes, protective socks (such as those made from thick cotton) solve the problem. Occasionally, one must order special shoes not containing the allergen.

Children can be sensitive to over-the-counter medications used to treat cuts, insect bites, sunburn, and the like. The preparations most frequently causing reactions are those with—*caine* in the ingredients (for example, benzocaine), topical antihistamines and antibiotics, and ethylenediamine (used as a solvent and emulsifier in a number of medical compounds).

Contact dermatitis around the mouth, often confused with atopic dermatitis, is commonly caused by licking the lips. Acid foods, such as oranges and juices, can dry around the mouth and irritate the skin. Rubber erasers can cause contact dermatitis around the lips.

URTICARIA AND ANGIOEDEMA

This topic is discussed in detail in chapter 12. The details of diagnosis and treatment are similar in children and adults. Chronic urticaria is much less common in children, but requires the same workup.

Children are more prone to a condition called papular urticaria, which is a persistent skin eruption representing an allergic reaction to insect bites (e.g., mites [other than dust mites], fleas, bedbugs, gnats, mosquitoes, animal lice). Papular urticaria usually occurs in atopic kids and is characterized by crops of small urticarial papules (hard small raised bumps) and wheals (welts) and transitional forms of these lesions, which may become secondarily infected or lichenified (thickened and hardened) as a result of rubbing and scratching.

Treatment is mild topical corticosteroid creams and oral antihistamines to relieve the intense itch. In rare cases, a short course of systemic steroids may be needed as well as topical or systemic antibiotics if the lesions become infected. The best treatment is prevention: the child should be protected with insect repellents.

Persistent papular urticaria may indicate serious illness and requires an extensive medical workup.

ALLERGIC RHINITIS-RELATED CONDITIONS IN CHILDREN

Allergic rhinitis is an all-too-common childhood disease. When combined with the usual quota of head colds in childhood, this one-two punch can leave kids with runny noses for a good portion of their young lives.

Children with allergic rhinitis tend to develop an "allergic look."

Their eyes may be dark circled, with so-called allergic shiners. Frequently there is a crease between the tip and bridge of the nose as a result of pushing up the snub of the nose in the "allergic salute," which is a vigorous wiping of the nose. The allergic cluck occurs when the tongue is placed against the roof of the mouth to form a seal and withdrawn rapidly in an effort to scratch the palate.

Serial sneezing, an itching palate, allergic conjunctivitis, and coughing round out the most-common symptoms.

The presence of fever, persistent one-sided nasal obstruction, persistent dark-colored discharge, and/or nasal discharge need medical attention as they are suggestive of nonallergic causes that could be serious.

Needless to say, the popularity of children with allergic rhinitis can be affected by these miserable symptoms. Some children who live with untreated allergies do well in school and sports and are well liked. But most need medical attention to be and do their best.

There have been studies done in Great Britain that showed that the incidence of asthma can be reduced by reducing mite exposure in children at high risk for developing asthma. Because of such studies, most allergists recommend the following for such children in high-risk families (families in which one or both parents have a history of allergic diseases—allergic rhinitis, asthma, or eczema): an important first step in most cases is to make the child's room allergen-free (see chapter 4). This sometimes leads to a dramatic improvement, whether the offending culprit is an indoor allergen such as a dust mite or whether it is pollen or mold from outside.

If a child already has rhinitis and cleaning up his is unhelpful, the child should be taken for medical diagnosis and treatment. How long to wait to take this step depends on how uncomfortable the child is and whether there is any improvement. With moderately severe symptoms, one should not wait more than a few days to two weeks. With intermittent or very mild symptoms, a slightly longer delay will probably do no harm, but you should not let any physical discomfort drag on for months without getting a diagnosis.

Ongoing symptoms warrant diagnosis and treatment. What parents may describe as "just" an allergy or "only" a cold may be more serious. Among the possible underlying causes of continuing rhinitis is a sinus infection.

In the first three months of life, a stuffy nose and nasal discharge may be due to a congenital defect (choanal atresia). This is usually spotted in the hospital just after the baby is born or by the child's pediatrician. Still, parents should be aware of it. The defect can usually be completely corrected by surgery.

Toddlers often stuff things up their noses. The result can be a smelly discharge from the affected nostril.

In severe cases of asthma or rhinitis, especially if there are nasal polyps or failure to grow normally, it is important to rule out cystic fibrosis. The sweat test, which is painless, can be done to analyze the amount of sodium in the sweat. Patients with cystic fibrosis have a higher amount of sodium than normal people do. The test is painless. Mild electrical stimulation to an extremity is performed over a thirty-minute period. Filter paper covered by paraffin is placed in the test area. The paper is weighed and the sodium content analyzed. The test is done twice, and if positive twice, this is definitive for a diagnosis of cystic fibrosis. It is important to diagnose cystic fibrosis as soon as possible as it is treatable but not curable.

Hay Fever

Hay fever, or seasonal allergic rhinitis, usually does not appear before age three because it takes several years for this sensitivity to develop. However, children who live in the most-southern areas of the United States or in any tropical or semitropical region may develop pollen allergies in the first year or two of life. The pollen season is essentially year-round, and so is the hay fever season. The more typical pattern in the United States is the appearance of symptoms between ages three and ten, with the disease getting worse for about three years and then stabilizing.

Children with hay fever can be helped by antihistamines. Cetirizine and desloratadine are approved for > six months of age, loratadine for > two years of age, and fexofenadine for > six years of age. But if a physician thinks it advisable, they may be used in reduced doses for younger children under the doctor's supervision.

It is important to keep in mind that in children, the side effects of medication not only appear at much lower doses but may also be different from the reaction in adults. All children taking medicine should be carefully observed and any changes reported to the doctor. Medicating a child with over-the-counter drugs can be risky. The treatment should be discussed with a doctor. When you are buying a drug, tell the pharmacist the age of the child who will be using it and ask if there are any warnings about which you should be aware. The first-generation antihistamines available over the counter usually have adverse cognitive effects (perception, thinking) due to their sedative side effect and, as a result, can impair learning. The second-generation antihistamines do not.

Leukotriene modifiers have a modest effect on nasal symptoms and are often used successfully to treat rhinitis.

Two nasal antihistamine sprays (azelastine [Astepro, Astelin] and olopatadine [Patanase]) are available but not below age twelve (unless a physician feels their use is warranted in a younger child), and the reader is referred to chapter 5 for further discussion of those sprays. However, they are first-generation antihistamines and, when used, can cause some cognitive impairment as well. They are very fast acting, often producing relief in fifteen to thirty minutes.

If all else fails, then the recommended treatment is with steroid sprays, which are the most effective therapy as they work on all the symptoms (even related to the eye); this should be done under the supervision of an allergist or ear, nose, and throat specialist. We now know that the newer medication such as budesonide (Rhinocort

AQ), ciclesonide (Omnaris), fluticasone (Flonase) and mometasone (Nasonex), and are all more effective with less side effects than the older medications: beclomethasone, triamcinolone, and flunisolide.

After age five, immunotherapy may be undertaken and, as we noted, is often successful.

MIDDLE EAR DISEASE

A complication of allergic rhinitis and other respiratory ailments that can be very serious for children is middle-ear disease (serous otitis media). It can also be caused by chronic exposure to some irritant, such as cigarette smoke.

Serous otitis media affects ten million children annually in the United States alone; it is the commonest reason for surgery among children here and the commonest cause of hearing loss. The disease is most frequently found among children under age five and may be hidden at that age because the child often feels no pain.

As discussed earlier, when hearing loss occurs as children are learning to understand language and to speak, the child may miss important steps in the development of language skills. This can lead to speech disorders and apparent learning disabilities.

Middle ear disease results from blockage of the Eustachian tube, which runs from the back of the throat to the ear. In children, the anatomy of the immature tube makes it more prone to infection, with material entering from the nose and throat. What parents can do to spot this disease is to consciously look out for any diminishment in hearing, especially in an infant or toddler. A child's hearing is normally very acute, and if a child does not turn toward or otherwise react to sounds as you would expect, notify your doctor. In addition, your child's hearing should be tested at least once a year.

Treatment depends on the underlying cause of the disease (see chapter 11). One type of therapy designed particularly for children is the insertion of tubes into the ears to drain them. The tubes are made to be extruded in a year or two, depending on what the doctor orders.

Children who have these tubes must follow their doctor's instructions carefully with regard to swimming, blowing their noses, and so on.

Ear-tube surgery is best reserved for cases in which fluid has been present in the inner ear for more than three months in both ears, or six months for one ear, despite antibiotic therapy.

SINUS DISEASE

Sinus disease can arise as a complication of allergic rhinitis or as an independent entity (see chapter 11). The most-worrisome aspect of sinus disease in a child, especially one younger than age five, is that like serous otitis media, the disease is often hidden. The child often feels no pain or discomfort. The main symptom may be coughing. Sometimes, following a virus infection in the upper respiratory tract, a sinus infection sets in, marked by a smelly clear-white to green nasal discharge. Again, coughing is common; there is often a barking cough at night, with apparent bronchitis. The child may run a low fever and be lethargic.

Although doctors today like to keep X-rays to a minimum, if no explanation can be found for coughing, fatigue, and so on, a sinus CT-Scan may be recommended.

The treatment is the same as for adults (see chapter 11).

COUGH

Cough is a common problem in children and children normally cough often. It has been demonstrated that a child can cough up to thirty-four times in a twenty-four-hour period and still be within the normal range. Even so, cough still can be annoying and should be dealt with.

The most common cause of cough in children is an acute viral upper respiratory tract infection (URI, or the common cold). The frequency of this problem increases when children first enter a daycare facility, because of the way these are spread. Cough from URIs can last up to three weeks. The next most-common cause of cough is upper-airway cough syndrome, which is usually caused by post-nasal drip. Sinusitis and allergic rhinitis often cause this problem.

There are many other causes of cough in children, most nonallergic, such as GERD. Usually, cough is dealt with by the pediatrician. Prolonged cough with wheezing should be treated with a trial course of several weeks of inhaled corticosteroids. If the cough disappears, then the diagnosis is bronchial asthma.

Cough following a choking episode is often caused by a foreign body, although sometimes there is no preceding choking episode.

HABIT COUGH

The most common types of cough in children are related to asthma and sinusitis. A relatively uncommon but important cause of cough in children is habit cough that typically starts after an upper respiratory tract infection and persists despite the absence of any apparent physical cause.

The cough is an explosive, croupy cough with a characteristic barking or honking sound. These young patients complain of "something" in the throat or a "tickle" in the throat. They sometimes adopt a chin-on-chest position, holding one hand against the larynx as if to support it.

The coughing is disturbing to parents and disruptive in school, although the child typically does not seem perturbed by the symptom (la belle indifference: *which is a medical term meaning "lack of concern"*) and also does not cough while asleep. Often the cough worsens in the presence of medical professionals and can be reproduced on request. The treatment is explanation, reassurance, and counseling, if necessary.

An extensive evaluation for the causes of cough, as discussed in chapter 9, should be done to be sure nothing is missed. All neurologic tic disorders including Tourette's syndrome must be ruled out as well.

Various pharmacological treatments for asthma, GERD, post-nasal drip, and other causes of cough are usually tried at first. The diagnosis of habit cough is a "diagnosis of exclusion," which means the other possible causes are ruled out when the treatments for these fail.

In our experience and in that of the pediatric literature, these children tend to be emotionally unhappy or under stress and to benefit from various forms of behavior modification. Various relaxation-therapy techniques as well as voice therapy have been successful. Hypnosis has been shown to be effective in some patients, and Dr. Young had one case that responded to hypnosis. Psychological counseling is advisable in these patients as well.

ASTHMA IN CHILDREN

In the United States as well as worldwide, childhood asthma continues to increase. In the United States in 2002, 8.9 million children (12.2 percent) had been diagnosed with asthma. Asthma is the most common cause of pediatric emergency room visits (887,000 per year), hospitalizations (166,000); and there are 10.1 million school days lost each year. Asthma is increasing in children worldwide at the same alarming rate as well.

The greatest increase occurs in urban areas, and we do not know all the reasons for the increase; but inadequate medical care, air pollution, and heavy exposure to allergens, including cockroach and dust mite allergens, seem to be likely contributors to the spread of asthma in inner cities.

Teenagers are particularly at risk from serious asthma attacks, in part because they naturally dislike the thought of being ill and may ignore symptoms of trouble. Education and reassurance are very important.

One of the great satisfactions of treating children of all ages with asthma is how much we can help these youngsters, many of whom are weakened and frightened by the disease. Most can learn to manage their symptoms and can attain outstanding accomplishments both athletically and academically.

Many children, about 50 percent of them, wheeze occasionally in infancy and early childhood; but only about a third of these go on to develop asthma. About twice as many boys as there are girls are affected in early childhood. But as they grow, boys tend to go into remission and girls tend to develop the disease. Among teenagers, boys and girls in equal numbers have asthma.

With infants and toddlers up to age five, the most common precipitating factor leading to asthma is a viral infection. The fact that the asthma has struck at such a young age, however, does not make the prognosis any worse or better.

The viruses most commonly implicated are respiratory syncytial virus, rhinovirus, and parainfluenza virus—in other words, bugs that cause colds. Why these viruses in some cases cause asthmatic wheezing is not known, but it may be because of actual damage done to the epithelium lining the respiratory tract. Genetics plays a role in some cases, as the young patients are likely to have an atopic history (that is, to suffer from hay fever or atopic dermatitis or have parents who have these diseases or have asthma). Currently, more than twenty-two loci on fifteen autosomal chromosomes have been linked to asthma.

Once the viral infection has set up the asthma, allergens, exercise, and other standard causes of asthma (see chapter 9) may become the precipitating causes of future attacks. It seems that allergies may play a greater role in provoking asthma attacks in children than in adults.

Among children, an allergy to cow's milk may provoke asthma, but this thesis is somewhat controversial. The role of cow's milk has not been fully delineated. Among infants, the risk, if it is there, can be avoided by breast-feeding.

Children who develop asthma and who also test positive in skin tests for allergies are less likely to outgrow the asthma than children who are not allergic. And children with both asthma and eczema are especially likely to be stuck with the asthma for most of their lives.

For the majority of children, the prognosis is quite good. In one large study of four hundred children with asthma, the majority had a mild intermittent form of the disease; and more than half of these were free of asthma by age twenty-one. A minority of these with mild asthma continued to have the disease all the way into adulthood.

Of the one hundred children with *severe* asthma, 20 percent were asthma-free by age twenty-one and 40 percent were improved by that age. The other approximately 40 percent remained quite sick or their asthma got worse.

In summary, the most-severe asthma is the least likely to go into remission, although most children can look forward to an improvement in their asthma.

One factor that we recognize as a danger for children with very severe asthma is depression, as shown in a study by Dr. Robert Strunk at National Jewish Health (formerly National Jewish Medical and Research Center in Denver). If your child is both asthmatic and depressed, extra care and attention are needed. Causes of depression in children include a recent divorce or death in the family, substance abuse or violence in the family, and continued unhappy experiences at school. Depression might be caused by the asthma drugs themselves. Signs of depression are lack of interest in life and adverse changes in sleeping and eating habits and in school performance.

Obesity is now recognized as a risk factor for both the development of asthma and for contributing to the severity of asthma.

DIAGNOSIS AND TREATMENT

Reaching a diagnosis of asthma in children is ordinarily not very different than with adults; but it can be more problematic with children under age five, who are too young to take a pulmonary-function test.

Many different terms are applied to episodes of wheezing during a respiratory infection: *wheezy bronchitis*, *asthmatic bronchitis*, and *pseudoasthma*. A common view is that three or more episodes of wheezing are adequate evidence for a diagnosis of asthma. Diagnosis is especially difficult in those infants with asthma who wheeze only when suffering from respiratory infections.

Sometimes, as with adults, a cough is the only sign of asthma. A history of coughing worsening after exercise or at night can lead to a diagnosis of asthma. The cough may occur and persist only after a viral infection.

In differentiating asthma from other conditions that might cause the symptoms, a doctor looks for somewhat different conditions than in adults. Disorders of the cartilage in the trachea, cystic fibrosis, foreign bodies aspirated into the lung, infections such as croup, and anxiety conditions are primarily of concern among children, as compared to adults.

The treatment of children with asthma who are older than age four is essentially the same as with adults, except that lower doses of most medicines are used. (See chapter 9 for more on the treatment of asthma in both children and adults.)

Younger children, however, often are not able to use the inhalers that deliver medicines topically to the respiratory tract. To open the airways, they are more dependent on oral medicines, including theophylline and beta$_2$-agonists (Proventil, Ventolin, Alupent). Oral cortisone (corticosteroids) may also be needed.

Medication-delivery devices, such as AeroChamber and InspirEase, have lowered the age at which children can take drugs by inhalation from about age four to about age three, which is very helpful because of the undesirable side effects of the oral drugs. Another device, which consists of a nebulizer and a mask, can be used with children as young as nine months.

Theophylline, which is related to caffeine, may improve the attention span of older children, but a 1986 study suggested that it may cause learning and behavioral problems. This contributed to a reassessment of theophylline use so that it is rarely used today at any age.

Statistically, theophylline does not seem to have significant negative effects, but individuals certainly may experience adverse reactions.

If in the rare case your child is taking theophylline and you suspect that it is causing your child difficulty, discuss the situation with your child's teachers so that they will understand the situation and report to you promptly if a problem is developing.

Cortisone must be used with great care and restraint in infants and children. Among other side effects, it can prevent bone growth, resulting in short stature. Every effort must be made to use this drug in the lowest possible doses and for the shortest possible period of time. Recent studies are encouraging as they show that the loss of growth is usually less than one inch.

Cigarette smoke in the house is bad for all children and especially for asthmatics. Areas your child frequents should be free of allergens, smoke, and other irritants that make the asthma worse.

As the child grows, your doctor should encourage him or her to live as fully as possible (see chapter 9). All asthmatic children can and should be taught to engage in some form of physical activity. Many athletes as well as successful people in all fields of endeavor have asthma and are very successful in dealing with it and leading normal lives—your child should not be the exception.

ASTHMA CLASSIFICATION AND TREATMENT

The classification of asthma in children is very similar to adults as discussed in chapter 9. However, there is a slight difference. The following classification is for patients under age five. (For patients older than five, the treatment is the same as for adults and the reader is referred to chapter 9.) In all the scenarios described below, the child is prescribed some sort of rescue inhaler or nebulizer or both. A rescue medication is a short-acting beta$_2$-agonist. (See chapter 9.)

MILD INTERMITTENT ASTHMA

The mildest form is characterized by daytime symptoms that occur twice a week or less and nighttime symptoms that occur less than twice a month. In this group, no medication on a daily basis is needed.

MILD PERSISTENT ASTHMA

Daytime symptoms occur more than twice a week and nighttime symptoms occur more than twice a month. The preferred treatment is a low-dose inhaled corticosteroid spray either delivered by nebulizer or MDI (inhaler) with a holding chamber with a face mask for children less than age four or without a face mask for older children. Alternatively, a leukotriene-receptor inhibitor can be given.

MODERATE PERSISTENT ASTHMA

Symptoms occur daily during the day and more than once a week at night. In this case, the child is treated with low-dose inhaled corticosteroids and long-acting inhaled beta$_2$-agonists or medium-dose inhaled corticosteroids. Alternatively, low-dose inhaled corticosteroids and a leukotriene-receptor antagonist or theophylline. In addition, if there are still recurring severe exacerbations, the inhaled steroid dose will be increased to a medium dose with a long-acting beta$_2$-agonist. The alternative treatment is also medium-dose inhaled corticosteroid and a leukotriene-receptor antagonist or theophylline.

SEVERE PERSISTENT ASTHMA

Finally, we get to severe persistent, where the daytime symptoms are continuous and the nighttime symptoms occur frequently. The preferred medication is high-dose inhaled corticosteroids in combination with a long-acting inhaled beta$_2$-agonist. When needed, corticosteroid tablets or syrup may be used. The dose should not exceed two milligrams per kilogram a day up to sixty milligrams of prednisone a day.

ASTHMA EMERGENCY

The following symptoms indicate that a child may be having a major asthma attack and should be seen immediately by a physician, either in the office or in an emergency room.

- Severe shortness of breath, coughing, wheezing, tightness in the chest
- Changes in breathing patterns (shallow and fast or slower than usual)
- Difficulty concentrating or talking
- Hunched shoulders
- Nostrils flare when breathing
- Refraction, which means that when the child breathes, muscles in the neck and between and below the ribs move inward
- A bluish tinge (cyanosis), especially in the lips and face

Chapter 17

PREGNANCY AND ALLERGIES

Pregnancy should be a happy time, and for many women it is very happy indeed. The joy, however, may be tempered by considerable discomfort—from morning sickness in the early weeks to aches and fatigue near the end. This is normal. Even though some women feel wonderful throughout pregnancy, the majority experience stress and strain from time to time.

Ideally, pregnancy is planned, with health taken into account. Even before conception, the woman should try to be as physically well as possible, avoiding medicines or drugs that might undermine her health or that of the baby.

If you intend to get pregnant, you should not indulge in alcohol, cigarettes, or any other recreational drugs from the time that conception may occur through birth. You will have a better chance of avoiding a miscarriage and delivering a healthy child if you are completely drug-free.

Among smoking's destructive effects on the fetus is an increase in the risk that the child will develop asthma or other respiratory difficulties early in life. Furthermore, a child who grows up in a home where there is cigarette smoke has a higher risk of developing asthma.

If you take medicines frequently or regularly for any reason and you want to become pregnant, you should discuss with your doctor how to manage medical matters prior to and during the pregnancy.

Among allergic diseases, the one that causes the most concern during pregnancy is asthma. But other allergies or their complications, such as sinus infections or skin infections, do pose problems for some patients.

Physical Changes in Pregnancy

The total impact of the myriad physical changes that occur in pregnancy, many of which are secondary to hormonal changes, can be difficult to predict with respect to allergies or asthma. With some patients, allergies and asthma clear up during pregnancy; with some, there is no significant change; and with some, the allergies or asthma gets worse.

In pregnancy, there is an increase in the production of estrogen, which is believed to be related to the need for a larger blood flow to accommodate the developing fetus. The additional estrogen, however, causes changes in the lungs that tend to decrease the pulmonary exchange of gases. So this is a potential negative for anyone with asthma.

Another effect of high levels of estrogen is to slow the clearance of cortisol from the body. Cortisol is the equivalent of cortisone, which is used to treat severe asthmatic and allergic reactions. So in theory, having more cortisol should help people prone to such reactions.

The hormone progesterone, produced by the placenta in pregnancy, has among its effects relaxation of the smooth muscle throughout the body. The sphincter muscle between the esophagus and stomach, therefore, may slacken, with a greater likelihood of reflux of stomach contents into the esophagus. This, as we have noted, can make asthma worse in some patients.

To help avoid this reflux and the resultant heartburn, doctors typically advise women in the latter stages of pregnancy to eat lightly (several small meals per day rather than one large one) and to avoid very spicy and fatty dishes. Sleeping with your head and shoulders raised on pillows or a bolster may also help.

Progesterone also increases the rate of respiration. The more rapid breathing (hyperventilation) tends to counterbalance the depressive effect of estrogen on gas exchange. But hyperventilation during pregnancy may cause a worsening of asthma in some women; the hyperventilation is similar to the heavy breathing that follows exercise, which in some people triggers asthma attacks.

All in all, the sum of the effects of estrogen and progesterone on respiration, especially in asthmatics, is not clear one way or another. As it happens, about one-third of asthmatics improve in pregnancy (especially if the asthma is mild), about one-third get worse, and one-third stay the same.

But any condition affecting respiration needs to be watched in pregnancy because of the increased respiratory burden in these nine months. The lungs must provide more oxygen for the baby and excrete more carbon dioxide. Similarly, the blood volume increases in pregnancy, requiring more work by the heart.

Hormonal changes also affect the lining of the nasal passages. The result is a condition known as vasomotor rhinitis of pregnancy. This causes nasal congestion, which is usually most noticeable in the last four to five months. It affects about one-third of pregnant women.

The fetus is, by immunological standards, a foreign invader (50 percent of its genes come from the father); and it takes important changes in the immune system during the pregnancy to prevent the rejection of the fetus. All the means by which the immune system adjusts and permits the baby to grow are not known, but researchers have demonstrated the following changes, among others: a decrease in one kind of antibody (IgG); variable changes in the allergy antibody (IgE); changes in the numbers of white blood cells (some kinds increase, some decrease); and changes in the levels of the chemical mediators of allergic reactions, including histamine.

With these alterations in the immune system, one would expect dramatic effects on allergies in pregnant women. But as is the case with the total effect of hormonal changes, the picture is not clear, and your doctor probably will not be able to predict if your allergies or asthma will get better or worse in pregnancy.

ALLERGIC RHINITIS

If you get hay fever seasonally and badly enough that you would be very uncomfortable without medication, you may want to try to plan your pregnancy so that the first trimester is not in the hay fever season. It is in these first three months that it is most important to take no medicines, or as few as possible and only those that have been cleared as safe for use during pregnancy. Because the fetus is so vulnerable during this first trimester, you should consult your doctor before taking medication during a time in which you might conceive. Find out whether the medicine poses any risk to a developing fetus.

If you have perennial rhinitis or severe seasonal rhinitis and anticipate that you would like to become pregnant in a year or so, you might consider starting immunotherapy. If you are a good candidate for this type of treatment (see chapter 6), it may be worthwhile to undertake it as a preventive so that you do not feel the need for medicine during pregnancy.

A large study of pregnant women has demonstrated the safety of immunotherapy during pregnancy. But immunotherapy should be started well before pregnancy, not only so that the patient will have improved by the time she becomes pregnant, but also so as to avoid the chance of an adverse reaction to a shot, less likely once a maintenance dose is achieved.

A woman who already suffers from allergic rhinitis may find that condition worsening during pregnancy. This may or may not be due to a worsening of the allergic rhinitis. Recall that vasomotor rhinitis is a common condition in pregnancy, even among women who ordinarily have no such symptoms.

About one-third of pregnant women with preexisting rhinitis experience a worsening of that condition. About one-fifth improve. Almost half experience no change.

A complication of rhinitis (sinusitis) is about six times more common in pregnant than in nonpregnant women.

Avoidance of allergens—that primary treatment in all allergy medicine—is especially important in pregnancy. Remove allergens from your home and keep allergens from making their way in from the out-of-doors. (See chapter 4.)

SINUSITIS

Acute bacterial sinusitis, according to a Finnish study, is six times more common in pregnancy than in the general population. Therefore, we need to be on the lookout for it during pregnancy especially after the common cold. The treatment is similar as in nonpregnant patients with several adjustments being made because of the pregnancy. Higher doses of antibiotics may be required to compensate for the increased clearance of antibiotics during pregnancy. X-rays and oral steroids should be avoided because of their potential to harm the developing fetus.

SAFE AND UNSAFE DRUGS

Although it is prudent to minimize medication in pregnancy, treatment is sometimes necessary. Infections should not be allowed to become established or to linger.

Many antibiotics are considered safe in pregnancy and are prescribed frequently and appropriately for pregnant patients. Certain antibiotics, however, must not be used, especially tetracycline and its derivatives minocycline and doxycycline. Iodides too should be shunned.

Tetracycline, a drug with many side effects, discolors the teeth of fetuses and children and therefore is not used in pregnancy or in children under age eight. Iodides tend to cause goiter in fetuses.

Certain antihistamines may be used, but with caution. Their use should be supervised by your doctor. Chlorpheniramine (Chlor-Trimeton and others) until recently was considered the safest antihistamine in pregnancy and has a category B rating. Loratadine (Claritin), cetirizine (Zyrtec), and levocetirizine (Xyzal) are also considered category B. However, one must consider that chlorpheniramine has been used for a much longer period of time, thus adding a layer of safety above and beyond the other category B drugs. So you have to weigh the risk of sedation from chlorpheniramine (Chlor-Trimeton and others) versus the more newly rated category B drugs.

Higher-than-recommended doses of antihistamines should not be taken, particularly near the end of pregnancy. There is a higher incidence of retrolental fibroplasia (which in its most severe form causes blindness in some premature babies) among women who have taken antihistamines on a regular basis and who give birth to premature or small babies weighing 1,500 grams (5.25 pounds) or less.

The jury is out on this; but if there is a known risk of prematurity, as for example when there are multiple fetuses, then antihistamine use, if any, should be carefully supervised by a physician.

The only oral decongestant considered safe in pregnancy is pseudoephedrine, but it should not be used during the first trimester as there have been reports of adverse effects on the fetus in the first trimester. Among topical decongestants, oxymetazoline in a nasal spray is not appreciably absorbed and is probably safe, although there are no data to substantiate this.

One of the better medicines in terms of safety and effectiveness in treating allergic rhinitis is cromolyn in topical form (Nasalcrom for the nose and Crolom or Opticrom for the eyes). The drawback is that this medicine is strictly a preventive and takes a couple of weeks to work and is not currently being manufactured (see section on asthma).

The research evidence on the safety of nasal steroids is mixed. In animal studies, an effect on fetuses has been observed. The apparent safety of inhaled steroids in pregnant women with asthma suggests that the nasal forms are safe, except for dexamethasone (Decadron), which can be absorbed systemically. (See the section below on asthma during pregnancy for more information on steroids.) Only one inhaled steroid has a category B rating, and that is budesonide (Rhinocort), although it is highly likely that as more data accumulates, the others will become category B.

With rhinitis, toughing it out through pregnancy without using antihistamines or other allergy medicines is often the best course. But you should also be guided by your doctor. Severe symptoms of rhinitis may warrant treatment, if only to prevent sinusitis or other infections. When drugs are used, topical medication is preferable to oral medication. If the worsening of rhinitis is felt to be from vasomotor rhinitis, then several nonpharmacologic treatments are available that can be of benefit. These are saline nasal sprays, exercise, and external nasal dilators (Breathe Right Strips, etc.) for nocturnal symptoms.

ASTHMA

When dealing with rhinitis, we suggested above that it is often better to bear the symptoms without using medications. This approach does not apply to asthma. The developing fetus needs a constant supply of oxygen through the mother's bloodstream. But as the fetus grows, it presses upward against the pulmonary cavity, reducing the volume of gas in the mother's lungs. So if blood oxygen is depleted by asthma attacks, the fetus may be deprived of some of the oxygen it needs.

The aim of pregnancy, therefore, is to maintain optimal oxygen in the mother's lungs. If you have asthma, treatment to maintain oxygen levels may be necessary, even including use of steroids.

Whether or not ongoing medication is needed, the outlook for the pregnancy is very good. It is essential, however, that the health of the woman and fetus be monitored throughout pregnancy by the appropriate doctors, normally an obstetrician and an allergy or pulmonary specialist.

There is conflicting evidence as to whether or not women with asthma have a greater incidence of complications in pregnancy, including toxemia, vaginal bleeding, and (in the first trimester) nausea and vomiting; but at any rate, the increase in risk is not dramatic.

There is probably no increase in the risk of death from asthma during pregnancy. Studies have shown that pregnant asthmatics that are monitored by asthma specialists show no increase in fetal mortality.

For some people with asthma, it is difficult to distinguish between an asthma attack and the effects of anxiety or fatigue that mimic asthma symptoms. Making the distinction can be more difficult in pregnancy because the increased blood volume and rate of respiration now and then cause breathlessness and a pounding heart even in the healthiest women. These sensations can be unsettling. Naturally you may wonder if you are having an asthma attack.

Discuss these changes with your doctor. If there is doubt as to whether the breathlessness is normal or abnormal, a pulmonary-function test or other lung assessment may be indicated.

There is sophisticated medical help available for coping with asthma-related problems in pregnancy. Asthma has been extremely well studied, with the result that many specialists (allergists or pulmonary specialists) have the expertise to guide the asthma patient. The outcome of any pregnancy cannot be guaranteed; but the authors of this book are among the thousands of physicians who can attest from personal experience that even severely asthmatic, steroid-dependent women can have healthy, normal babies.

SAFE MEDICATIONS

Ideally, if you have asthma, before conception, you should discuss with both an asthma specialist and an obstetrician how to manage the pregnancy. If you can find a team that has worked together successfully before, all the better.

To minimize the need for drugs, avoidance of asthma triggers such as dust mites or cockroaches should be conscientiously attempted.

Another aim is to attain optimal treatment prior to conception. The goals of asthma treatment in pregnancy are the same as they are for asthma in general, which include prevention of attacks, maintaining normal activity and sleep, and keeping the pulmonary-function test normal or close to normal. The major difference is in the selection of medications. We want to choose the drugs with the most data showing safety in pregnancy. Albuterol HFA (ProAir, Proventil, and Ventolin) is the rescue medication with the longest history of use in pregnancy and therefore is our first choice. Budesonide (Pulmicort) is the inhaled steroid with the most-comforting data in pregnancy and is thus the first choice in this class. But if a patient has been doing well on another inhaled steroid before pregnancy, then it may be continued as there is no negative pregnancy data with the other inhaled steroids.

In addition to frequent, regular visits with physicians who are specialists in asthma management, regular medications are sometimes required except for the mildest of asthmatics. Peak-flow monitoring at home might be helpful in the patient who has trouble differentiating the normal breathlessness of pregnancy (from compression of the chest) and those with shortness of breath related to anxiety. The first line of treatment for mild persistent asthma in pregnancy is an inhaled corticosteroid, with cromolyn (if still available), leukotriene antagonists, or a long-acting theophylline preparation being second choices. A step-up approach as described in the "Asthma" chapter is then followed, with increasing numbers and/or doses of medications for moderate persistent and severe persistent asthma. Oral steroids should be avoided if possible and only used for the most severe of patients and for acute attacks. The appropriate oral steroids are prednisone and methylprednisolone. Dexamethasone (Decadron) should not be used. Decadron, even in nasal-spray and inhaler forms, may be absorbed and affect the fetus.

Cromolyn inhaler (Intal) and nedocromil (Tilade) have recently been discontinued because of the expense of changing them to HFA-propellant inhalers, but we include them as there is a slight possibility one or both may be manufactured by another company. A cromolyn (Intal) trial may be in order several months before conception. This drug has tested as very safe in pregnancy (it has a category B rating—see the chart below), and it can eliminate or decrease the need to use other drugs. But it may take up to two months to become fully effective, so you need to get started early with it.

Mild intermittent asthma can usually be adequately controlled with short-acting inhaled beta$_2$-agonists. These are also called rescue inhalers. Of the choices, albuterol is considered safest and considered the drug of choice during pregnancy, although there is no adverse pregnancy data with the other rescue inhalers (Maxair or Xopenex).

Oral forms of beta$_2$-agonists (albuterol, metaproterenol, and terbutaline) should be avoided.

Theophylline, as we mentioned, is not used much anymore. Testing indicates that theophylline (which is related to caffeine) has a good safety record, but it does not rate as high as cromolyn on the safety scale (it has a C rating, compared to cromolyn's B). Many doctors are cautious about using it during pregnancy. A patient who is well controlled on theophylline may be left on it during pregnancy.

Inhaled steroids can be extremely helpful. Data suggests that their use by asthmatics in pregnancy does not increase the incidence of fetal malformations or abortions (miscarriages), although animal data shows a slight adverse tendency.

Inhaled steroids are absorbed only minimally in the bloodstream. We have the longest experience with budesonide (Pulmicort), which is the only one that has a category B rating and thus is the preferred inhaled steroid in pregnancy, but a close second is beclomethasone (Beclovent, Vanceril, and Qvar).

Triamcinolone acetonide (Azmacort) has a lower safety rating and probably should be bypassed unless you are intolerant of the other drugs. It was recently discontinued but is included in case another manufacturer starts manufacturing it again. None of the inhaled steroids, however, has been unequivocally demonstrated to be harmful to the human fetus.

Omalizumab (Xolair) is used in more-severe asthma patients, is considered to be safe in pregnancy (category B) and therefore should be continued. There is a potential for side effects (particularly anaphylaxis), which do pose a threat to the fetus, but again we have to carefully weigh the risk versus the benefit of using it.

Even oral steroids can be used successfully in pregnancy, although the careful medical supervision that is always important with these drugs must be even more scrupulous when the patient is pregnant.

Atrovent, a form of atropine used to treat certain types of asthma, is also considered safe. It is in category B.

A word on the pregnancy safety-rating system: The Food and Drug Administration gives drugs grades, ranging from A to D, with an X at the bottom rank, based on trials with pregnant animals and data accumulated in humans. For ethical reasons, we cannot do human-pregnancy clinical trials. These ratings are not always as definitive as one would like and are sometimes out-of-date. Also, not all drugs are rated. But the rating system provides some guidelines. As a rule, if two drugs are available in the same class but with different ratings, the drug with the better rating should be used.

The rating system is set up as follows:

ADMINISTRATION (FDA) PREGNANCY CATEGORIES

Category	Animal Studies	Human Data	Benefit May Outweigh Risk
A	Negative[*]	Studies[†] negative	Yes
B	Negative	Studies not done	Yes
	Positive[‡]	Studies negative	Yes
C	Positive	Studies not done	Yes
	Not done	Studies not done	Yes
D	Positive or negative	Studies or reports positive	Yes
X[§]	Positive or negative	Studies or reports positive	No

* No teratogenicity (fetal defects) demonstrated.

† Adequate and well-controlled studies in pregnant women.

‡ Teratogenicity demonstrated.

§ Drug contraindicated during pregnancy.

*Negative means that when the drug was used during pregnancy, no more fetal malformations or abortions appeared than would be expected on average without the drug. During pregnancy, it is recommended to avoid a drug with an X rating. Unless the benefits outweigh the risks, D-rating drugs should also be avoided. Note that there are no category A drugs because we cannot ethically do studies in pregnant females.

ECZEMA AND HIVES

Atopic dermatitis, or eczema, is sometimes of concern in pregnancy. About 50 percent of women get worse, 25 percent get better, and the other 25 percent remain the same. It is wise to try to avoid triggers of eczema during pregnancy so that less medication is needed. Also, being especially careful to keep the skin moisturized is important. Nevertheless, because research with animals has shown fetal defects associated with the most-potent steroid creams and ointments—as yet there is no evidence from studies of humans—it seems prudent to use the lowest-potency topical medicine that will work. If the patient has widespread, severe skin disease, it may be preferable to use oral steroids rather than lavish amounts of high-potency topical steroids. The calcineurin inhibitors tacrolimus (Protopic) and pimecrolimus (Elidel) are rated category C. However, corticosteroids (also rated category C) have been in use for much longer and, in general, are preferred.

Hives, or urticaria, with swelling (angioedema) also are not usually a major concern in pregnancy. Sometimes, hives are triggered by an underlying infection, such as hepatitis, or an autoimmune disease such as lupus or Hashimoto's thyroiditis; so of course, undiagnosed hives should be seen by a doctor and diagnosed, before conception if possible.

About one woman in one hundred, usually in her first pregnancy, will develop an urticaria-like rash around abdominal stretch marks. A mild cortisone cream often takes care of the problem.

The woman who suffers from frequent hives or from severe chronic hives should be supervised by an allergist during pregnancy. Antihistamines rated safe for pregnant women should be tried first. Rarely, in severe urticaria, oral steroids may be needed.

The woman who suffers from urticaria triggered by cold may have to avoid cold during pregnancy as far as possible. The second-generation antihistamines ordinarily used to control the disease, fortunately, are considered safe in pregnancy.

Delivery rooms and operating rooms tend to be rather chilly. So if you suffer from hives induced by cold, be sure that your obstetrician knows this. A special effort should be made to keep you warm during labor and delivery.

ANGIOEDEMA AND ANAPHYLAXIS

A major medical concern at any time is angioedema, or swelling, associated with anaphylaxis.

Anaphylaxis, described in chapter 13, is a systemic allergic reaction in which the airways swell and close and the patient may go into shock and die. Naturally, the aim in pregnancy is to prevent anaphylaxis from occurring. If it does occur, aggressive emergency treatment must be taken. Delay or diminishment of standard treatment only adds to the danger for both fetus and mother.

Exercise-induced anaphylaxis is sometimes associated with particular foods, as described earlier. The remedy is simple in such cases: avoid the food, or better yet, avoid the food and do not exercise after eating anything else until several hours have passed.

If exercise alone has induced anaphylaxis in the past, then exercise anywhere near that level should not be done in pregnancy. Apparently, the rigors of labor will not induce an anaphylactic episode; but if antibiotics are required during labor, care must be taken to avoid any that the patient may be allergic to.

Idiopathic anaphylaxis, which means anaphylaxis for which no cause has been discovered, is also very rare and not well studied. Patients who have had episodes of such anaphylaxis are sometimes treated with oral steroids, and it has not been shown one way or the other whether it is better to continue this treatment during pregnancy or abandon it.

If you suffer from either of these disorders, you should ask your doctor, preferably before conception, to help you find a specialist or specialized care center with experience in treating these disorders.

Hereditary angioedema, which can lead to throat swelling and death, is also a dangerous and rare disease but better studied than the two disorders just mentioned. It tends to recede in pregnancy. In one study, twenty-five of twenty-five women experienced markedly fewer or no attacks during pregnancy.

This condition used to be managed by giving hormones that had the potential to damage the fetus. Fortunately, we now have the ability to give injections of the actual blood protein, which is missing in this disease. This is described in the chapter on skin diseases (chapter 12).

A caesarean section can precipitate an episode of severe angioedema in someone with hereditary angioedema. Prior to surgery, the patient can be treated (see chapter 12) to prevent such episodes. Local anesthesia is preferable to general anesthesia since putting a tube into the lungs can trigger an attack. Vaginal delivery seldom leads to an attack.

CHILDBIRTH

If you have asthma or another condition that may require medication during and after childbirth, then sometime in the seventh or eighth month of pregnancy, talk over with your doctor what medicines you should take with you to the hospital. Some women with asthma carry inhalers right into the labor room, but this sort of thing is best arranged ahead of time.

Asthma symptoms during labor and delivery occur in 10 to 20 percent of well-managed asthmatic women. Fortunately, this does not usually adversely affect the outcome of labor and delivery.

Your doctor and allergist should consult, and one of the two should advise the hospital staff what medicines you will take and who is responsible for administering them. The arrangements should cover caesarean as well as vaginal delivery.

Similarly, if you are going to be breast-feeding—and this is normally the healthiest means of feeding for both mother and baby—your doctor may want to recommend some adjustments in your medicines.

A discussion of potential ways that alterations in diet during pregnancy can affect the allergic status of the child is included in chapter 16.

Chapter 18

Surgery and Allergies

Allergies rarely complicate surgery, and surgery is rarely needed to treat allergies.

Chronic sinusitis is the only allergy-related disorder for which surgery is likely to be recommended. You should be very certain before committing yourself to the operation that such aggressive treatment really is needed. Get a second opinion from an ear, nose, and throat specialist affiliated with a teaching hospital, preferably not the same hospital with which your original doctor is associated.

Anytime that you must enter a hospital or clinic for any surgery, it is very important that your doctor and the staff know of any allergies that you may have to drugs, dyes used in taking X-rays or scans, and food. If you have a relative, friend, or nurse who will be with you in the hospital, this person should be aware of your allergies and watch what drugs and food you are given. Unfortunately, special notes regarding allergies are sometimes overlooked by hospital staff, even by doctors.

Allergic Rhinitis

If you suffer from seasonal or perennial allergic rhinitis, coughing and sneezing can complicate recovery from surgery on the nose or face (including, of course, cosmetic surgery), hernia surgery, or any abdominal surgery. Depending on the severity of your symptoms, it may be advisable to have elective surgery in a season when you can count on not being afflicted with rhinitis.

If you are considering immunotherapy, it might be best to get this treatment under way and your symptoms under control before having an operation. This issue of timing comes up fairly often with young adolescents, who tend to suffer from frequent colds and allergies, and a number of whom have corrective or cosmetic surgery in their teenage years.

If there is no sure way to avoid a flare-up of rhinitis or if the surgery is urgent, then consult your doctor to be certain that you have on hand adequate medication to suppress those sneezes and coughs. A series of sneezes or a hacking cough can open up a surgical incision.

ASTHMA

If you have asthma, it is important that the surgeon know about it, even in emergency surgery. This is one more reason to wear a MedicAlert bracelet or carry such medical information in your wallet with your identification and your medical-insurance card (which you can be sure hospital personnel will be looking for).

The risk of surgical and anesthesia complications is elevated in people with asthma. Therefore, it is important that the asthma be under good control before elective surgery in order to reduce the risk.

The best course is to arrange preoperative planning between your asthma doctor and your surgeon. Most preoperative evaluations require a recent chest X-ray, which is probably even more important in someone with asthma. All asthmatics should have a pulmonary-function evaluation at least a week before surgery so that any alterations in medication can be made to get you into an optimal state. If the asthma is not in good control and medication changes are necessary, the pulmonary function should be repeated closer to the date of surgery to verify improvement. If you are currently taking steroids to control asthma or have taken them in the eighteen months prior to surgery, your own adrenal gland output may be suppressed. Not only oral steroids but also high doses of inhaled steroids may inhibit the adrenal glands.

Normally, the adrenal glands respond to the stress of surgery with a surge of hormone production. If your response is blunted, you may need steroid supplementation before and during surgery.

This will be administered intravenously during the time that you are not allowed to eat or are anesthetized. It is important that your surgeon and anesthesiologist are aware of your asthma as well as your steroid history so that they can make the appropriate decisions about steroid supplementation before, during, and after surgery.

After the operation, any additional steroids that have been given will be tapered down quickly to your usual dose or to zero, if you can do without them.

The anesthetic gases used in surgery, such as halothane and enflurane, fortunately, tend to dilate the bronchial tubes. Enflurane may be preferable for the rare patient on theophylline because it is less likely to cause irregular heartbeats when used in conjunction with theophylline. Propofol and ketamine, which are often used in anesthesia, are bronchodilators.

Some patients wonder whether their doctor will realize the danger if their asthma worsens during an operation. The anesthesiologist can monitor lung function and detect changes that require treatment.

The use of epidural or spinal anesthesia is not necessarily safer than general anesthesia, although until recently it was thought that it was best for an asthmatic patient to avoid general anesthesia that requires insertion of a tube into the trachea (windpipe). It is crucial in elective surgery for your asthma to be under optimal control prior to surgery. That being said, most asthmatics should do as well with anesthesia and surgery as any other person of their age and sex should.

If you have asthma and still smoke, you must give up smoking before surgery. If you cannot do this on your own, ask your doctor for help or for a referral to a doctor, clinic, or program through which you can learn to kick the habit. The American Cancer Society (www.cancer.org) is another source that you can use for information on where to find help in breaking your habit.

HIVES AND ANGIOEDEMA

Precautions for pregnant patients who suffer from a couple of very rare allergic disorders are reviewed in the chapter on pregnancy. Some of these apply to all such patients about to undergo surgical procedures.

If you break out in hives when your skin is exposed to the cold, a special effort should be made to keep you warm before, during, and after surgery. Your doctor and the staff should be aware of the problem. As it happens, keeping patients warm during surgery appears to aid in recovery, so this is probably a good idea in any case.

If you lack C1 esterase inhibitor or if it does not function properly, special steps must be taken to protect you during both minor and major surgery, including oral surgery or even minor dental work. (Even the injection of a local anesthetic into the gums can precipitate an attack.)

The lack of C1 esterase inhibitor underlies the formerly extremely dangerous condition of hereditary angioedema (see chapter 12). People with this disease are prone to attacks of angioedema and, in the past, often died young. Today, the disease can be treated with very-effective treatments with minimal risk of side effects compared to the male hormone treatments that used to be used.

Patients with hereditary angioedema must be specially prepared for surgery by a physician with expertise in dealing with this condition. See chapter 12, where newer treatments are discussed. One of these modalities is probably what will be used when you have surgery.

Chapter 19

QUESTIONABLE THEORIES
AND TREATMENTS

Many times in this book, you have been advised that the physiology of certain allergy reactions is "not fully understood" or is "not completely known" or is "not entirely clear." The immune system is extremely complex, and substantial research remains to be done to bring doctors to the point of being able to diagnose and treat all allergies and related immune system malfunctions with ease and confidence. There is an unwritten rule in medicine that whenever there is a void in our understanding of illnesses or in our ability to cure illnesses, unscrupulous practitioners rush in to fill that void.

Since allergy was first discovered, the range of symptoms found to be related to allergic sensitivity has been impressively wide, from mild sniffles associated with hay fever, to stomach disorders and skin rashes, to the life-threatening choking of anaphylaxis. Given this variety of symptoms, it is understandable that allergy might be suspected as the cause of almost any unexplained ailment.

Most of us occasionally or even frequently experience mysterious discomforts that we cannot link to any particular infection, trauma, or other cause. These may be headaches, fatigue, nervousness, muscle and joint aches, and the like. It is not surprising that doctors and laypeople alike have wondered whether undiagnosed allergies are the cause of such symptoms. But what is surprising—at least to most ordinary doctors and researchers—is that speculation about the role of allergy has led to an array of popularly accepted claims about allergy that are based on little if any scientific evidence.

In the last fifty years, an influential nonscience of allergy has grown up alongside the main branch of allergy medicine. Called clinical ecology, or bioecology, this approach is based largely on unproven or unprovable hypotheses and treatments.

Clinical ecologists include some doctors trained in allergy medicine, but most are not.

The bad repute that surrounds clinical ecology does not mean that every idea put forward by clinical ecologists is unsound. Some of their concepts should receive and are receiving attention from research scientists. The problem arises when unproven hypotheses are presented as facts and consumers are induced to invest time and money on untested evaluation procedures and treatments.

Proof of a hypothesis in medicine usually involves testing according to scientific methods that minimize the chance of error. For example, there are statistical rules to follow: often a double-blind procedure is used, in which neither the researcher nor the patient knows whether what is being administered is the substance being tested or a placebo, and the study should be reproducible by anyone who wants to double-check the results. Indeed, before any medical claim is accepted as fact, the key studies should be repeated several times.

On some points in the theory of clinical ecology, there is no scientific evidence, or only disputed evidence supporting the claim. On other points, the evidence is clearer: certain tests and treatments have been studied and shown to do no good. Yet they are still sold to the public.

One reason that it is so easy to keep selling worthless remedies is that no matter how ineffective the treatment, it will often seem to work. A significant portion of patients who receive a sugar pill or other placebo from a health-care provider will report some therapeutic benefit or improvement in symptoms. So when a new drug is being tested, it is not enough that it helps patients; it must yield better results, statistically, than ones obtained with the placebo.

In scientific, clinical drug studies, one group of patients gets a placebo and another group of similar patients gets the actual drug being tested. The study must take a double-blind form; that is, neither the patient nor the provider knows which group is getting the placebo.

Most alternative therapies either have not been rigorously tested in double-blind trials, or if tested, they have not been shown to be effective. Of course, to be fair, if an alternative treatment proves itself effective, it is usually accepted into mainstream medicine and thus is no longer alternative. Nevertheless, we do advise caution in experimenting with alternative approaches. An important point to keep in mind about the untested theories mentioned in this chapter is that whenever one of them is subjected to double-blind testing, they almost never pass muster, often failing badly by being equal to the placebo.

Use common sense. Massage therapy has obvious benefits, usually improving one's sense of well-being. There are any numbers of illnesses, however, that will not improve significantly with massage therapy alone. So-called therapeutic-touch massage is unlikely to confer any benefits at all apart from the placebo effect. Therapeutic touch does not actually involve touching, but rather sensing an aura or field around the patient. Recently, one of the world's most prestigious medical journals, the *Journal of the American Medical Association,* published the results of a study of therapeutic touch, showing that practitioners in a blind situation could not determine whether or not their hands were near a patient's hand; in other words, they were not able to tell whether an aura was present or not. The principal investigator in this study was a girl just eleven years old!

THEORIES UNDERLYING CLINICAL ECOLOGY

In the 1940s, one of the pioneers in clinical ecology, Theron Randolph, suggested that maladaptation to the environment may result in a comprehensive "immune system dysregulation." Underlying this dysregulation is a hypersensitivity to several or many substances in the environment, often including food and water.

Typically, according to clinical-ecology theory, overexposure to one or more substances leads to an initial sensitivity, and this initial sensitivity flowers into a state of chronic or near-total hypersensitivity to numerous environmental factors.

The substances that may trigger symptoms, according to clinical ecologists, are almost infinitely numerous: air pollutants; chemicals in building materials; food additives; many, many foods; synthetic fabrics; standard allergens such as pollen and mold spores; perfumes and aftershave lotions; water from most sources; viral infections; fungal infections, including excess growth of the *Candida albicans* organism; and so on.

The symptoms said to be traceable to environmental origins cover just about every problem a human being can have: behavior disorders, gastrointestinal discomfort, fatigue, depression, urinary complaints, sexual malfunction, hyperactivity, schizophrenia, respiratory difficulties, acne, headaches, arthritic pain, learning and memory disabilities, weight gain and weight loss, bed-wetting, nagging cough, high blood pressure, and so on.

Even the symptoms of multiple sclerosis and cerebral palsy have been treated as allergy related. Some clinical ecologists claim to treat food allergies with immunization. Mainstream physicians do not consider this an effective method for handling sensitivities to foods or chemicals; in fact, immunization to food allergens is downright dangerous and potentially life threatening.

The claims of clinical ecologists put mainstream doctors in a quandary. No one rules out the possibility of adverse effects arising from exposure to substances in the environment, including chemicals and food. This is a critical problem, and medical researchers in the past twenty years have made important discoveries relevant to it.

For example, in the 1980s researchers demonstrated that ozone (a common air pollutant in metropolitan areas on sunny days) has much more of an effect on respiration than had previously been thought. This finding is of great importance to asthma and cardiac patients.

There have been hundreds, if not thousands, of reports in the medical literature of exposure to chemicals leading to adverse effects on the skin, respiratory system, liver, and other organs. Most reactions are categorized as due to an intolerance, rather than an allergy. But a few chemicals, such as toluene 2,4-diisocyanate, or TDI (used in plastics, foam, and adhesives), have been linked to allergic or other immunologic mechanisms. (TDI is associated with allergic asthma and hypersensitivity pneumonitis.)

As for adverse effects from food, despite numerous claims and warnings in popular literature, there is as yet no strong evidence that food allergies are a major health problem or have any connection to neurological diseases, such as multiple sclerosis, or any other chronic diseases other than eczema and the gastrointestinal illnesses mentioned in the chapter on food allergy. There is, in fact, no known cure for multiple sclerosis, and the National Multiple Sclerosis Society is in constant conflict with healers and doctors, licensed and unlicensed, who use untested cures or palliatives to treat the disease.

In the five decades since it was first posed, no scientific proof has been found of the central hypothesis of clinical ecology: that environmental maladaptation causes immune system dysregulation as described in the literature of clinical ecology.

There have been some reports that suggest that chronic exposure to certain chemicals and elements (for example, heavy metals and polychlorinated biphenyls) and perhaps even low-level magnetic fields can cause immune dysfunction. But this is not the extreme, comprehensive dysfunction described in clinical ecology.

Another general syndrome "discovered" by clinical ecologist A. H. Rowe in the 1940s is cerebral allergy. This is a kind of food allergy that affects the central nervous system, causing fatigue, confusion, irritability, depression, and so on. In one form or another, the concept of cerebral allergy continues to attract a popular following. But given the lack of proof that it exists, treatment, in the form of restrictive diets or other measures, is difficult to justify medically or financially.

Another concept in clinical ecology is that maladapted patients develop an addiction to the substances to which they are sensitive. It has been suggested that a water-addicted patient should treat this problem by drinking from four to five different water sources each day. Finally, there is the dramatic suggestion that there may be certain people who suffer from total immune-disorder syndrome. To borrow a phrase from Dr. Elliott Middleton Jr., editor of a distinguished allergy textbook, these patients would be "allergic to the twentieth century." Such people are termed universal responders—they are adversely affected by everything.

MULTIPLE CHEMICAL SENSITIVITY

Dr. Randolph died in 1995, but his theories live on in a variety of forms. Today, we speak of it in terms of "multiple chemical sensitivity" (MCS), "environmental AIDS," toxic chemical encephalopathy, and in line with Dr. Middleton's comment, the "twentieth-century disease," which has now become the "twenty-first-century disease."

These all refer to a presumed comprehensive immune system disorder, almost identical to that described by Dr. Randolph decades ago—and still mysterious and controversial.

Recently, the American Council on Science and Health published a report (*Unproven "Allergies": An Epidemic of Nonsense*) warning that these so-called disorders are highly speculative and untested. They pointed out that when common symptoms such as headaches, sneezes, and stomach upsets are diagnosed as caused by pervasive chemicals, this interpretation validates some patients' "view of the world as a hostile place filled with harmful chemicals and contaminated foods." The World Health Organization suggested using the term *idiopathic environmental intolerances* or *IEI*, and we use this term. This term is more accurate since MCS suggests a cause-and-effect relationship between chemical exposure and the symptoms mentioned. However, no such cause and effect has been established.

Nevertheless, the number of people claiming to suffer from IEI continues to grow, and the issue of whether this is a medically valid diagnosis is being litigated nationwide as patients seek compensation for disabilities that they believe have been caused by exposure to chemicals of various sorts.

These are often hard cases because there are indeed numerous chemicals in our environment that may be causing ills that we do not understand. Even expert study may fail to decide a claim one way or another. Think, for example, of Gulf War syndrome. Researchers have yet to determine with certainty whether there are one or more chemical or biological causes of the veterans' complaints or even whether some may be psychogenic in nature.

Repeatedly in recent decades, chemicals originally described as safe and harmless have proved to be dangerous. On the other hand, in many cases, people suffering from IEI appear to be physically normal according to standard tests; and their symptoms are often similar to symptoms of depression, agoraphobia, and anxiety associated with panic attacks.

People who are, or believe that they are, adversely affected by all synthetic substances are likely to withdraw from the day-to-day world in order to live in a sheltered environment constructed of all-natural materials.

It is unlikely that IEI is a bona fide immune system disorder. But in all fairness, we need more research to determine whether it is, and patients who complain of such symptoms should be studied carefully to rule out a valid diagnosis. We can certainly agree that we need to know more about what effect the chemicals in our environment do have on our bodies and health.

The patients themselves should be wary of doctors, or others offering care, who claim to understand exactly what the problem is and how it should be treated. There is no reliable evidence as to what sort of treatment is appropriate. Beware of health-care practitioners who are affiliated with the American Academy of Environmental Medicine. This is the organization that was renamed from the original Society for Clinical Ecology, cofounded by Theron Randolph.

Attorneys have had some success establishing IEI as a valid disorder. The cases labeled IEI range from recognized allergic reactions, such as latex allergy, to questionable cases of total sensitivity, to just about everything. At the same time, some courts are reluctant to accept scientific testimony in favor of IEI plaintiffs because the disorder is still hypothetical at best.

The claims of clinical ecologists are essentially regarded as unacceptable by essentially all allergists; by the professional organizations of allergists (the American Academy of Allergy, Asthma & Immunology and the American College of Allergy, Asthma and Immunology); by other medical organizations, such as the American College of Physicians and the American Medical Association; and by the Food and Drug Administration.

IMMUNE SYSTEM DISEASE RELATED TO FOOD

The only known connections at this time between diseases related to the immune system and the ingestion of food have little clinical application, although they are worth further study.

There have been a few reliably reported cases of a connection between eating alfalfa seeds and the appearance of an illness resembling lupus, which is an immune system disease, or flare-ups of existing lupus. (More precisely, lupus is an autoimmune disease, which means a disease in which the patient's own immune system is causing the damage.)

In the early 1980s in Spain, contaminated cooking oil (the exact contaminant was never discovered) caused three hundred deaths and twenty thousand cases of a multisymptomatic disease with fever, cough, rashes, gastrointestinal symptoms, and blood abnormalities. Among the last was an increase in the level of eosinophils in the blood, a type of blood cell often elevated in patients with allergies and other immunological disorders.

Later, some of these patients developed an illness resembling scleroderma, an autoimmune disease with multiple organ involvement. Certain patients were more at risk than others, and genetic analysis revealed that these people were also more at risk of developing other autoimmune diseases such as lupus or rheumatoid arthritis.

More recently, it was recognized that the dietary supplement tryptophan (or at least some sources of it) could cause a serious disease characterized by muscle pain and high eosinophil counts. Tryptophan, an amino acid, is present naturally in most foods, especially meat, fish, poultry, and some cheeses, and is considered harmless since it is naturally found in the body. Whether there was a contaminant in the pills or whether an altered form of tryptophan caused the illness is still not known.

These discoveries, which are of interest to research scientists, may eventually lead to useful insights into links between certain foods or additives and autoimmune diseases. Clinical ecologists, however, are not particularly interested in studying or treating such diseases. The only exception would be rheumatoid arthritis, which has been treated with just about every legitimate and illegitimate therapy the human mind has been able to devise. Food allergy has been suggested as a cause, and complicated diets are sometimes prescribed by doctors of marginal status as arthritis experts.

Several studies have shown that elimination of certain foods may benefit some patients with rheumatoid arthritis. The benefit, however, may only be short-term. These studies are small in number, and further research in this area is certainly needed. Both the cause and cure of rheumatoid arthritis remain to be discovered; and by far, the best course for the patient is to follow the therapy prescribed by an arthritis specialist or rheumatologist, which can often alleviate its effects. One thing is certain: beware of practitioners who claim to treat rheumatoid arthritis through dietary manipulation alone.

HOMEOPATHY AND NATUROPATHY

Practitioners of these alternative approaches to medicine sometimes invoke principles of allergy medicine but then stray far from proven types of treatments.

Homeopathy was developed around 1900 by Dr. Samuel Hahnemann of Leipzig. It is based on the notion that "like cures like." The key idea is that certain drugs, such as quinine, produce symptoms similar to the diseases that they cure. Homeopathy is practiced by giving patients extraordinarily dilute amounts of plant or animal extracts that are supposedly curative. It appears that in homeopathic medicine, the smaller the dose, the more claims are made for it, giving rise to the joke about the homeopathic doctor who forgot to take his medicine and died of an overdose.

Naturopathy is based on the idea that the human body will naturally cure itself, given appropriate natural foods and drugs, massage, rest, and so on.

No studies of either of these therapies has demonstrated efficacy beyond that from a placebo effect. So the question is, how much you are willing to pay for a placebo or sugar pill? Insurance companies are certainly not interested in paying for these or any other unproven techniques.

The main danger to patients who turn to these disciplines is that they may fail to seek expert medical help when needed, and this delay in dealing with it may allow it to worsen.

Reliance on herbal remedies can also be risky. Use of herbs, like use of any drug, may have serious negative side effects (including allergy reactions, by the way).

Finally, there is a question whether some practitioners may be deliberately or at least recklessly exploiting vulnerable patients. While we were working on this book, we were asked to intervene in a case of a woman attending a naturopath who claimed to have discovered that she had numerous food allergies and who had put her on such a restricted diet that her friends feared for her health. In addition, this woman, who was in the midst of a divorce, appeared seriously depressed.

There is actually not much that outsiders can do in such cases. Direct attacks on the questionable practitioner are usually counterproductive. Emotional support from family and friends, plus gentle skepticism, may help.

QUESTIONABLE TESTS AND TREATMENTS

Presently, a number of questionable testing methods for allergies are being marketed and recommended to the public. Many are associated with the clinical-ecology approach.

Some irresponsible doctors give patients expensive, esoteric tests of immune function that are not relevant to their symptoms, along with various marginal or useless tests and perhaps some standard tests as well. Exorbitant prices are charged for the evaluation, to say nothing of the treatment. Unfortunately, such abuses are not rare, and many of the physicians implicated are involved in ongoing legal battles with state health authorities and medical organizations.

CYTOTOXIC TESTING

Testing for and diagnosing food allergies is frequently a difficult, frustrating process. Not surprisingly, therefore, a number of questionable tests are directed toward food allergies.

One of these procedures, cytotoxic leukocyte (white blood cell) testing, or cytotoxic testing, was excluded from Medicare and other insurance coverage in the 1980s for lack of proof that it is effective. The test kits have been outlawed by the Food and Drug Administration.

Cytotoxic leukocyte testing is based on the idea that there will be changes in a patient's leukocytes or a drop in their count after exposure to a food or other substance to which the patient is allergic. The test can be done in vivo, by exposing the patient to the substance and then drawing blood, or in vitro, by mixing the suspected substance with a blood sample. The latter method is more convenient and more widely used. Neither will be reliable. Consumers should avoid these tests and the doctors or other practitioners who advocate them.

FOOD IMMUNE COMPLEX ASSAY

This is another blood test designed to detect "hidden" food allergies. A measure is made of food immune complexes (antibodies coupled with food antigens) in the patient's serum. But actually, food immune complexes cannot be correlated with any known disease and appear to be present normally.

Although there may be some future insight to be derived from this line of research, as of now, absolutely no useful information can be obtained from this assay.

INTRADERMAL TITRATION FOR INHALANT ALLERGENS

Some early allergists, including H. Rinkel, believed that intradermal injection of inhalant allergens (such as pollen or dander) in varying strengths would not only reveal existing allergies but also determine an optimal dosage (the lowest effective dosage producing symptoms) for treating these allergies through immunotherapy. Unfortunately, the Rinkel method results in treatment with very low doses, which does not work. Higher doses are needed to attain immunity.

INTRADERMAL PROVOCATION TECHNIQUE

The intradermal provocation technique is an adaptation of the Rinkel method used to detect food allergies. Long regarded as useless, it was decisively discredited in an article in the *New England Journal of Medicine*. The method is based on injecting food allergens into the skin to provoke symptoms, such as restlessness or fatigue. Once the alleged allergy and an optimal dosage level has been identified, then further food injections once or twice a week are used to neutralize the response.

The research published in the *New England Journal of Medicine* found that statistically, subjects could not distinguish between injections of placebo and injections of food in terms of symptoms produced or in terms of diminishing the supposed allergy. Moreover, intradermal injection of food can be extremely dangerous. One might be dealing with a patient with a genuine food allergy who could even die from an overwhelming anaphylactic reaction.

SUBLINGUAL PROVOCATION AND NEUTRALIZATION

The sublingual provocation and neutralization approach to testing and treatment is similar to that just described above, except that drops of food extracts are placed under the tongue. The neutralizing doses are also administered sublingually.

Defenders of this approach sometimes point to penicillin desensitization, which is occasionally successfully done in emergency situations through sublingual administrations of carefully regulated doses of the drug. But intermittent sublingual administration of food drops has been studied and does not have any beneficial effect.

This approach should not be confused with recent studies documenting desensitization to certain foods using a sublingual approach. This approach is similar to sublingual immunotherapy to inhalant allergens, which is discussed in chapter 6. However these studies are only being done at university hospitals.

URINE AUTOINJECTION

Readers will no doubt be happy to hear that using injections of the patient's own urine to detect and treat allergies is not recommended. It is a useless and dangerous procedure that enjoyed a vogue in the 1930s and 1940s.

ELECTRODERMAL TESTING

This method applies a device to measure currents of electricity in the skin. A vial of substance to be tested (food, pollen, etc) is placed in the circuit and the resistance to electrical flow is measured. Proponents claim that testing for food is done on the legs, testing for pollens on the arms or trunk, and testing for allergens affecting the nose or sinuses should be done on the scalp. A recent study showed this technique to be useless.

APPLIED KINESIOLOGY

This method of "testing" uses patient muscle strength as an indicator of allergy. A patient holds a vial of an offending food in an outstretched arm or on their chest while lying down with outstretched arms. The arm weakens quicker if the vial contains a food to which they are allergic to. Not surprisingly, a controlled study demonstrated that the results are random and not reproducible.

OTHER INAPPROPRIATE TESTS

Here is a list of additional tests that are inappropriate for diagnosis of allergic diseases. However, some of them are legitimate tests used for other conditions, particularly to assess immune function. But keep in mind that abnormalities in immune function typically result in serious, life-threatening infections, not fatigue, headaches, muscle aches, and the like.

1. Antigen leukocyte cellular antibody test (ALCAT)

This is a variation of the cytotoxic test that uses electronic manipulation and computer analysis of the sample.

2. Total serum immunoglobulin

This test is normally used to measure immunity. In the evaluation of allergic illness, it really doesn't provide any useful information.

3.   Specific IgG antibodies

This test is used in the diagnosis of hypersensitivity pneumonitis. Low levels of these antibodies to foods are normally present, and their significance is not known.

4.   Lymphocyte subset counts

This test measures levels of the various subsets of lymphocytes in the blood. It is useful in the analysis of certain immunodeficiency states such as HIV infection.

5.   Lymphocyte function assays

These tests are used to evaluate immune-deficiency states but are not abnormal in patients with allergic illness.

6.   Cytokine assays and cytokine receptor assays

These tests (interleukins, interferons, etc.) measure levels of proteins that normally allow communication between white blood cells and are used in research in immunology. Their measurement in the diagnosis of allergic illness is speculative.

7.   Chemical analysis of body fluids, hair, and tissue

Chemicals present in our environment are present in our body fluids and in our tissues and hair. Newer technologies now exist to measure their presence at extremely low levels. The meaning of these tests is not known.

8.   Food immune complex assay

Complexes of food proteins and antibodies are present in low levels in our blood. It is felt these levels are normal and represent metabolism of foods we are exposed to.

9.   Pulse test

This test measures the pulse rate after exposure to a food by either oral, injection, or sublingual routes. An increase in ten beats per minute is considered positive. Pulse rates vary for many reasons. There is no correlation between small changes in pulse rate and exposure to a food to which we are allergic except in the case of an anaphylactic reaction in which case the pulse rate would be expected to double along with other symptoms.

QUESTIONABLE ALLERGIC DISORDERS

YEAST HYPERSENSITIVITY

One of the liveliest allergy controversies is whether a sensitivity to yeast in the patient's body accounts for a multitude of symptoms, from fatigue to hyperactivity, headaches to flatulence.

The common yeast organism *Candida albicans*, normally present in the body, sometimes proliferates excessively, usually after a course of antibiotics that kill off organisms controlling yeast in most circumstances. In women, the excess *Candida* (thrush or yeast infection) may cause vaginal burning and itching, which can be treated with an antifungal drug. Around 1980, Drs. C. O. Truss and William Crook popularized the idea that excess yeast may impair the immune system, causing a general feeling of illness and symptoms that may affect any or every organ system. Particularly appealing was the idea that this infestation might account for otherwise unexplained exhaustion, irritability, difficulty concentrating, depression, and anxiety.

A craving for sweets and/or alcohol is said to be related to yeast hypersensitivity. Patients supposedly also feel bad on damp or moldy days, or when exposed to smoke or chemical odors.

The tests run to evaluate yeast levels include a *Candida* skin test and a stool test. These are almost always positive—they are so in over 90 percent of all people. (Keep in mind that in mainstream medicine, the test for *Candida* is used to evaluate immunity. A positive test is considered normal. Also, *Candida* is normally present in the stool.) The treatment by the "Crook disciples" is by medication to kill yeast organisms (usually the drug nystatin), as well as special diets and environmental controls.

Unfortunately, there have been no scientific studies to document the legitimacy of the theory or the efficacy of the treatment. Furthermore, in a study in the *New England Journal of Medicine*, the question of whether a treatment for the so-called candidiasis hypersensitivity syndrome was effective yielded interesting results. Women with fatigue, premenstrual tension, gastrointestinal symptoms, depression, and other symptoms that fit the diagnostic criteria for this syndrome were treated with nystatin (an anti-*Candida* drug used by clinical ecologists to treat the syndrome). There was no difference in outcome when a similar group of women were treated with a placebo (sugar pill). The authors concluded that therapy for such women with nystatin was unwarranted.

There is not ordinarily any danger involved in the treatment, and the placebo effect of finding a doctor who seems to understand and care can be very helpful. Oftentimes, these patients have depression and other psychological conditions, and they have been to many doctors and finally find a doctor who understands. The danger then is from not addressing the true problem. For these patients and for others suffering from other medical conditions, there may be more appropriate treatment. Also, of course, the unproved treatment is not done for free; and some unscrupulous health-care providers recommend numerous additional tests and treatments of little worth.

HEADACHES

Many people, including some doctors, ascribe headaches to food allergies. But although sensitivity to certain foods does cause headaches in some cases, allergy is not usually involved.

Foods may play a role in some patients in producing migraine, cluster headaches, and some other headaches. It may be worthwhile for the patient to keep a food diary to see if the headaches and any type of food are linked. The following are the most likely known culprits: Alcohol can precipitate migraines and cluster headaches in some individuals. Migraines may also be related to tyramine in aged cheese, herring, liver, dates, and figs. Chocolate contains a related chemical, phenylethylamine, which may also cause headaches. Sodium nitrate used in processed deli meats and monosodium glutamate often used in Chinese food may also cause headaches in some people.

Certainly, poor eating habits may result in headaches. Any sudden reduction in one's customary caffeine intake is likely to cause a headache from caffeine withdrawal. But if you have a problem with chronic headaches, beware of the doctor who thinks exclusively in terms of food allergy as the answer. Headaches are serious enough to warrant careful diagnosis.

The first step is to find out what kind of headache you have. The classic migraine headache is not just a severe headache. It is preceded by an "aura," a sensation that indicates the headache is coming on. There may be disturbances in vision at this time, such as perception of a flashing light or shimmers in the visual field. The headache itself consists of a deep, throbbing ache, often behind one eye. The patient is extremely sensitive to light or noise while the headache lasts, and this may be a few hours or even a couple of days. There may be nausea and vomiting. There is often a family history of migraines. The underlying condition in migraines is a widening of the blood vessels to the brain. Most migraines should be treated by a specialist.

Other vascular disorders may cause cluster headaches, which are extraordinarily painful. Characteristically, there are long periods of remission and then the headaches come back in "clusters."

Sinus headaches may be associated with allergic rhinitis or any infection that causes inflammation and blockage of the sinuses (see chapter 11). The pain may be over the eyes, in the cheekbones, near the tear ducts, in the teeth, or in the top rear of the skull.

High blood pressure may be associated with headaches, but remember that high blood pressure can also have no symptoms.

Tension and disorders involving the joint of the jaw (the temporomandibular joint) may cause aches on both sides of the back of the neck and a bandlike ache around the head.

Severe headache may be caused by meningitis (inflammation of the tissue covering the brain). Associated symptoms may include fever, a stiff neck, and/or a rash.

Sudden, severe headaches may be a sign that a stroke is occurring.

There is treatment available for almost all types of headache, but a reliable diagnosis must first be reached. Sudden, severe headaches should be evaluated immediately. A trip to the emergency room is in order if there is no other medical help available. Recurring, severe headaches should also be taken seriously. Usually, a neurologist is the specialist of choice in such cases.

HYPERACTIVITY

The popular notion that food additives or other elements in food may cause hyperactivity in children dates back to the mid-1970s and a book by Dr. Ben Feingold, *Why Your Child Is Hyperactive*. Dr. Crook, one of the authors of the *Candida*-allergy theory, proposed that a sugar allergy causes hyperactivity.

Some people are indeed adversely affected by certain food additives; and as many parents have observed, sugar may stimulate adrenaline production, especially in children. (See chapter 7.) But this is a transient reaction, and allergy is not involved. The cure is to limit sugar intake.

Chronic hyperactivity associated with difficulties in academic work and social adjustment is a serious problem that requires expert evaluation. The causes may range from use of cocaine by the mother during pregnancy to frustration and aggression arising when a learning-disabled child is not appropriately diagnosed and helped. (Some students with learning difficulties are also extremely bright, which only adds to their restlessness and anger.) Allergy testing is not, however, a useful diagnostic tool in cases of hyperactivity.

Children with ADD (attention deficit disorder) and ADHD (attention deficit/hyperactivity disorder) must be treated as soon as the diagnosis is established. Early intervention is key to how successful treatment will be—and treatment can be very successful in these patients. It is important to involve the pediatrician, educators, and psychopharmacological experts in treatment. The use of unproven methods in treatment of these children prior to utilizing known, effective mainstream treatment thereby causing delay in appropriate therapy is unconscionable.

DANGER SIGNS

Certain types of treatments for alleged allergies may cause harm and should sound an alarm as to the physician's method of practice. These are the following:

- Highly restricted diets. Most people are allergic to only a few foods, if any, and do not need to eat only organic foods or only vegetables or large quantities of red meat, etc. Children and elderly people are particularly at risk if the diet is unbalanced or inadequate.

- The use of allergy treatments for symptoms that may indicate a serious health problem. These would include severe headaches, severe joint pains, chronic gastrointestinal disturbances, depression, and learning handicaps.
- Allergy or diet treatments for presently incurable diseases, such as multiple sclerosis or rheumatoid arthritis.
- Expensive nonstandard tests and treatments.

We have not listed all the questionable methods in allergy medicine, just those that are more common and long-lived. When in doubt of a practitioner's method of testing or treatment, we urge you to use a website designed to reduce health-care fraud in the United States. It is www.quackwatch.com and is useful for allergy as well as other areas of medicine. Share this useful website with your friends.

Chapter 20

COMPLEMENTARY AND ALTERNATIVE MEDICINE

This is a new chapter appearing in our books for the first time. We decided to devote a whole chapter to this subject because Americans go to complementary practitioners of medicine more than they go to conventional doctors.

Over the past twenty years, patients have become increasingly interested in complementary medicine. As a result, conventional medicine researchers have begun to study complementary medicine in order to determine which treatments are helpful, what might be harmful, and what might be ineffective. Sometimes it's difficult to study complementary medicine with methods used to study conventional medicine. Usually, there is no financial incentive to study a treatment (such as there is with a new drug), and even worse is the possibility that some providers do not want studies to be done should they disprove a technique.

Nonetheless, the government has been studying complementary medicine since 1993. The National Center for Complementary and Alternative Medicine (NCCAM, www.nccam.nih.gov/) is the main government organization that evaluates complementary medicine and provides useful information to the public.

In the past, the FDA has not closely regulated the manufacture of dietary supplements. Recently, new FDA regulations require compliance with manufacturing practices that guarantee the quality and safety of supplements. The FDA provides alerts about harmful dietary supplements at their website (www.fda.gov/Food/DietarySupplements/Alerts/default.htm).

Since this book was last published in 1998, there have been extraordinary gains in knowledge in the treatment of allergic disorders, enabling us to use conventional medicine successfully in 99 percent of our patients.

Yet there is that small percentage of patients where either the conventional methodology does not work, the side effects are unacceptable, or the patient prefers to utilize alternative medical methods. It is in that group of patients that an integrative approach with complementary medicine can be used.

Breakthroughs in research are shedding light on various alternative medical techniques, some positive and some negative. One of the authors of this book (SHY) published a study of the successful use of hypnosis in the prevention of exercise-induced bronchospasm. Dr. Young has found hypnosis useful in some of his patients and is discussed below. Recently, researchers at Mount Sinai Hospital in New York City have demonstrated great promise in the use of a combination of three Chinese herbs in the treatment of asthma. These herbs were shown to be as effective as prednisone (and without the side effects) in the treatment of asthma!

In fact, the American Academy of Allergy, Asthma & Immunology recently appointed a committee to evaluate the use of complementary and alternative medicine in our field. For the rest of this chapter, complementary and alternative medicine will be called by its acronym, *CAM*. One author, SHY, is on this committee.

It is important for patients utilizing complementary medicine to let your physician know that you are doing so, as herbs and other alternative therapies can have an impact on the conventional treatment your physician is offering you. In addition, there are potential interactions with prescription medications and harmful potential side effects to your health that your physician will be aware of. Don't be afraid that your physician will criticize you for utilizing complementary medications—nor should they.

And if you do utilize chiropractic methods, acupuncture, or other alternative methods, be sure that your practitioner is licensed and has the highest credentials available in her field.

Although much of alternative medicine is safe the significant risks are the following:

1. Heavy metal contamination of some herbs
2. Some botanicals can be toxic, especially to the liver and kidneys
3. Interactions between CAM therapies (e.g., botanicals, micronutrients, other dietary supplements) and other drugs, although usually not a problem in those CAM therapies used to combat allergies or asthma
4. Use of alternative medicine during a time that conventional medicine is known to be efficacious (e.g., an herbal mix as the sole treatment for a life-threatening attack of asthma)

Since we believe that there can be some merit in alternative methods, we need to discuss the various types of complementary medicine available. We will not list or advocate any herbs that are used to treat allergic disease (with the exception of the Mount Sinai Division of Clinical Immunology studies) as that is beyond the scope of this book. The reader is referred to her own physician for this advice as well as the government website that we have listed above and the CAM database listed in the appendix.

So first, a few definitions would be helpful:

In Western culture, complementary and alternative medicine (CAM) includes various healing approaches and therapies that are not based on conventional Western medicine. These therapies are called alternative medicine when they are used alone and complementary medicine when they are used with conventional medicine. Integrative medicine refers to the use of all appropriate therapeutic approaches.

So what's the difference? The distinction between conventional medicine and alternative medicine is that conventional medicine generally defines health as the absence of disease or dysfunction. The main causes of disease and dysfunction are various factors, such as pathogens (bacteria or viruses), biochemical imbalances, trauma, and of course, aging. Treatment usually utilizes drugs, surgery, or rehabilitative techniques; and treatments have, for the most part, been studied and proven to be effective. Another term for conventional medicine is evidence-based medicine.

In contrast, alternative medicine practices often define health holistically, that is, as a balance of systems—physical, emotional, environmental, social, and spiritual—involving the whole person. Disharmony between these systems is believed to cause illness. Treatment involves strengthening the body's own defenses to restore these balances. Furthermore, treatments have not been subjected to scientific study. Indeed, when a treatment is studied and shown to be effective, it is then incorporated into conventional or evidence-based medicine.

There are many alternative modalities. We will only list and discuss the various modalities that have relevance to the treatment of allergic disorders and that have supportive literature suggesting that they may be of some use in treating allergic disorders. This is a very controversial and evolving field.

We will divide the discussion into the three general categories of CAM: those dealing with mind-body interaction, which are formally known as mind-body interventions, energy-based methods, and biologically based therapy.

MIND-BODY INTERVENTIONS

The mind-body-intervention group has the most-scientific evidence to support its use in medical treatment. In fact, one author (SHY) utilizes hypnosis successfully in his practice. However, many of these methods have not been proven to have validity in the treatment of asthma and allergies.

We will start with hypnosis, which involves a complex alteration of consciousness, the exact mechanism of which is unclear. It is not a sleep state; and in reality, the hypnotic subject, when entering the trance state, becomes more alert and awake than usual. She enters a state of intense concentration with diminution of peripheral awareness as well as becoming more focused and centrally aware. It is widely and incorrectly believed that the subject is under the complete control of the hypnotist, whereas the converse is true. It is the subject's awareness, focus, and control that enables them to channel extraordinary healing power in the natural trance state to control the syndrome the subject is dealing with. Patients are put into a state of attentive and focused concentration. They become absorbed in the images presented by the hypnotherapist and can be relatively unaware, but not entirely unconscious, of their surroundings; they tend not to register experiences as a part of their conscious awareness.

The author (SHY) has found hypnosis to be a very helpful modality in the treatment of asthma since it induces a very powerful state of relaxation in any subject. Therefore, whatever part stress may be contributing to the patient's asthma is lessened. But what is crucial is that the subject can exert some degree of control of their autonomic nervous system and perhaps lessen the immune system malfunction that is related to their illness. In fact, SHY participated in a study published in the *American Review of Respiratory Diseases* that demonstrated hypnosis can be of benefit in reducing exercise-induced asthma.

Hypnosis essentially induces a trance state, which is a natural state. This is not psychotherapy in any way and is more akin to guided imagery, which is discussed later in this chapter. The hypnotist is the guide, but the subject is in control. The subject can enter and leave the trance state with very little training.

Hypnosis has become much easier to use medically than previously because of a breakthrough in the quantification of the hypnotizablity of the subjects. The method developed by Herbert Spiegel, MD, a professor of psychiatry at Columbia Presbyterian Hospital, is called the HIP (hypnotic induction profile). It appears that there is a correlation with the degree of eye roll and hypnotizablity. The eye roll is a measure of the amount of visible sclera (the white of the eye) between the lower border of the iris and the lower eyelid when the subject is asked to gaze up as high as he can and then close his eyes slowly. The more white of the eye that shows with this maneuver, the more the person can be hypnotized. The next step is to measure various other functions of hypnotizablity such as how long it takes to get the subject to raise their arm while hypnotic suggestion is utilized by the operator. There are various other modalities that are tested, and the whole procedure takes less than ten minutes. Simultaneously, the subject is learning how to go into a state of self-hypnosis.

Biofeedback involves the use of instrumentation that can measure biological functions and their variations of which an individual would not be aware. These measurements are fed back to the individual, informing her of biological functions so that she can learn to control them. An example is forehead tension, where the subject is taught (using sensors on the forehead that measure muscle tension) to intentionally reduce that tension. This technique can be utilized to reduce blood pressure or minimize or eliminate migraine headaches. Similar techniques can be used to alleviate bronchospasm in asthma.

So in essence, biofeedback is a process that enables an individual to learn to change physiologic activity for the purpose of improving health. This allows a person to alter their physiological response, such as bronchospasm, initially with instrumentation but eventually on their own without any instrumental crutch.

Guided imagery. This method utilizes imagery developed in the subject's imagination to direct their thoughts toward a relaxing or peaceful scene. This is usually a pleasant, idyllic scene, and the subject imagines they are there. There is a stepwise relaxation program to induce relaxation. The mental images are used to promote healing of a particular condition including asthma. The images can utilize any of the senses and can be self-guided or guided by an instructor. It appears to be similar to self-hypnosis. There are anecdotal reports of success in allergy.

Meditation. Meditation is the intentional self-regulation of attention or a systematic mental focus on particular aspects of inner transcendental experience. Most meditation techniques utilize repeating certain meaningless sounds while sitting quietly and comfortably for a period of time. Often, breathing exercises are added and focusing on breathing is emphasized. In effect, this will produce relaxation and can theoretically reduce bronchospasm.

Relaxation technique. A method to reduce stress, it is usually done in a formalized progressive relaxation of various muscle groups. These techniques are specifically designed to elicit a psychophysiologic state of hypoarousal. They may be aimed at reducing sympathetic nervous system activity and blood pressure, easing muscle tension, slowing metabolic processes, or altering brain wave activity.

A popular method is progressive relaxation developed by Edmund Jacobson. His method is to train the subject to progressively tense and relax groups of muscles starting in the extremities and moving first to the torso and then to the head and neck. When this method is used, a deep state of relaxation is induced in most individuals. It is similar to yoga meditation and hypnosis. All the above methods have anecdotal reports of success. However, there are no definitive studies—and certainly no scientific double-blinded studies to demonstrate their efficacy.

ENERGY-BASED METHODS

The next category is energy-based methods, and the most studied and useful method is acupuncture.

Acupuncture. Specific points on the body are stimulated by inserting thin needles into the skin and underlying tissues. Stimulating these specific points is believed to unblock the flow of qi (loosely described as vital energy) along energy pathways (meridians) and thus restore balance between yin and yang. The procedure is not painful but may cause a tingling sensation. A variation of acupuncture, called acupressure, uses localized massage instead of needles to stimulate acupuncture points.

Research has shown that acupuncture releases various neurotransmitters (e.g., endorphins) that act as natural painkillers. Adverse effects are rare if the procedure is done correctly. Worsening of symptoms (usually temporary) and fainting are the most common. Infection is extremely rare as most practitioners use disposable needles.

There is much anecdotal evidence that acupuncture is useful in asthma and allergies, but there are no very clear-cut double-blind studies to back this up. Nevertheless, the work done in this field is encouraging.

We mention some of the other methods in this category but do not describe them in depth as there is no evidence currently to substantiate their use in allergy and asthma. These include magnetism (there is ongoing research concerning moving magnets but no clear answer yet); therapeutic touch (mentioned elsewhere in this book and has been debunked in a study published in the *Journal of the American Medical Association*); and Reiki—a formalized therapeutic touch developed in the early 1900s in Japan that in some forms may use remote touch or distant healing. Reiki is sometimes referred to as Oriental medicine.

Biologically Based Therapy

Biologically based therapy includes dietary-based therapy, orthomolecular medicine, and chelation therapy. Currently, there is no evidence to support their use in the treatment of asthma and allergy, but there is ongoing work of interest in dietary therapy.

Manipulative and body-based therapy. Chiropractic, reflexology, rolfing, and massage therapy. Currently, there is no evidence to support their use in the treatment of asthma and allergy.

The following are alternative medical systems that are widely utilized, but their validity in allergic and asthmatic disease has not been demonstrated at this point.

Ayurveda. An ancient Indian medical system that uses herbs, massage, yoga, and therapeutic elimination to restore balance within the body. It is based on balancing the three bodily qualities (*doshas*): *vata*, *pitta*, and *kapha*. Efforts have been made to organize this method in India. Outside India, it is not subjected to such regulation. The National Center for Complementary and Alternative Medicine spends a portion of its annual budget studying Ayurvedic medicine, but conclusions about efficacy are still pending.

Homeopathy. Developed in Germany during the late 1700s, homeopathy is a system of medicine based on the law of similars. The theory is that a substance that causes certain symptoms of a disease, when used in high concentrations, can be used to treat that disease and its symptoms when given in a very dilute concentration or miniscule dose. So a substance that causes nausea at very high doses will be used to treat nausea at very low doses. Studies both here and in the United Kingdom have shown that homeopathic treatments are no more effective than placebo.

Naturopathy. Founded on the healing power of nature, this system uses a combination of therapies (including acupuncture, applied kinesiology, chelation therapy, colonic enemas, hair analysis, nutrition, and many others) most of which do not appear to have any benefit in the treatment of asthma and allergies. Some such as acupuncture have already been discussed in this chapter.

Diet therapies. There are many specialized dietary regimens; a well-known example is the macrobiotic diet. There have been studies to evaluate various diets and food stuff such as primrose oil, fish oil, and many other foods. And because of the great interest in these, there is ongoing research of these substances. Even though there are anecdotal reports of benefits, there have not been clear-cut studies demonstrating efficacy so far.

SUPPLEMENTS

Dietary supplements are also known as food supplements or nutritional supplements. They include vitamins, minerals, herbs and other botanicals, amino acids, and even some hormones (DHEA and melatonin). As with pharmaceuticals or drugs, they are regulated by the FDA in the United States. However, unlike drugs, dietary supplements can enter the marketplace without efficacy studies. There are many scientific studies demonstrating various effects of everything, from vitamin C to fish oil, on one aspect of the immune system or another. But there is a dearth of studies showing beneficial effects in humans. Therefore, we cannot recommend any specific supplements for allergic illnesses.

There are ongoing studies and great interest in these supplements, so perhaps this will change for the next edition of our book. The scientific research that shows effects on the immune system creates untoward effects on the usage of these substances. An example is vitamin C. Years ago, scientific studies demonstrated that vitamin C can boost the function of certain cells of the immune system. As a result of these studies, claims were made that vitamin C, in high doses, can reduce the duration of the common cold. Further studies in humans failed to prove this. The moral of this story is that just because something happens in a test tube does not mean you can extrapolate that into an effect on living human beings.

There is a multitude of alternative treatment methods, from rolfing, which manipulates and stretches the fascia (connective tissue), to align muscles and ligaments, to utilization of shark cartilage. All these have their proponents, but there is certainly no evidence linking any of these methods to usefulness in allergy and asthma treatment.

Although there is no clear-cut evidence that alternative methods work, we have described above those where there is strong anecdotal evidence that they work. Certainly, hypnosis, biofeedback, relaxation therapy, meditation, and acupuncture may have some use in treating allergies and asthma. At the very least, these can reduce stress and contribute to an overall feeling of well-being.

We believe that more careful studies of the above methods should be done. Physicians should integrate the methods that show promise with the conventional therapies that they utilize. We all should be vigilant against charlatans who utilize methods that clearly demonstrate no benefit except to the pocketbook of the practitioner who utilizes the method.

Finally, the National Center for Complementary and Alternative Medicine as well as specialty committees such as the CAM committee of the American Academy of Allergy, Asthma & Immunology should continue their study of all these methods to give us the knowledge to choose what methods have validity in the treatment of allergic disease.

Chapter 21

THE FUTURE IN ALLERGY MEDICINE

Mark Twain once said that making predictions can be very difficult especially when dealing with the future. In allergy, however, the immediate future is easy to predict. The advances that have been made in the last decade will continue.

Allergy extracts, although very pure now, will continue to improve in quality.

Allergens for immunotherapy will continue to be modified so that they will not induce an allergic reaction and will be more effective in desensitizing and will do so in a much-shorter time than currently is.

Sublingual and oral allergy extracts will be utilized to treat both environmental as well as food allergies.

Xolair (omalizumab) is a monoclonal antibody that selectively binds to human immunoglobulin E (IgE). Monoclonal antibodies have been developed to treat a whole host of diseases, including infections, cancers, and inflammatory conditions. In allergy medicine, these monoclonal antibodies are as of now only available to treat asthma but in the near future will be used to treat other allergies, including food allergies such as peanut allergy, in a safe and effective manner. Monoclonal antibodies will also be effective in the treatment of hives, angioedema, sinusitis, and possibly eczema.

Elidel (pimecrolimus) and Protopic (tacrolimus) are topical medications used for the treatment of atopic dermatitis (eczema). These medications, called topical calcineurin inhibitors (TCIs), were the first nonsteroid topical medications developed to treat eczema. Their use is limited today because of fears that they can cause lymphoma. These drugs are very effective and virtually without side effects. This type of medication will be made safe to use and will be very effective in treating eczema.

Work will continue on the mind-body interaction. Hypnosis, biofeedback, meditation, and relaxation therapies will become important adjuncts in the treatment of allergic disease. See chapter 20 on CAM (complementary alternative medicine). Our understanding of these complementary and alternative therapies will continue to improve.

We discussed the use of Chinese herbs in the treatment of allergies and asthma. This is discussed in the chapter on CAM, especially the work of researchers at the Mount Sinai Medical Center in New York. Herbal remedies will be studied and introduced into our armamentarium of treatments.

In the more-distant future, greater than ten years from now, there will be medications that will attack allergy reactions at a fundamental level—stopping them before they start. These medications will be able to alter inflammatory pathways and directly alter allergic disease.

With respect to food allergy in particular, another approach being studied is manipulation of the helper T cells, which are white blood cells that assist in immune system reactions. There are two types of helper T cells, TH1 and TH2. The former, TH1 (the "good" ones), appears to release chemicals that suppress the formation of allergic antibodies to foods and other allergens. The TH2 cells (the "bad" ones) have the opposite action and stimulate the development of the allergic response.

The reason for the effectiveness of current allergy immunotherapy (allergy shots) may be that it shifts the balance between TH1 and TH2 so that TH1 dominates and the allergy antibodies are suppressed. However, we cannot yet, as we have said, use food extracts for allergy shots because of the danger of anaphylaxis.

A solution to this dilemma that researchers are now investigating is to use a slightly altered version of the DNA of a particular food allergen, say peanut allergen, as a vaccine. The vaccine, ideally, will create immunity without risk of a full-blown systemic allergic reaction (anaphylaxis). Vaccines are now being tested with peanut-allergic mice.

We are in the early stages of our understanding of genetics. Eventually, as our understanding of the genetics of allergy and other diseases deepens, we will be able to treat diseases at the cellular level and eventually prevent the development of disease through intervention at the genetic level.

Our ability to diagnose drug allergies will greatly improve as we understand the genetic nature of these reactions and can use this information to develop tests to find out who is susceptible and who is not.

We are in the early stages of understanding how the environment interacts with the expression of the genes. So for example, if a baby is born to a mother or father who has asthma, we will eventually be able to predict whether that baby will develop asthma and even prevent or reduce the likelihood of asthma developing. And if the child develops asthma, we will be able to predict which medications or treatments will work the best and which ones will cause side effects. In summary, and probably the most significant of future advances, is that based on gene testing we will be able to predict which medications and treatments will be tolerated and effective in which patients.

Appendix A

ASTHMA INHALATION DEVICES

THE METERED-DOSE INHALER (MDI)

This little metal pressurized container—the metered dose inhaler, or MDI—contains medications for treating and/or preventing asthma.

How to Use Your MDI

(1) Shake the MDI vigorously, or you may not get the proper dose of medication.

(2) Depending on your doctor's advice, hold the canister mouthpiece about two inches from either your open mouth or in your mouth with your lips sealed around it. (If you are using a spacer that accomplishes the same effect as the two-inch distance, then the mouthpiece of the spacer must be in your mouth with your lips around it.) Patients on high-dose inhaled steroids may have to use a spacer. This is dependent on which medication you are on as some medications (Qvar and Dulera, with their unique delivery systems, produce particles that are small enough to deposit in the small airways of the lungs and do not require a spacer.)

(3) Exhale all the air out of your lungs.

(4) As you start to take a deep breath in, actuate the canister to discharge a puff of medication and continue breathing in, sucking the medication into your lungs.

(5) Try then to hold your breath for ten seconds before breathing out so that the medicine has time to settle in your lungs. Then resume normal breathing.

(6) If the MDI that you use first is a bronchodilator (and you should use the bronchodilator first if it is one of two or three inhalers being used at a given time), wait five minutes before taking the second puff (if instructed to take a

second puff) or before using your other medication (e.g., inhaled steroid) so that your airways open up and subsequent puffs get deeper into the lungs (into the smaller airways that are susceptible to inflammation).

(7) The number of puffs to be used of each medication is as prescribed by your doctor. If you need more puffs of your bronchodilator or it is not relieving your symptoms, you must contact your doctor.

How to Determine If Your MDI Is Empty

There is no reliable way to tell if your MDI is empty. Some newer inhalers, particularly the dry powder inhalers but also some of the metered-dose inhalers, come with a counter that keeps track of the number of doses left. If the MDI has no counter, then the only way to know when to replace it is by keeping track of the number of doses you use on average per week. For example, if you use an average of four puffs per week of your rescue inhaler and the canister has two hundred sprays in it when you bought it, then replace it after fifty weeks. We recommend erring on the conservative side so you don't run out of the medication. Therefore, we would recommend replacing it in about forty-five weeks.

How to Care for Your MDI

To prevent the valve from clogging with medication, rinse it with warm water every couple of days that you are using it.

Medications available for the MDI are (1) the rescue inhalers (beta$_2$-agonists), including albuterol HFA (ProAir HFA, Proventil HFA, and Ventolin HFA), pirbuterol (Maxair), and Xopenex HFA, and (2) corticosteroids, including budesonide (Pulmicort), ciclesonide (Alvesco) fluticasone (Flovent), mometasone (Asmanex), beclomethasone dipropionate (Beclovent, Qvar, and Vanceril), and anticholinergics such as ipratropium (Atrovent HFA).

The Spacer

The spacer or holding chamber, referred to above, is a plastic tubelike device that can be attached to the MDI. There are many types of spacers, including the commonly used AeroChamber, InspirEase, and OptiHaler. Typically, children under age five cannot use an MDI correctly, but the spacer lowers the age to about four. Spacers decrease the amount of the drug deposited in the throat, which is important, when corticosteroids and even beta$_2$-agonists are being used, to avoid absorption of the drug into your system. The larger spacers may improve the MDI's delivery of the medication to the lungs. A spacer may be as effective as a nebulizer (see below) in delivering high doses of beta$_2$-agonists during an asthma flare-up.

Breath-Actuated MDI

The standard MDI, often called the pump, can be difficult to use, especially for children and older patients. The new breath-actuated MDI delivers medication when you inhale. Only one short-acting beta$_2$-agonist (Maxair) is available in this form, and spacers are not necessary when using it. Consult your doctor for the latest information.

Nebulizers

The nebulizer runs on electricity from an outlet or battery. The device aerates a liquid medicine, which is delivered as a mist through a mask or plastic mouthpiece. The mask type can be used to treat young children who cannot use a mouthpiece. The medicine is best inhaled with slow regular breaths plus occasional deep breaths. For adults, a nebulizer may be recommended for high-dose beta$_2$-agonists and anticholinergics when asthma symptoms become severe. Nebulizers generally deliver medication efficiently but are relatively large and clumsy to carry and use. Smaller, more portable units are available. Different models vary considerably in efficiency. A variety of bronchodilator medications are available for use with a nebulizer. The corticosteroid budesonide (Pulmicort Respules) is particularly useful in younger children and even infants when used with a mask. Nebulizers are more commonly used for children with all grades of asthma and in adults who have more severe asthma.

Appendix B

How to Use Your Peak Flow Meter

If you have asthma, your doctor may recommend that you monitor your airflow to keep track of your condition. You should record the results in an asthma diary as your doctor instructs. The following instructions are courtesy of the National Institutes of Health's *Guidelines for the Diagnosis and Management of Asthma*.

Ask your doctor or nurse to show you how to use a peak flow meter and to periodically check on your technique.

Do the following five steps with your peak flow meter:

1. Move the indicator to the bottom of the numbered scale.
2. Stand up.
3. Take a deep breath, filling your lungs completely.
4. Place the mouthpiece in your mouth and close your lips around it. Do not put your tongue inside the hole.
5. Blow out as hard and fast as you can in a single blow as if you were trying to blow out a large piece of burning newspaper.

- Write down the number you get. But if you cough or make a mistake, don't write down the number. Do it over again.
- Repeat steps 1 through 5 two more times and write down the best of the three blows in your asthma diary.

Find Your Personal-Best Peak-Flow Number

Your *personal-best* peak-flow number is the highest peak-flow number you can achieve over a two—to three-week period when your asthma is under good control. Good control is when you feel good and do not have any asthma symptoms.

Each patient's asthma is different, and your personal-best peak flow may be higher or lower than the peak flow of someone of your same height, weight, age, and sex. There are no normal or expected values for you or for your particular peak flow meter. This means that it is important for you to find your personal-best peak-flow number when you first get your peak flow meter. And in the case of a child, the personal best will typically increase as the child gets older. Therefore, the personal best will have to be reassessed every year or so.

- To find out your personal-best peak-flow number, take peak-flow readings: at least twice a day for two to three weeks; when you wake up and between noon and 2:00 p.m.; before and after you take your short-acting inhaled beta$_2$-agonist (albuterol HFA, Proventil HFA, ProAir HFA, or Ventolin HFA), pirbuterol (Maxair), levalbuterol (Xopenex HFA) for quick relief, if you take this medicine as instructed by your doctor.

THE PEAK-FLOW-ZONE SYSTEM

Once you know your personal-best peak-flow number, your doctor will give you the numbers that tell you what to do. The peak-flow numbers are put into zones that are set up like a traffic light. This will help you know what to do when your peak-flow number changes. For example, ***green zone*** (more than *a number expresses as* L/min [which is 80 percent of your personal-best number]) signals good control. No asthma symptoms are present. Take your medicines as usual.

Yellow zone (50 percent to 80 percent of your personal-best number) signals caution. You must take your short-acting inhaled beta$_2$-agonist right away. Also, your asthma may not be under good day-to-day control. Ask your doctor if you need to change or increase your daily medications.

Red zone (below 50 percent of your personal-best number) signals a medical alert. You must take your short-acting inhaled beta$_2$-agonist right away. Call your doctor or emergency room and ask what to do or go directly to the hospital emergency room.

Record your personal-best peak-flow number and peak-flow zones in your asthma diary.

Appendix C

FOOD GROUPS

- Food allergy: *Guidelines for the Diagnosis and Management of Food Allergy in the United States*, published by the National Institute of Allergy and Infectious Diseases (a branch of the National Institutes of Health) in December 2010. The reference here is intended for physicians. Guidelines for the layperson are expected to be released sometime in 2011.
  - http://www.niaid.nih.gov/topics/foodAllergy/clinical/Pages/default.aspx

FOOD GROUPS

Researchers have found that if you are allergic to a particular food, there is a chance that you may be allergic to other foods related to it. Table C1 lists groups of food that share similar allergens; table C2 lists foods alphabetically and provides a group reference number so you can quickly locate and avoid related foods that might trigger an allergic reaction.

SOURCE: ADVERSE REACTIONS TO FOODS

American Academy of Allergy, Asthma & Immunology Committee on Adverse Reactions to Food. National Institute of Allergy and Infectious Diseases. U.S. Department of Health and Human Services. Public Health Service. National Institutes of Health. NIH Publication No. 84-2442, July 1984.

TABLE C1.

FOOD PROTEINS CLASSIFIED ACCORDING TO SIMILAR ALLERGIC POTENTIAL
(See alphabetical list of foods that follows this table.)

ANIMAL GROUPS

1. **AMPHIBIANS**
   - frog
2. **BIRDS (flesh and organs)**
   - chicken
   - Cornish hen
   - duck
   - goose
   - grouse
   - guinea hen (fowl)
   - partridge
   - pheasant
   - pigeon
   - quail
   - squab
   - turkey
3. **CRUSTACEANS**
   - crab
   - crayfish
   - lobster
   - prawn
   - shrimp
4. **EGGS (bird)**
   - ovomucoid
   - ovovitellin
   - white
   - whole
   - yolk
5. **FISH (representative families)**
   - Acipenseridae:
     - sturgeon (caviar)
   - Anguillidae:
     - eel
   - Argentinidae:
     - smelt
   - Carangidae:
     - pompano
   - Centrarchidae:
     - black bass
     - crappie
     - sunfish
   - Clupeidae:
     - herring
     - sardine
     - shad
     - sprat
   - Cyprinidae:
     - carp
   - Esocidae:
     - muskellunge
     - pickerel
     - pike
   - Gadidae:
     - cod
     - haddock
     - hake
     - pollack
     - scrod
   - Mugilidae:
     - mullet
   - Percidae:
     - perch
   - Pleuronectidae:
     - flounder
     - halibut
   - Salmonidae:
     - grayling
     - salmon
     - trout

- whitefish
- Scienidae:
  - croaker
  - drum
  - redfish
  - sea trout
  - weakfish
- Scombridae:
  - bonito
  - mackerel
  - tuna
- Serranidae:
  - grouper
  - rockfish
  - white bass
- Siluridae:
  - bullhead
  - catfish
- Soleidae:
  - sole
- Sparidae:
  - porgy
  - red snapper
- Stolephoridae:
  - anchovy
- Xyphidae:
  - swordfish

6. **RED MEATS** (flesh and internal organs)
  a. Bovidae (cattle):
  - beef
  - calf
  - steer
  - veal
  - gelatin
  - goat
  - ox
  - sheep
    - lamb
    - mutton
  - sweetbread
  b. Suidae (pig):

- bacon
- boar
- ham
- hog
- pig
- pork
- sausage
- scrapple
- sow
- swine

7. **MILK PRODUCTS** (cow, goat):
  - butter
  - buttermilk
  - casein
  - cheese
  - cream
    - sour
    - whipped
  - ice cream
  - lactalbumin
  - milk
    - condensed
    - evaporated
    - homogenized
    - powdered
    - raw
    - skimmed
  - selected infant formulas
  - yogurt

8. **MOLLUSKS:**
  - abalone
  - clam
  - cockle
  - mussel
  - octopus
  - oyster
  - quahog
  - scallop
  - snail (escargot)
  - squid

9. **REPTILES:**
  - alligator

- crocodile
- rattlesnake
- terrapin
- turtle

PLANT GROUPS

10. APPLE FAMILY
- Apple
  - cider
    - vinegar (apple cider))
- crabapple
- pear
- quince
- quince seed

11. BANANA FAMILY
- banana
- plantain

12. BEECH FAMILY
- beechnut
- chestnut
- chinquapin

13. BIRCH FAMILY
- filbert
- hazelnut
- wintergreen

14. BUCKWHEAT FAMILY
- buckwheat
- rhubarb
- sorrel

15. CASHEW FAMILY
- cashew
- mango
- pistachio

16. CITRUS FAMILY
- citron
- grapefruit
- kumquat
- lemon
- lime
- orange
- tangelo

- tangerine

17. COLA NUT FAMILY
- chocolate (cocoa)
- cola (kola) nut

18. FUNGI
- mushroom
- truffle
- yeast:
  - baker's
  - brewer's
  - distiller's
  - Fleischmann's
  - lactose-fermenting
  - lager beer

19. GINGER FAMILY
- cardamon (cardamom, cardamum)
- East Indian arrowroot
- ginger
- turmeric

20. GOOSEFOOT FAMILY
- beet
- lamb's quarters
- spinach
- Swiss chard

21. GOURD (MELON) FAMILY
- cantaloupe (muskmelon)
- casaba (winter muskmelon)
- Chinese watermelon
- citron melon
- cucumber
- gherkin
- honeydew melon
- Persian melon
- pumpkin
- summer squash
- watermelon
- winter squash

22. GRAPE FAMILY
- champagne
- grape
- raisin
- vinegar (wine)

- wine (grape)

23. GRASS (CEREAL) FAMILY

- bamboo
- barley
- corn (maize)
- hominy
- malt (germinated grain)
- millet
- oat
- popcorn
- rice
- rye
- sorghum
- sugar cane
- wheat:
  - bran
  - germ
  - gliadin
  - globulin
  - glutenin
  - leucosin
  - proteose
  - whole

24. HEATH FAMILY

- black huckleberry
- blueberry
- cranberry
- wintergreen

25. LAUREL FAMILY

- avocado
- bay leaf
- cinnamon
- sassafras

26. LECYTHIS FAMILY

- Brazil nut

27. LILY FAMILY

- aloe
- asparagus
- chives
- garlic
- leek
- onion

- sarsaparilla
- shallot

28. MADDER FAMILY

- coffee

29. MALLOW FAMILY

- cottonseed
- marshmallow
- okra (gumbo)

30. MINT FAMILY

- balm
- basil
- catnip
- horehound
- Japanese artichoke
- lavender
- marjoram
- mint
- oregano
- peppermint
- rosemary
- sage
- savory
- spearmint
- thyme

31. MORNING GLORY FAMILY

- sweet potato
- yam

32. MULBERRY FAMILY

- breadfruit
- breadnut
- fig
- hop

33. MUSTARD FAMILY

- broccoli
- Brussels sprouts
- cabbage
- cauliflower
- collards
- garden cress
- horseradish
- kale
- kohlrabi

- mustard
- radish
- rutabaga
- turnip
- watercress

34. MYRTLE FAMILY

- allspice
- clove
- guava
- myrtle
- pimento

35. NIGHTSHADE FAMILY

- bell pepper
- cayenne pepper
- chili (paprika, red pepper)
- eggplant
- ground cherry
- melon
- pear
- potato (white)
- strawberry tomato
- tobacco
- tomato
- tree tomato

36. NUTMEG FAMILY

- mace
- nutmeg

37. OLIVE FAMILY

- jasmine
- olive

38. ORCHID FAMILY

- vanilla

39. PALM FAMILY

- cabbage palm
- coconut
- date

40. PAPAYA FAMILY

- papain
- papaya

41. PARSLEY FAMILY

- anise
- caraway

- carrot
- celeriac
- celery
- coriander
- dill
- fennel
- parsley
- parsnip

42. PEA (LEGUME) FAMILY

- acacia
- alfalfa
- black-eyed pea (cowpea)
- broad bean (fava bean)
- carob bean (St. John's bread)
- chick pea (garbanzo)
- common bean:
    - kidney
    - navy
    - pinto
    - string (green)
- Jack bean
- lentil
- licorice
- lima bean
- mesquite
- pea
- peanut
- soybean
- tamarind
- tragacanth

43. PEPPER FAMILY

- black pepper

44. PINE FAMILY

- juniper
- pine nut (Pignolia)

45. PINEAPPLE FAMILY

- pineapple

46. PLUM FAMILY

- almond
- apricot
- cherry
- peach, nectarine

- plum, prune

47. POPPY FAMILY
- poppy seed

48. ROSE FAMILY
- black raspberry
- blackberry
- boysenberry
- dewberry
- loganberry
- red raspberry
- strawberry

49. SAXIFRAGE FAMILY
- currant
- gooseberry

50. SUNFLOWER (COMPOSITE, ASTER) FAMILY
- absinthe (sagebrush, wormwood)
- artichoke
- camomile
- chicory
- dandelion
- endive, escarole

- Jerusalem artichoke
- lettuce
- oyster plant (salsify)
- safflower
- sunflower seed
- tansy
- tarragon

51. TEA FAMILY
- tea

52. WALNUT FAMILY
- black walnut
- butternut
- English walnut
- hickory nut
- pecan

TABLE C2.

FOOD GROUPS CLASSIFIED ACCORDING TO SIMILAR ALLERGIC POTENTIAL

Food	Group	Food	Group
As listed in Table C1 Above		• Jerusalem	50
		• asparagus	27
• Abalone	8	• avocado	25
• absinthe	50		
• acacia	42	• bacon	6b
• alfalfa	42 *	• balm	30
• alligator	9	• bamboo	23
• allspice	34	• banana	11
• almond	46	• barley	23
• aloe	27	• basil	30
• anchovy (Stolephoridae)	5	• bass, black	
• anise	41	• (Centrarchidae)	5
• apple	10	• bass, white (Serranidae)	5
• apricot	46	• bay leaf	25
• arrowroot. East Indian	19	• bean	42
• artichoke		• broad (fava)	
• Japanese	30	• carob (St. John's bread)	

Food	Group	Food	Group
• common		• Brussels sprouts	33
• kidney		• buckwheat	14
• navy		• bullhead (Siluridae)	5
• pinto		• butter	7
• string (green)		• buttermilk	7
• Jack		• butternut	52
• lima		• cabbage	33
• beechnut	12	• cabbage palm	39
• beef	6a	• calf	6a
• beet	20	• camomile	50
• blackberry	48	• cantaloupe	21
• blueberry	24	• caraway	41
• boar	6b	• cardamon	19
• bonito (Scombridae)	5	• carp (Cyprinidae)	5
• boysenberry	48	• carrot	41
• Brazil nut	26	• casaba	21
• breadfruit	32	• casein	7
• breadnut	32	• cashew	15
• broccoli	33	• catfish (Siluridae)	5

Food	Group	Food	Group
• catnip	30	• citron	16
• cattle	6a	• citron melon	21
• cauliflower	33	• clam	8
• caviar (Acipenseridae)	5	• clove	34 •
• celeriac	41	• cockle	8
• celery	41	• cocoa	17
• champagne	22	• coconut	39
• cheese	7	• cod (Gadidae)	5
• cherry	46	• coffee	28
• cherry, ground	35	• collards	33
• chestnut	12	• cola (kola) nut	17
• chicken	2	• coriander	41
		• corn	23
• chicory	50	• Cornish hen	2
• chili	35	• cottonseed	29
• chinquapin	12	• cowpea	42
• chives	27	• crab	3
• chocolate	17	• crabapple	10
• cider	10	• cranberry	24
• cinnamon	25	• crappie (Centrarchidae)	5

Food	Group	Food	Group
• crayfish	3	• eggplant	35
• cream	7	• endive	50
• sour		• escargot	8
• whipped		• escarole	50
• croaker (Scienidae)	5		
• crocodile	9	• fennel	41
• cucumber	21	• fig	32
• currant	49	• filbert	13
		• flounder	
• dandelion	50	• (Pleuronectidae)	5
• date	39	• frog	1
• dewberry	48		
• dill	41	• garbanzo	42
• drum (Scienidae)	5	• garden cress	33
• duck	2	• garlic	27
		• gelatin	6a
• eel (Anguillidae)	5	• gherkin	21
• Egg:	4	• ginger	19
• white		• goat	6a
• whole		• goose	2
• yolk			

Food	Group	Food	Group
• gooseberry	49	• hop	32
• grape	22	• horehound	30
• grapefruit	16	• horseradish	33
• grayling (Salmonidae)	5	• huckleberry, black	24
• grouper (Serranidae)	5	• ice cream	7
• grouse	2	• infant formulas	7
• guava	34		
• guinea hen (fowl)	2	• jasmine	37
• gumbo	29	• juniper	44
• haddock (Gadidae)	5	• kale	33
• hake (Gadidae)	5	• kohlrabi	33
• halibut (Pleuronectidae)	5	• kumquat	16
• ham	6b		
• hazelnut	13	• lactalbumin	7
• herring (Clupeidae)	5	• lamb	6a
• hickory nut	52	• lamb's quarters	20
• hog	6b	• lavender	30
• hominy	23	• leek	27
• honeydew melon	21	• lemon	16

Food	Group	Food	Group
• lentil	42	• mullet (Mugilidae)	5
• lettuce	50	• mushroom	18
• licorice	42	• muskellunge (Esocidae)	5
• lime	16	• muskmelon	21
• lobster	3	• mussel	8
• loganberry	48	• mustard	33
		• mutton	6a
• mace	36	• myrtle	34
• mackerel (Scombridae)	5		
• maize	23	• nectarine	46
• malt	23	• nutmeg	36
• mango	15		
• marjoram	30	• oat	23
• marshmallow	29	• octopus	8
• melon pear	35	• okra	29
• mesquite	42	• olive	37
• milk	7	• onion	27
• millet	23	• orange	16
• mint	30	• oregano	30
• mulberry	32	• ovomucoid	4

Food	Group	Food	Group
• ovovitellin	4	• black	43
• ox	6a	• cayenne	35
• oyster	8	• red	35
• oyster plant	50	• peppermint	30
• papain	40	• perch (Percidae) •	5
• papaya	40	• Persian melon	21
• paprika	35	• pheasant	2
• parsley	41	• pickerel (Esocidae)	5
• parsnip	41	• pig	6b
• partridge	2	• pigeon	2
• pea	42	• pike (Esocidae)	5
• pea, black-eyed (cowpea)	42	• pimento	34
• pea, chick	42	• pine nut (Pignolia)	44
• peach	46	• pineapple	45
• peanut	42	• pistachio	15
• pear	10	• plantain	11
• pecan	52	• plum	46
• pepper		• pollack (Gadidae)	5
• bell	35	• pompano (Carangidae)	5
		• popcorn	23

Food	Group	Food	Group
• poppy seed	47	• rattlesnake	9
• porgy (Sparidae)	5	• red snapper (Sparidae)	5
		• redfish (Scienidae)	5
• pork	6b	• rhubarb	14
• potato:		• rice	23
• sweet	31	• rockfish (Serranidae)	5
• white	35	• rosemary	30
• prawn	3	• rutabaga	33
• prune	46	• rye	23
• pumpkin	21		
		• safflower	50
• quahog	8	• sage	30
• quail	2	• sagebrush	50
• quince	10	• salmon (Salmonidae)	5
• quince seed	10	• salsify	50
• radish	33	• sardine (Clupeidae)	5
• raisin	22	• sarsaparilla	27
• raspberry:		• sassafras	25
• black	48	• sausage	6b
• red	48	• savory	30

Food	Group	Food	Group
• scallop	8	• squash:	
• scrapple	6b	• summer	21
• scrod (Gadidae)	5	• winter	21
• sea trout (Scienidae)	5	• squid	8
• shad (Clupeidae)	5	• steer	6a
• shallot	27	• strawberry	48
• sheep	6a	• sturgeon(Acipenseridae)	5
• shrimp	3	• sugar beet	20
• smelt (Argentinidae)	5	• sugar cane	23
• snail	8	• sunfish (Centrarchidae)	5
		• sunflower seed	50
• sole (Soleidae)	5	• sweetbread	6a
• sorghum	23	• swine	6b
• sorrel	14	• Swiss chard	20
• sow	6b	• swordfish (Xyphidae)	5
• soybean	42		
• spearmint	30	• tamarind	42
• spinach	20	• tangelo	16
• sprat (Clupeidae)	5	• tangerine	16
• squab	2	• tansy	50

Food	Group
• tarragon	50
• tea	51
• terrapin	9
• thyme	30
• tobacco	35
• tomato	35
• tomato, strawberry	35
• tomato, tree	35
• tragacanth	42
• trout (Salmonidae)	5
• truffle	18
• tuna (Scombridae)	5
• turkey	2
• turmeric	19
• turnip	33
• turtle	9
• vanilla	38
• veal	6a
• vinegar (apple cider)	10

Food	Group
• vinegar (wine)	22
• walnut:	52
• black	
• English	
• watercress	33
• watermelon	21
• watermelon, Chinese	21
• weakfish (Scienidae)	5
• wheat:	23
• bran	
• germ	
• gliadin	
• globulin	
• glutenin	
• leucosin	
• proteose	
• whole	
• whitefish (Salmonidae)	5
• wine (grape)	22

Food	Group	Food	Group
• winter muskmelon	21	• baker's	
• wintergreen:		• brewer's	
• Betula spp.	13	• distiller's	
• Pyrola spp.	24	• Fleischmann's	
• wormwood	50	• lactose-fermenting	
		• lager beer	
• yam	31	• yogurt	7
• yeast:	18		

Appendix D

LIST OF ORGANIZATIONS AND HOSPITALS

The following are resources for information on allergies, asthma, and other less-common conditions. See also appendix E for allergy information on the Internet.

1. American Academy of Allergy, Asthma & Immunology
    o   (414)272-6071
    o   Physician's referral and information line: (800) 822-ASMA (2762)
    o   www.aaaai.org
2. National Institute of Allergy and Infectious Diseases
    •   (301)496-5717
    •   www.niaid.nih.gov
3. American College of Allergy and Immunology
    •   (800) 842-7777
    •   www.acaai.org
4. National Jewish Health in Denver Colorado(formerly National Jewish Medical and Research Center)
    •   (800) 222-LUNG (5864)
    •   www.nationaljewish.org
5. Allergy and Asthma Network: Mothers of Asthmatics Inc.
    •   800-878-4403
    •   www.aanma.org
6. American Lung Association
    •   (800) 586-4872
    •   www.lungusa.org
7. Asthma and Allergy Foundation of America

- • (800) 727-8462
- • www.aafa.org
8. National Asthma Education Program
   - • (301)951-3260
   - • www.nhlbi.nih.gov/about/naepp/

Appendix E

ALLERGY INFORMATION ON THE INTERNET

- **Find a board-certified allergy, immunology, and asthma specialist**
  - www.acaai.org/allergist/Pages/locate_an_allergist.aspx
  - www.aaaai.org/physref/
- **Websites of the authors**
  - Bruce S. Dobozin, MD
    - www.nyallergyasthma.org
  - Stuart H. Young, MD
    - www.allergynewyork.com
- **Allergy—and immunology-related organizations**
  - American Academy of Allergy, Asthma & Immunology (AAAAI)
    - http://www.aaaai.org—a useful list of related organization compiled by the AAAAI
      - www.aaaai.org/members/resources/health_related_sites.stm
  - American College of Allergy, Asthma and Immunology (ACAAI)
    - www.acaai.org
  - Joint Council of Allergy, Asthma and Immunology
    - www.jcaai.org/
  - European Academy of Allergology and Clinical Immunology
    - http://eaaci.net/
  - National Heart, Lung, and Blood Institute (NHLBI)of the National Institutes of Health
    - http://www.nhlbi.nih.gov/
  - NHLBI Asthma Control Initiative
    - www.nhlbi.nih.gov/health/prof/lung/asthma/naci/

- ○ National Institute of Allergy and Infectious Diseases (NIAID) of the National Institutes of Health
  - ▪ www.niaid.nih.gov/
- ○ Pan American Aerobiology Association
  - ▪ www.paaa.org/
- ○ International Food Information Council
  - ▪ www.foodinsight.org/
- ○ The American Lung Association
  - ▪ www.lungusa.org/
- ○ MedicAlert Foundation (ID bracelets plus jewelry)
  - ▪ www.medicalert.org/

ALLERGY AND IMMUNOLOGY: SUPPORT GROUPS

- Allergy and Asthma Network: Mothers of Asthmatics Inc.
  - ○ www.aanma.org
- Asthma and Allergy Foundation of America
  - ○ www.aafa.org/
- National Eczema Association
  - ○ www.nationaleczema.org/
  - ○ Eczema and sensitive-skin-education site from the above organization: www.easeeczema.org
- American Partnership for Eosinophilic Disorders (includes gastrointestinal, lung, and whole Body or hypereosinophilia)
  - ○ www.apfed.org/
- The Food Allergy and Anaphylaxis Network (FAAN)
  - ○ www.foodallergy.org/
- Food Allergy Initiative
  - ○ www.faiusa.org/
- Food Allergy Initiative has a useful page listing various online tools and mobile phone apps:
  - ○ www.faiusa.org/?page=Online_tools_and_apps
- Hereditary Angioedema Association
  - ○ www.haea.org/
- Immune Deficiency Foundation
  - ○ www.primaryimmune.org
- Latex allergy
  - ○ American Latex Allergy Association: www.latexallergyresources.org/
- Mastocytosis Society
  - ○ www.tmsforacure.org
- Yahoo! groups: various online support groups for allergy and asthma. Patient and family support groups but not monitored for medical accuracy:

- o www.groups.yahoo.com/
- Find an allergist plus general information on allergies:
  - o http://www.allergyandasthmarelief.org/

ALLERGY-CONTROL PRODUCT STORE

There are numerous companies that sell products to help control allergies. We refer to these products as environmental-control products (see chapter 4). We include one such company that is physician owned and physician operated and sells high-quality products. We do refer our patients to this company and its website, but there are alternatives as well.

- o Mission Allergy: (877) 662-5537www.missionallergy.com

GENERAL MEDICAL ORGANIZATIONS

- The American Medical Association
  - o www.ama-assn.org
- The U.S. Food and Drug Administration
  - o www.fda.gov
- Centers for Disease Control and Prevention
  - o www.cdc.gov
- National Institutes of Health
  - o www.nih.gov/
- American College of Physicians
  - o http://www.acponline.org/
- American College of Healthcare Executives
  - o www.ache.org/
- American College of Physician Executives
  - o www.acpe.org
- American College of Chest Physicians
  - o www.chestnet.org/

GOVERNMENTAL SITES

- Alerts on dietary supplements
  - o www.fda.gov/Food/DietarySupplements/Alerts/default.htm
- Health Care Financing Administration (HCFA)
  - o www.hcfa.gov/
- National Health Information Center
  - o www.health.gov/nhic/
- U.S. Department of Health and Human Services
  - o www.hhs.gov/

- National Center for Complementary and Alternative Medicine (NCCAM)
  - www.nccam.nih.gov/
- National Library of Medicine Consumer Health site:
  - www.nlm.nih.gov/medlineplus/
- The National Council against Health Fraud Inc.
  - www.ncahf.org/
- U.S. House of Representatives
  - www.house.gov/
- U.S. Senate
  - www.senate.gov/
- The White House
  - www.whitehouse.gov/WH/Welcome.html
- How did the politicians vote?
  - www.vote-smart.org/

HOSPITALS WITH NOTABLE ALLERGY—AND IMMUNOLOGY-RELATED DEPARTMENTS

Many hospitals, medical centers, and medical schools have developed websites that have valuable information related to the illnesses they research or treat. We urge you to use these. We list several related to allergy and asthma. The National Jewish site has particularly useful patient information, and these can be downloaded.

- National Jewish Health (formerly known as National Jewish Medical and Research Center)—this hospital (where both authors of this book trained at) is a global leader in treatment and research of lung disease, allergic disease, and immune system disease and is located in Denver, Colorado).
  - www.nationaljewish.org/
  - National Jewish's patient-education downloads:
    - www.nationaljewish.org/education/patient/print-multimedia/online-materials.aspx
- Mount Sinai Hospital Jaffe Food Allergy Institute
  - www.mssm.edu/research/programs/jaffe-food-allergy-institute
- Johns Hopkins Allergy and Asthma Center
  - www.hopkinsmedicine.org/allergy/AAC.html

PHARMACEUTICAL COMPANIES

Here we list the websites for many of the major pharmaceutical companies that manufacture drugs related to allergies or asthma. Each medication available usually has its own website and is often the "name of the drug.com" or for example, www.claritin.com.

- U.S. Pharmacopeia: The official public-standards-setting authority for prescription and over-the-counter medicines and other health-care products manufactured or sold in the United States. USP also sets widely recognized standards for food ingredients and dietary supplements. USP sets standards for the quality, purity, strength, and consistency of these products—critical to the public health.
  - www.usp.org/
- Abbott Laboratories
  - www.abbott.com/
- Alcon Labs
  - www.alcon.com/en/
- ALK Laboratories
  - http://allergy.mcg.edu/ALK/insect.html
- Autoepinephrine injectors
  - http://www.adrenaclick.com
  - http://www.epipen.com/
  - http://www.twinject.com/
- Ciba Pharmaceuticals
  - www.ciba.com
- Genentech
  - www.gene.com
- GlaxoSmithKline
  - www.gsk.com/
- GlaxoSmithKline (asthma-control test)
  - www.asthmacontrol.com/
- Ista
  - www.istavision.com/
- MEDA
  - www.astepro.com/
- Merck and Company
  - www.merck.com/
- Novartis
  - www.novartis.com/
- Pfizer
  - www.pfizer.com
- Sanofi-aventis
  - www.sanofi-aventis.us/live/us/en/index.jsp
- Schering-Key (recently became part of Merck)
  - www.claritin.com/
- Sepracor
  - www.sepracor.com/

- Teva
  - http://www.tevausa.com/

LITERATURE AND GENERAL INTERNET SEARCH

- Google, Yahoo! Lycos, AltaVista, and Bing are all search engines through which one can find information and literature references. However, the authors caution the reader that all sorts of unreliable information can show up on regular search engines. Therefore, going to a reputable site and using their links is recommended.
- Medscape
  - www.medscape.com
- PubMed: National Library of Medicine search
  - This website searches the medical literature and the articles can be highly technical, but it eliminates the unreliable information that a Google search can generate.
  - www.ncbi.nlm.nih.gov/PubMed/
- Wikipedia (online encyclopedia)
  - www.wikipedia.org/
- Doctor's Guide to Allergies, Information and Resources
  - www.pslgroup.com/Allergies.htm

GENERAL MEDICAL INFORMATION

- Many hospitals, medical centers, and medical schools have developed websites that have valuable information related to the illnesses they research or treat. We urge you to use these.
- National Center for Complementary and Alternative Medicine (NCCAM)
  - www.nccam.nih.gov/
- Natural Medicines Comprehensive Database
  - www.naturaldatabase.com
- Ophthalmology website, free text
  - www.ophthobook.com
- Breastfeeding and medications info: American Academy of Pediatrics:
  - www.aap.org
- Consumer Labs.com: Their stated mission is "to identify the best quality health and nutritional products through independent testing." They test products related to health, wellness, and nutrition, such as vitamins and supplements for contents and other quality measures.
  - www.consumerlab.com/
- Info on medications and pregnancy: **Teratology Society**—useful information as well as links to research data and the names of consultants in the field

o   http://teratology.org

MEDICAL NEWS

o   Reuters Medical News: www.reutershealth.com

POLLEN COUNTS

- The National Allergy Bureau (General information on outdoor allergies, pollen counts, and actual pollen-count levels.)
  o   www.aaaai.org/nab/index.cfm
- Pollen.com (can set up e-mail alerts for your area)
  o   www.pollen.com

SORTING OUT THE INFORMATION:

We add this section because there is a lot of incorrect information as well as quackery both on the Internet. Also, there are unscrupulous providers of allergy care as well. There are two useful sites on the Internet that can help someone sort out this information.

- Quackwatch: Your Guide to Quackery, Health Fraud, and Intelligent Decisions is a very useful online site of an organization founded in 1969 by a physician (Stephen Barrett) and now comprises a worldwide network of volunteers to help advise persons about quackery and health-care fraud. They maintain a whole host of related websites to help people sort through questionable theories and practices of medicine.
  o   www.quackwatch.com/
- Quackometer: This is a clever website developed by Andy Lewis. On this site, a user can enter the address of a website and give it the Quackometer Test. After analyzing the contents of the entered website, the Quackometer will give a result stating the likelihood that the entered website is legitimate or not.
  o   www.quackometer.net

Appendix F

SUMMER CAMPS FOR
CHILDREN WITH ASTHMA

- The Consortium on Children's Asthma Camps
  - o www.asthmacamps.org/asthmacamps/

Note that the camps are listed at their request; and neither the consortium nor any of its members nor we make any representation, warranty, or guarantee or assume any duty, liability, or responsibility respecting the operation of any such camp or the conduct of any person or firm associated with any such camp.

It is very likely that your own allergy or asthma doctor will have more detailed information about camps near where you live. For further information, visit the website or contact them directly: Consortium on Children's Asthma Camps, 490 Concordia Ave St. Paul, MN 55103. Phone: 651-227-8014

Appendix G

REFERENCES AND "OTHER STUFF"

CHAPTER 4 REFERENCES ON TOXIC MOLD

- AAAAI (American Academy of Asthma Allergy and Immunology) Position Paper: "The medical effects of mold exposure. Bush, R.K, MD, Portnoy, J.M, MD, Saxon, A, MD, Terr, A.I., MD and Wood, R.A, MD. J Allergy Clin Immunol Volume 117 Number 2 pp 326-333
- Damp Indoor Spaces and Health. Committee on Damp Indoor Spaces and Health. Board of Health Promotion and Disease Prevention. Institute of Medicine of the Nation Academies. Copyright 2004 National Academy of Sciences. Summary of Findings Regarding the Association Between Health Outcomes and the Presence of Mold or Other Agents in Damp Indoor Environment

The references in Appendix G are for the sophisticated reader, who is interested in learning more about the controversy of environmental manipulation which is far beyond the scope of this book. The authors' experience with environmental control is extensive and our instructions to patients are often based on those suggestions and instructions that are offered in our book. However once the clinical situation of each of our patients is analyzed it is almost never clear as to what effect the indoor environment really has on an allergic individual. And when scientific studies are done to try to sort out what manipulations are helpful, there are so many variables that the studies are often difficult to interpret or give inconclusive results. The controversy is discussed in the above references and is reflected in the allergic literature in general. A detailed and careful reading will reflect just how controversial this subject is and how things are often done to correct the indoor environment that are based on little evidence. However, allergy treatment is a complex algorithm and therefore we issue general instructions in the book to each of our readers whom we have never met. In practice we have the advantage of skin testing and detailed reviews of our patient's specific situation to further enhance our ability to make recommendations and on that basis we treat our patients.

Author Biographies:

Stuart H. Young, M.D., has practiced allergy in Manhattan for over 30 years. He received his training in allergy and Immunology at the National Jewish Hospital/ National Asthma Center (now known as National Jewish Health) in Denver. He is the author of numerous books, textbooks and scientific articles on allergy and immunology. He is an Attending Physician, Division of Allergy and Immunology at the Mount Sinai Medical Center and is on the faculty at the Mount Sinai School of Medicine all in New York City. He is the former Chief of Allergy Clinics at Mount Sinai Medical Center. He has been listed for the last 14 years in the Castle Connolly Guide of America's Top Doctors and has been picked as a top Doctor in New York City by New York Magazine. He has mentored numerous allergists-in-training and is considered a role model by those physicians. He is currently in private practice in Manhattan and lives in Northern New Jersey with his wife and family.

Bruce S. Dobozin, MD was born in Buffalo, NY. He graduated from The Nichols School, SUNY Buffalo, and SUNY Stony Brook Medical School. He completed a specialty residency at the Mount Sinai Hospital of New York and then a sub-specialty fellowship at the National Jewish Hospital/National Asthma Center (now known as National Jewish Health) in Denver. For the past 13 years, *U.S. News & World Report* has ranked National Jewish the #1 respiratory hospitals in the nation. His practices in Manhattan and Woodstock NY are affiliates of National Jewish Health. He is on staff at NYU Langone Medical Center, teaches at NYU School of Medicine, and attends the Allergy/Immunology clinic at Bellevue Hospital. Bruce and his wife, the acclaimed artist, Devorah Sperber, live in Manhattan.

INDEX

Printed in Great Britain
by Amazon